Core Conditioning for Horses

Yoga-Inspired Warm-Up Techniques

Increase Suppleness, Improve Bend, and Unlock Optimal Movement

Simon Cocozza

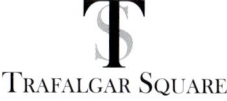

First published in 2019 by
Trafalgar Square Books
an imprint of The Stable Book Group
Brooklyn, New York

Copyright © 2019 *Simon Cocozza*

All rights reserved. No part of this book may be reproduced, by any means, without written permission of the publisher, except by a reviewer quoting brief excerpts for a review in a magazine, newspaper, or website.

Disclaimer of Liability
The author and publisher shall have neither liability nor responsibility to any person or entity with respect to any loss or damage caused or alleged to be caused directly or indirectly by the information contained in this book. While the book is as accurate as the author can make it, there may be errors, omissions, and inaccuracies.

Trafalgar Square Books encourages the use of approved safety helmets in all equestrian sports and activities.

Library of Congress Cataloging-in-Publication Data
Names: Cocozza, Simon, Visconte, 1970- author.
Title: Core conditioning for horses : yoga-inspired warm-up techniques that
  increase suppleness, improve bend, and unlock optimal movement / Visconte
  Simon Cocozza.
Description: North Pomfret, Vermont : Trafalgar Square Books, 2019. |
  Includes index.
Identifiers: LCCN 2018037118 | ISBN 9781570768040
Subjects: LCSH: Horses--Exercise. | Horses--Training.
Classification: LCC SF287 .C62 2019 | DDC 636.1/0835--dc23
LC record available at https://lccn.loc.gov/2018037118

Photographs and illustrations by *Paul Barber* except: p. xiii (Can/AdobeStock); pp. 6–7, 114–5 (Anton Rostovsky/AdobeStock); pp. 8, 10, 25 left–27, 34, 216 (Wikicommons); pp. 11, 18, 22, 29, 36, 64, 66–7, 70, 73, 77, 80, 88, 92, 95, 100–2, 104, 112, 118, 138, 248, 289 (Pixabay); p. 12 (Wellcome Images V0050695); pp. 13, 124, 196, 286 (Pexels); p. 25 right (Matt Cornock); p. 28 (Montanabw); p. 33 (Jenny Lee and Trigger by Veronica Lee); pp. 38, 94 (Gabriela Placco); p. 59 (Laila Klinsmann/Pexels); p. 60 (Whole Horse Dissection); p. 63 (4DDI Equine); p. 69 (Svetlana Zakarova); pp. 84, 129 (Tiia Tuulivaara and Kanada); p. 105 (Belinda Hankins Miller); p. 120 (Terri Walker); p. 150 (Jan Laugesen/Pexels); pp. 158, 170, 188, 200–1, 212, 224, 240, 252, 267, 276 (Alison Robertson Yoga); pp. 174, 176, 178, 180, 290 (courtesy of Dana & Ollie); p. 204 (courtesy of Dr. Doychin Lyudov); pp. 228, 230, 232 (courtesy of Debbie & Chaussette); pp. 256, 258 (courtesy of Marina Kallioniemi)

Book design by *Katarzyna Misiukanis–Celińska*
Cover design by *RM Didier*
Index by *Andrea Jones (JonesLiteraryServices.com)*
Typefaces: *Adobe Garamond Pro, Roboto* and *Libre Baskerville*

Printed in China

10 9 8 7 6

dedication

/ I dedicate this book to: /

*Nutty, Willow, Cracker, Campari, Boswell,
Winnie, Chance, Flox, Summertime, Archie, Quadria,
Joyeuse, Jet, Lancelot, Magda, Minerva, Skovvangs, Jeep,
Deera, Wall Street, Shanghai, Silver, and Dagwood.*

Thank you for your kindness, *my dearest friends.*
One day we will meet again, somewhere down the trail.

Look out for me.

CONTENTS

Mother Nature's Perfect Design 10

The Dark Side of the Core 54

Releasing the Natural Athlete 28

INTRODUCTION	1
PART ONE: UNDERSTANDING THE HORSE'S CORE	**7**

CHAPTER 1
THE BACK: WHERE ALL MOVEMENT BEGINS — 9
The Magic Inside Every Horse — 9
Mother Nature's Perfect Design — 10
The Silent Language of the Herbivore — 20
Riding "Feels" — 22
Taming the "Snorting Beast" — 24
Releasing the Natural Athlete — 28

CHAPTER 2
THE SOURCE OF THE FORCE IN THE HORSE: THE CORE — 37
The Power of Three Will Set You Free — 44
The Dark Side of the Core — 54

CONTENTS

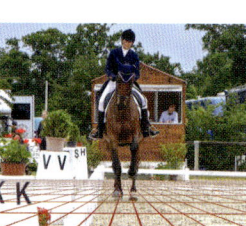
▼ *Yoga: Kind to the Core*

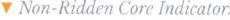
▼ *Non-Ridden Core Indicators*

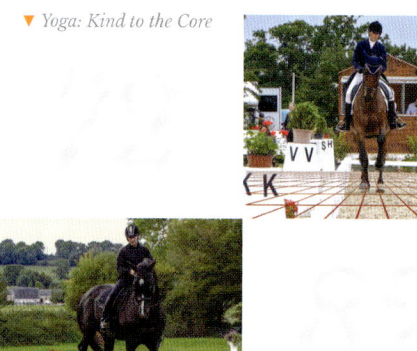

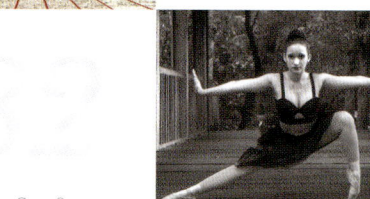
▲ *The Core Score*

CHAPTER 3	**HORSES ARE PEOPLE, TOO**	**65**
	The Human Touch	66
	Using the Warm-Up to Condition the Core	68
	Yoga: Kind to the Core	72
CHAPTER 4	**ASSESSING THE HORSE'S CORE AND CHOOSING A WARM-UP PLAN**	**81**
	The Core Score	82
	Non-Ridden Core Indicators	100
	Choosing Your Core Warm-Up Plan	107
	Putting It All Together	110
	Special Considerations	111

PART TWO: THE CORE CONDITIONING EXERCISES   115

CHAPTER 5	**HOW TO RIDE FROM THE HORSE'S CORE**	**117**
	Building Blocks: What You Need to Know for the Core Exercises	119
	The Three Exercise Levels: Release, Coordination, and Tone	123
	Head-and-Neck Positions (HNP)	130
	Yoga-Inspired Warm-Up Aids	136

CONTENTS

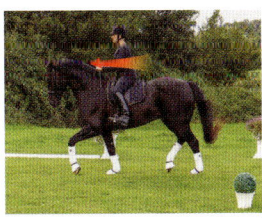

▼ *Getting Started* 151
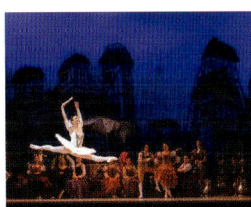
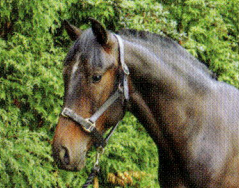
▲ *Yoga-Inspired Warm-Up Aids* 136
▲ *Practice Makes Perfect* 288

CHAPTER 6 — 10 CORE EXERCISES FOR THE HORSE — 151
Getting Started — 151
Exercise 1: ♣ *The Half-Moon Pose* ♞ *The Core Release Volte* — 156
Exercise 2: ♣ *The Yoga Half-Split* ♞ *The Turn on the Forehand* — 169
Exercise 3: ♣ *The Cat Pose* ♞ *Forward, Down, and Out (FDO)* — 186
Exercise 4: ♣ *The Balancing Table to Tiptoe Chair Poses* ♞ *Forward and Back* — 198
Exercise 5: ♣ *The Chair Pose* ♞ *The Driving Seat* — 211
Exercise 6: ♣ *The Garland Pose* ♞ *The Rounding Rein-Back* — 223
Exercise 7: ♣ *The Revolved Triangle Pose* ♞ *The Limbering Leg-Yield* — 238
Exercise 8: ♣ *Thread the Needle Pose* ♞ *The Perfect Pirouette* — 250
Exercise 9: ♣ *The Cat to Cow Pose* ♞ *Forward, Down, and Out to Competition Outline* — 264
Exercise 10: ♣ *The Revolved Half-Moon Pose* ♞ *La Giravolta Longe* — 274

CHAPTER 7 — HAPPY BENDY HORSEY! — 287
Practice Makes Perfect — 288

ACKNOWLEDGMENTS — 291
INDEX — 293

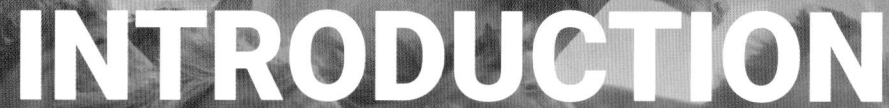

INTRODUCTION

> *Riding a horse is an incredible privilege.*
> *The opportunity to dance*
> *with such a magnificent creature*
> *can elevate your soul and bond you,*
> *in balance and spirit,*
> *with this truly wonderful animal.*

Riding a horse is an incredible privilege. The opportunity to dance with such a magnificent creature can elevate your soul and bond you, in balance and spirit, with this truly wonderful animal.

Riding, however, is not *always* like that. A serious rider will have earned that elevated soul with sweat and sacrifice, and will, without doubt, be on a first-name basis with his or her local pharmacy.

So what is the difference between the ride that "danced" and the ride that didn't?

It is all down to the horse's posture in motion. This is the horse's ability to use the powerful mechanisms already built into his body and relies not upon the strength you can see on the outside but the strength on the *inside*.

This invisible and complex arrangement of internal "core" muscles controls the way a horse's back functions and dictate his overall posture. A horse with a strong core and good posture will feel athletic and "round" underneath you, as if you are riding a slowly bouncing ball. If, on the other hand, the horse's posture is poor and his back is "hollow," the "horse ball" can't bounce, and the whole riding experience loses its ease and beauty.

INTRODUCTION

> *The human discipline of yoga, in particular, resonates beautifully with the horse's physiology and psychology, giving his body and mind the same benefits that we ourselves find in its practice.*

Core muscles are very difficult to isolate in normal equestrian training, and this can leave them weaker than they should be, even in very fit horses, as only very specific movements will engage them. The perfect solution lies in our extensive knowledge of the human core and how it functions and feels, as fortunately this know-how transfers easily to our vertebrate cousin—the horse. The human discipline of *yoga*, in particular, resonates beautifully with the horse's physiology and psychology, giving his body and mind the same benefits that we ourselves find in its practice. With a wonderful blend of gentleness and focus, the principles behind yoga are very effective in helping your riding partner with the unique demands made upon his back.

Yoga helps the horse to:

- Feel good when you ride him.
- Be physically supple enough to perform.
- Feel free in body and mind.
- Find his own, personal form of agility, rather than yours.

The specific yoga-inspired exercises in this book can help the horse owner to transform any horse or pony's body into the most supple and athletic version of itself. By conditioning areas of the equine body that may be a little rusty, we can release the horse's natural "dance" into every stride.

INTRODUCTION

> *I've organized this book into two parts:
> You will begin with introductory material
> that will help you understand
> the horse's core and how to "score" it.
> In Part Two, you will learn the key exercises
> to improve your horse's core condition.*

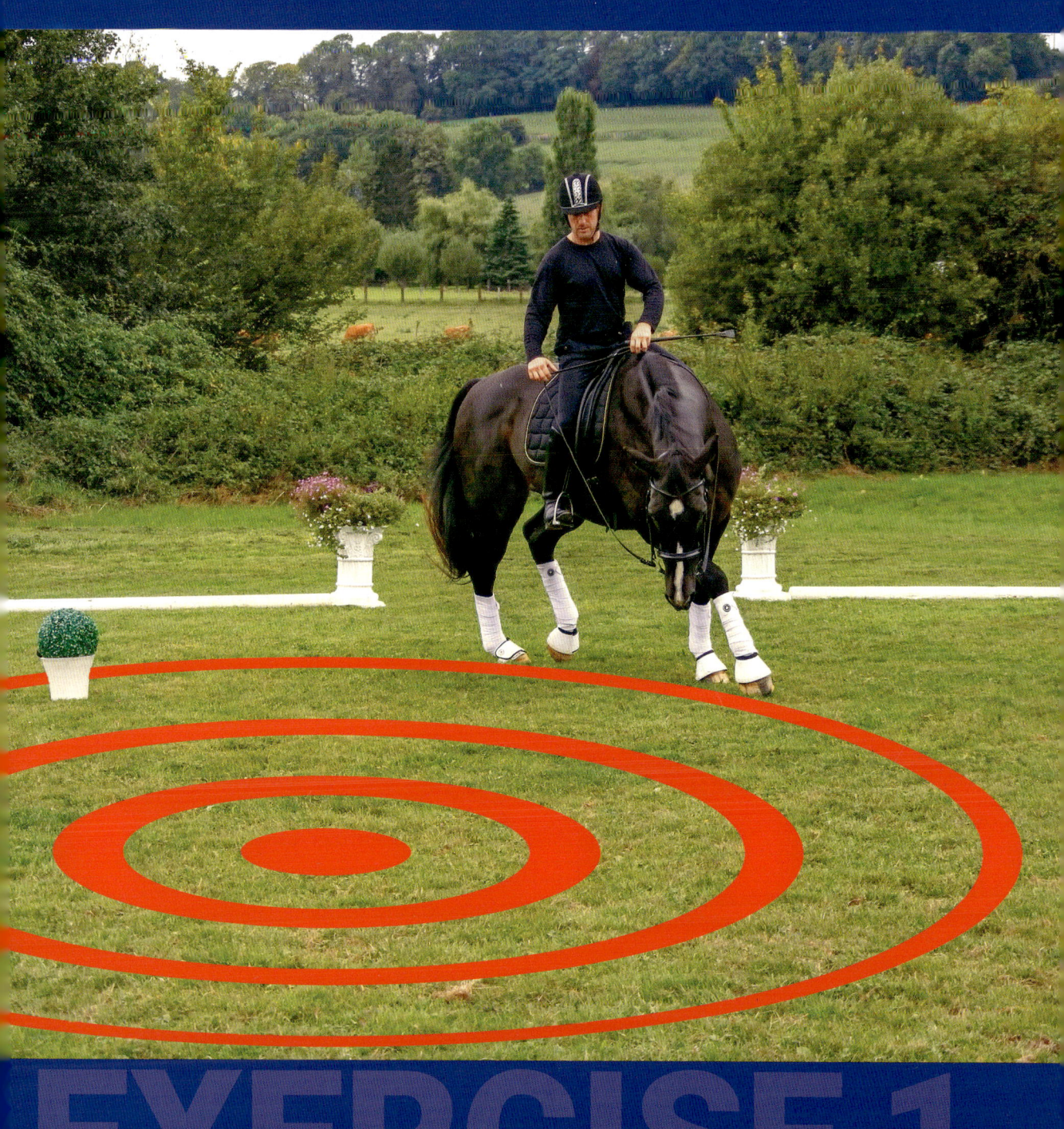

EXERCISE 1

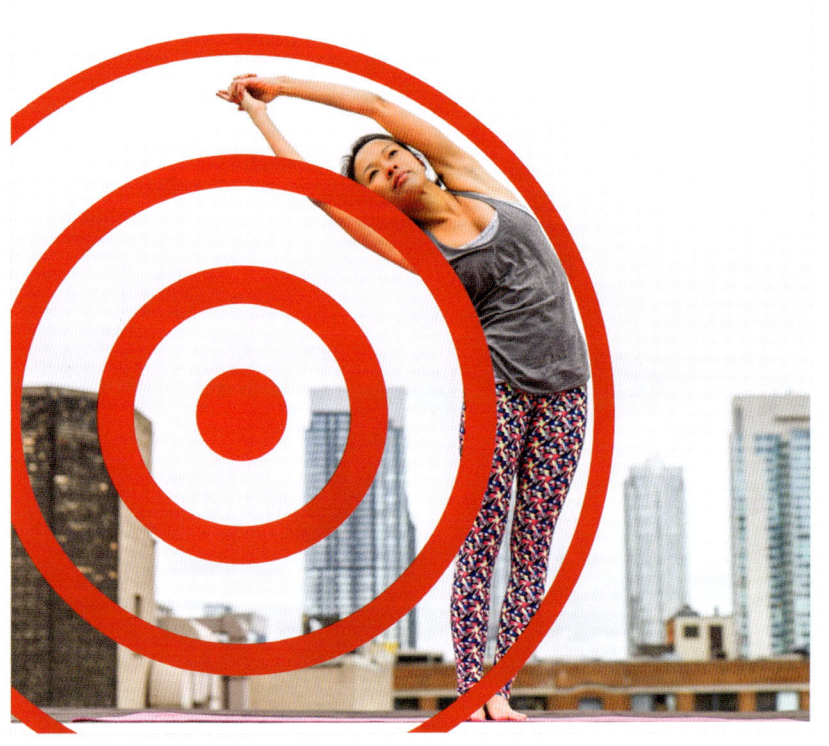

/ 6.6 / *The Yoga Half-Moon Pose gently bends the body through the back, releasing tension along the thoracic spine.* ▶

🪷 / The Half-Moon Pose

This exercise helps the human by:

- Stretching the shoulders, chest, hamstrings, calves, and lower and middle back.
- Strengthening the abdomen, thighs, buttocks, ankles, and oblique muscles.
- Improving flexibility through the spine.
- Easing tension and promoting circulation.
- Improving coordination and balance.

- Relieving stress.
- Improving digestion.

"The Half-Moon Yoga stretch creates traction for the spine, lengthening the vertebrae away from each other," explains Laura Phelps, ISSA fitness trainer and champion powerlifter. "It will stretch the muscles on both sides of the body as the spine needs to maintain an optimal range of motion in all directions" (fig. 6.6).

/ The Core Release Volte

The *Core Release Volte* is a wonderfully natural and simple exercise (fig. 6.7). It is also the most important back stretch a horse can do as

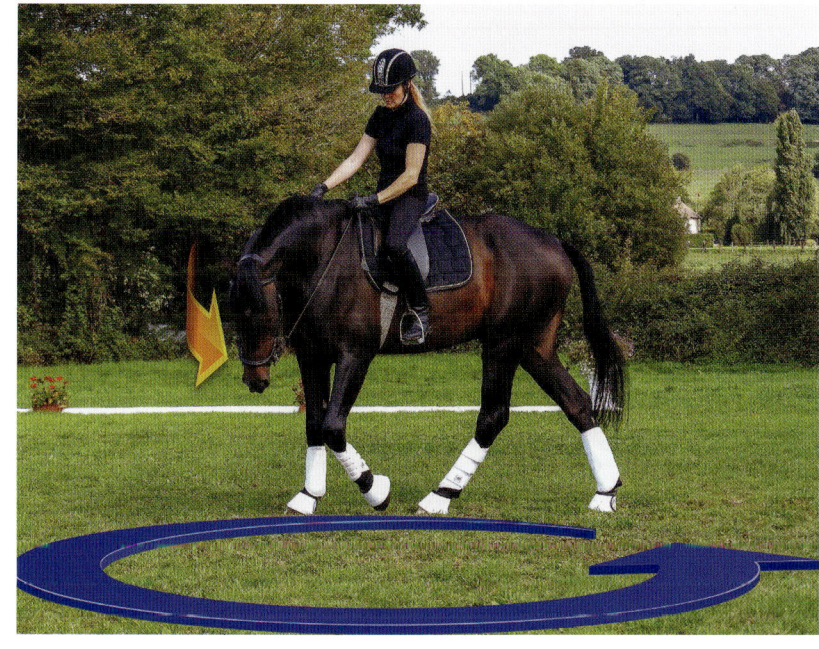

◀ / 6.7 / *Releasing the core: The Stretching Flexion brings the horse onto a volte and aligns his spine.*

it gives us a reliable and relaxed Long-and-Low HNP that you can use in almost all the other exercises.

It couldn't be easier: two circles on a figure of eight with a Stretching Flexion (see p. 139) may seem too easy, but it creates both lateral and vertical back flexions, making it an excellent body-confidence-building exercise, particularly when the back already shows some signs of being weak or sensitive. In any situation, this go-to exercise can alleviate mental and physical tension in very little time. The Long-and-Low Outline we achieve with this exercise leads naturally into the full back stretch of the Forward, Down, and Out, which is the all-important Exercise 3 (see p. 186).

/ *6.8* / *Longer and lower: When aligned well, Wardance can stretch naturally from the Long and Low HNP to the Forward, Down, and Out HNP to voluntarily stretch his own back.* ▶

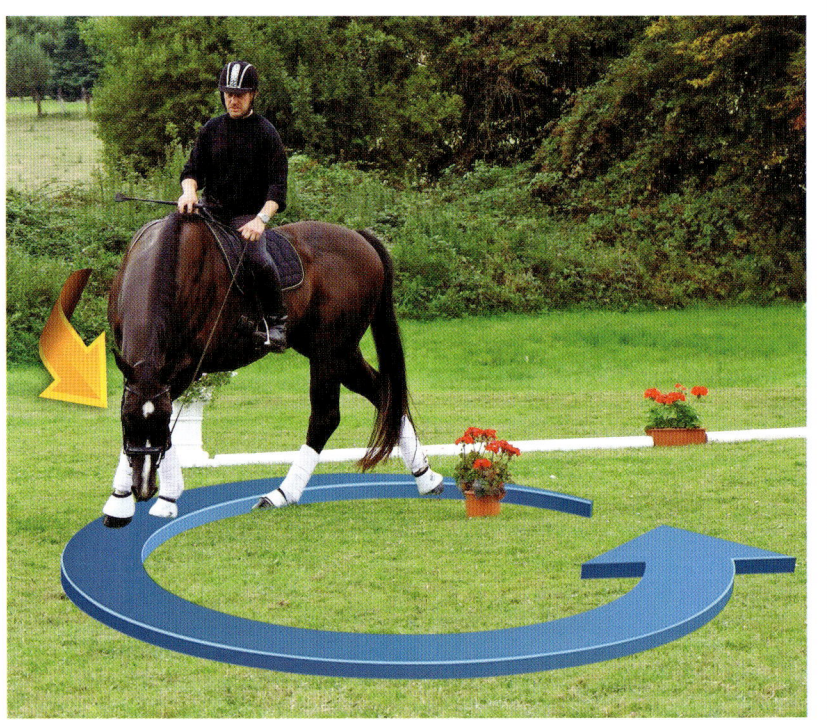

This exercise helps the horse:

- Align the spine and release the core.
- Stretch the *longissimus* to release the topline.
- Awaken the three Core Powers, particularly the Nuchal and Thoracic Lifts.
- Relieve tightness or spinal discomfort.

This exercise helps solve these issues under saddle:

- Falling in/out.
- Heavy contact.
- Stiff, unbending back.
- High head.
- Rushing.
- Uncomfortable seat.
- Hollow jumping style.

What It Does Inside the Horse

The bend of the 6-meter (20-foot) volte circle creates the ideal spinal angle to release the horse's core and round the back. The core releases as the spine drops into its correct alignment, allowing the Nuchal and Thoracic Lifts to activate. This gives the spine ideal conditions to release and mobilize through its entire length.

The 6-meter volte is a vital training tool requiring the horse to make his own body changes and round himself naturally. During this exercise the horse must think for himself and experiment with bending throughout

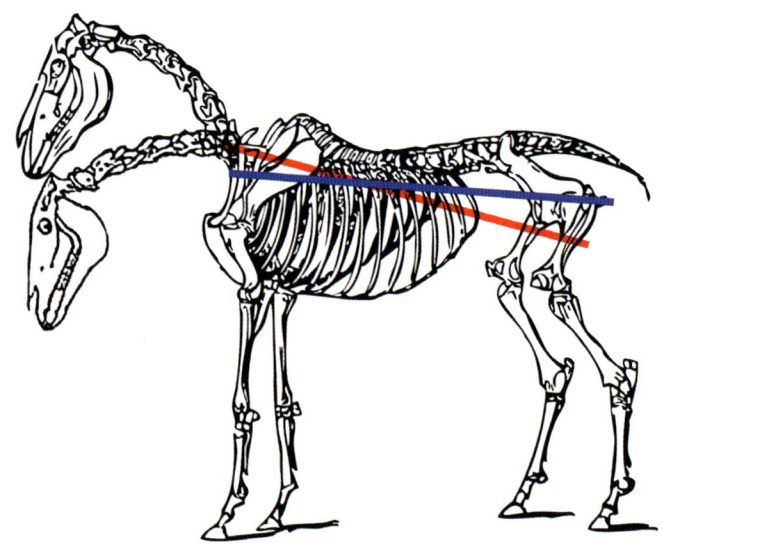

/ 6.9 / *Achieving Core Release lightens the forehand. By lowering the horse's head and activating the Nuchal Lift, this exercise helps to shift the horse's weight toward the rear and into a better balance.* ▶

the back (thoracic spine) evenly, so we don't really need to teach the horse anything, other than to maintain the bend around the volte and let him find a better way to balance himself.

As this exercise is purely a low-impact stretch, it is an ideal starting place for all horses, particularly for those that need to relax in the back, round a little more, and think about bending into in a softer outline.

Core Score, Level, and Head-and-Neck Position

If your horse has a Core Score of:

- **4–5**, then do this exercise at the **RELEASE LEVEL.**
- **2–3**, then do this exercise at the **COORDINATION LEVEL.**
- **0–1**, then do this exercise at the **TONE LEVEL.**

In the Core Release Volte we use two small circles to create a lateral and longitudinal stretch for the horse's back (fig. 6.10). Aim for a soft contact in Long-and-Low HNP until Core Release is felt before either encouraging a Forward, Down, and Out HNP or riding a more challenging exercise in the Warm-Up Plan.

- **RELEASE LEVEL** (Free-Walk with a Long-and-Low HNP): The walk reaches deeper than any other gait, which is why it is important to get this exercise right in the free-walk before moving up to the Coordination Level.

- **COORDINATION LEVEL** (*Trot d'École* with a Long-and-Low HNP): The Core Release Voltes in *trot d'école* are a wonderful way to establish a soft, natural way of going. The Stretching Flexion and body bend combine to coordinate core, limb, and spirit. Most healthy horses with a Core Score of 3, 2, or 1 can start the Core Release Voltes at this Level.

- **TONE LEVEL** (*Petit Galop* with a Long-and-Low or Forward, Down and Out HNP): This is a marvelous combination of coordination and fine muscle control. Once the horse is very soft in the Coordination Level, picking up the *petit galop* teaches the horse the very delicate management of his center of balance. The horse will, at some point, ask to lower into Forward, Down, and Out. This is a wonderful milestone for your horse's back—*bravissimo!*

When the horse is performing well in the *petit galop* Tone Level, those horses and riders capable of advancing the exercise can introduce slow, relaxed, long-and-low canter lead changes where the two voltes touch.

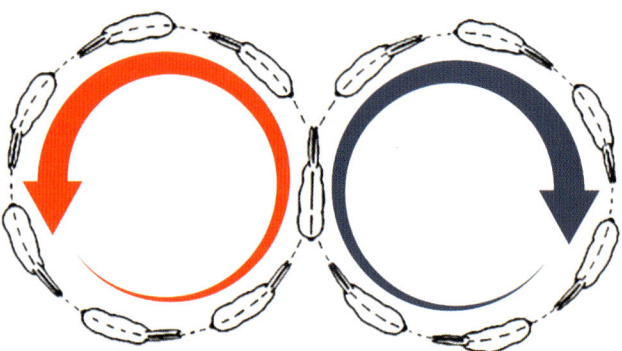

/ 6.10 / A figure of eight made of two voltes changes bend and direction so regularly that it gently releases many of a horse's back stiffnesses. ▶

Start with a simple change (through walk); then, when fluid, introduce the flying change. You will be surprised how much this will improve your horse's canter.

How to Do It

This is the number one exercise for simplicity. As a deliberately non-confrontational back relaxation exercise, great results are achievable for all horses in a short time, if ridden correctly. Consider author and renowned dressage coach Jane Savoie's words: "The stiff side is not the problem. Your horse feels stiff to the right because the muscles on the left side of his body are shortened and contracted. The solution to this problem is to stretch those shortened muscles on the left side by riding your horse with too much bend until you feel the muscles on his left side elongate."

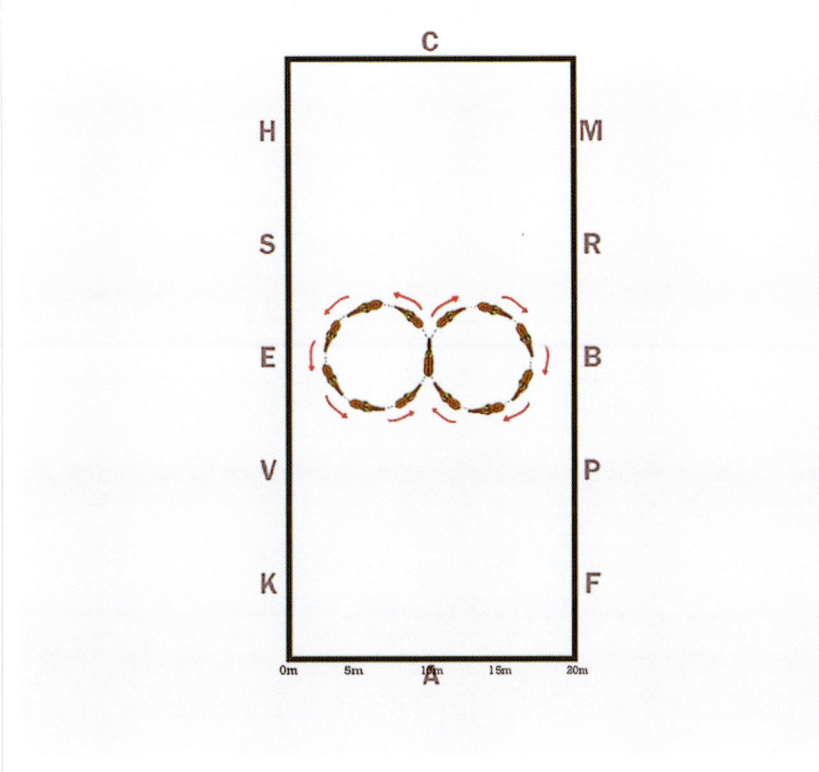

◄ / **6.11** / *Performing the voltes over the centerline helps you keep their size and shape.*

OVERVIEW: Ride a figure eight made from two 6-meter (20-foot) voltes, changing the Stretching Flexion (see p. 139) and direction where they touch (fig. 6.11).

- **STEP /1/** Choose a location with free space around you—X is ideal if in an arena.
- **STEP /2/** Begin riding the figure eight with an inside Stretching Flexion.
- **STEP /3/** Establish a rhythm and change the rein where the circles meet, gently plodding from a left to right volte.

- **STEP /4/** When Core Release happens, immediately allow the horse to stretch down as much as he wishes by letting the reins slip and lengthen through the fingers. The exercise can continue in this new Forward, Down, and Out.
- **STEP /5/** When working in Tone Level, change direction at random rather than every time to avoid anticipation.

When Core Release is achieved the horse's gait will slow dramatically. This is normal. Even though the horse's body can be felt as having have a better internal balance thanks to his rounder back, the newly active muscles will take time to gain grace and fluidity—but they will.

Common Problems and Solutions

Remember, if you experience any problem or difficulty, drop a Level until it is easy again before retrying.

- *No core release.* Not enough inside Stretching Flexion or the Level is too high.
- *The horse falls in or speeds up around the circle.* Also not enough Stretching Flexion.
- *A strong inside rein contact.* The outside of the horse is tight in the back. Continue with the exercise at Release Level until the core releases. This will release the inside rein to you.

If the horse has a bad back, this exercise will take time to achieve, yet the Core Release Volte always produces excellent results.

Core Score Zero Goal

At its highest Level, this exercise is no longer about stretching; it is about balancing. Once the horse can bend through the body both laterally and vertically without feeling any restriction, the paces become wonderfully measured, balanced, and elastic. ■

END OF EXERCISE 1
The Half-Moon Pose / The Core Release Volte

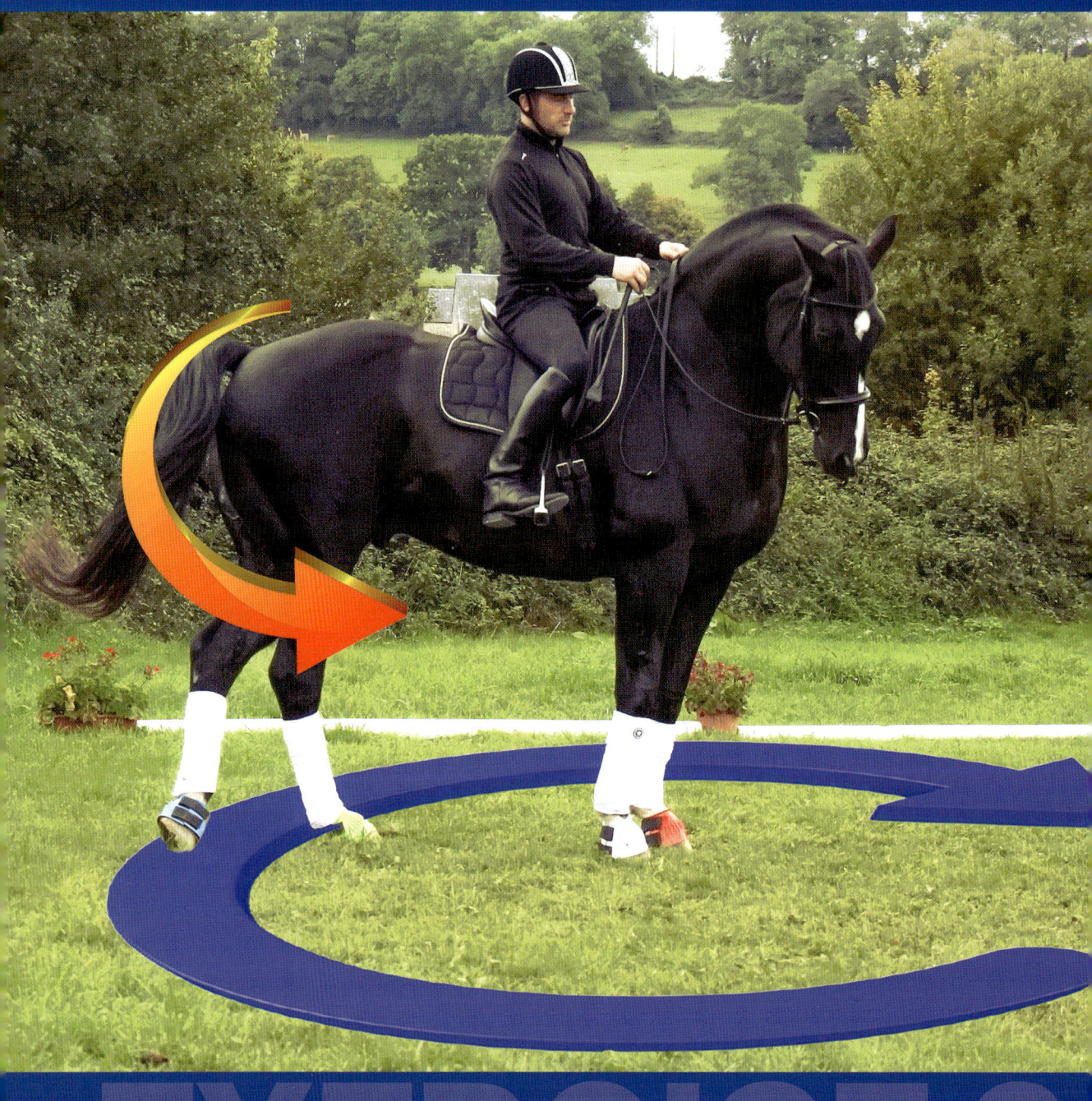

EXERCISE 2

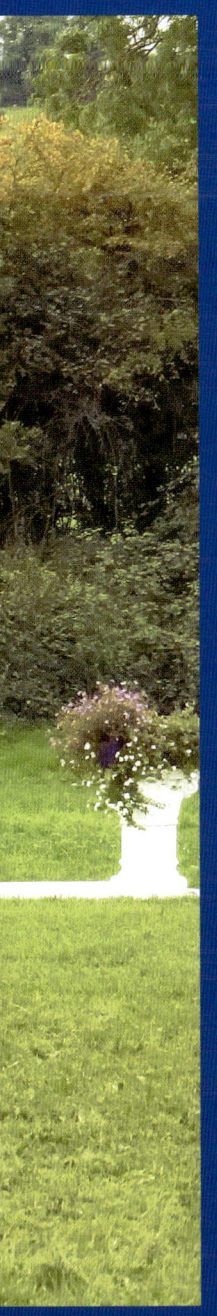

◀ / 6.12 / In the Turn on the Forehand the horse's hind legs cross, making the hindquarters describe a large circle around the pivoting forehand.

Exercise 2

🕉 / **The Yoga Half-Split**
🐴 / **The Turn on the Forehand**

The *Half-Split* is all about the lower back and legs. Its equine alter ego is the *Turn on the Forehand*, which can work miracles inside the horse's body (fig. 6.12). This movement isolates, liberates, and activates the deepest parts of the lumbar back in a way no other movement can, giving quick and permanent improvements when performed just right.

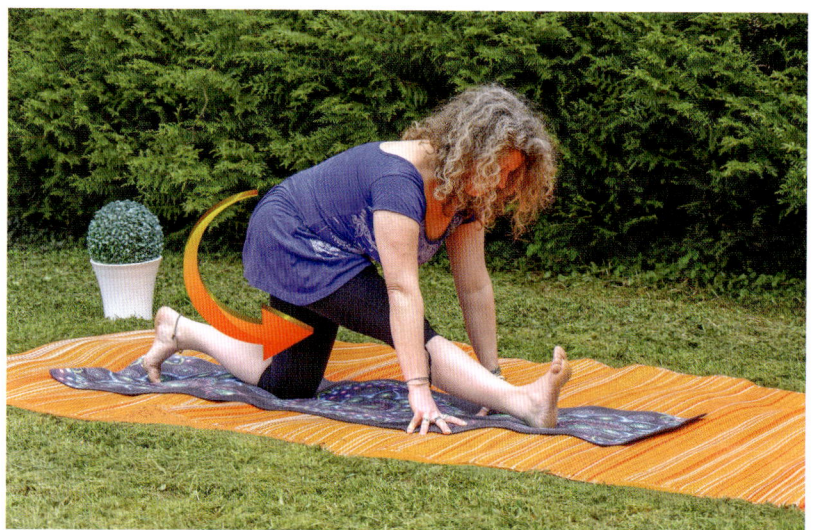

/ 6.13 / *The yoga Half-Split Pose brings your leg forward and under your body to stretch the lower back.* ▶

🧘 / The Half-Split Pose

The *Half-Split Pose* is a forward stretch that focuses on your pelvis' ability to place your leg under the body while rounding and rotating the lower back (fig. 6.13). It is even harder than it sounds. It is, though, a very effective exercise for stretching out the lower half of the body as a warm-up for advanced poses.

This exercise helps humans by:

- Stretching hips, hamstrings, calves, back, and hips.
- Relieving back and sciatic pain.
- Toning the abdominal muscles.
- Improving balance.
- Enhancing concentration and coordination.
- Helping to calm the anxious mind.

The *Half-Split Pose* stretches the hamstrings and opens the hips, which often relieves trapped nerves in the lower body that usually originate from muscular tightness in the lower back.

/ Turn on the Forehand

Good for opening gates? Certainly. Yet Turn on the Forehand is so, so much more. It's a rider favorite for how quickly a horse learns to engage the hind legs all on his own. Used naturally by horses in the stable and field to turn around, this completely natural movement, practiced to perfection and smoothly performed, will unlock a defensive back, engage the hind limbs, and guarantee a smile on the part of the rider (fig. 6.14).

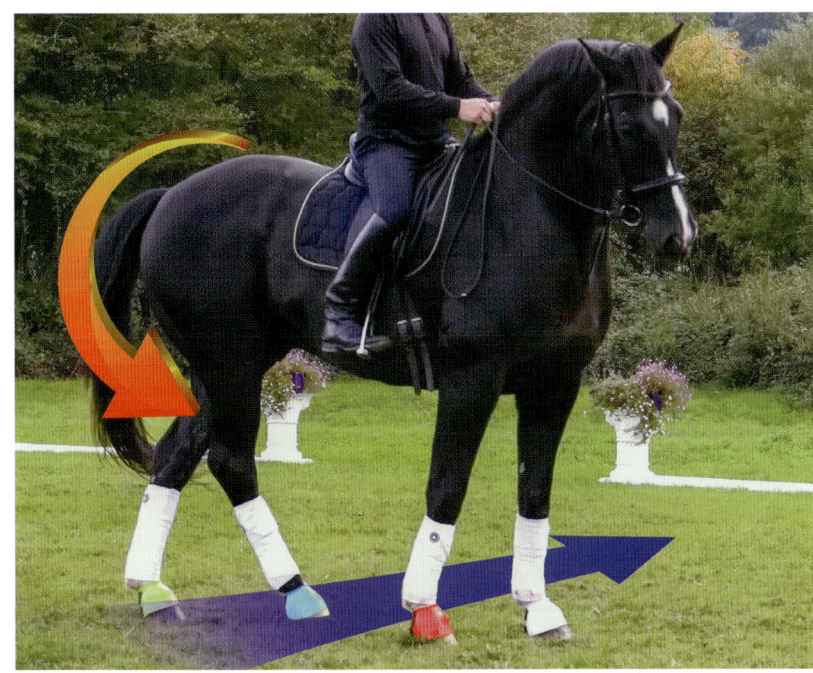

◄ / 6.14 / *Bringing the inside hind under the horse's body with each Turn on the Forehand stride activates the Pelvic Tilt Core Power.*

This exercise helps the horse:

- Mobilize through the pelvis and hind legs.
- Gain flexibility through the lower back.
- Tone core muscles including the *multifidus, abdominals,* and *iliopsoas.*
- Increase the range of motion of the hind limbs.
- Improve the transfer of weight from inside to outside hind.
- Improve balance.

This exercise helps solve these issues under saddle:

- Stiffness to inside bend.
- Poor engagement.
- Poor balance.
- A four-beat or disunited canter.
- Falling in/out.
- Crooked gaits.
- Poor inside leg response.

What It Does Inside the Horse

Having a similar effect to an "oblique crunch" for humans, the *Turn on the Forehand* is an incredibly simple combination of suppling, mobilizing, coordinating, and strengthening, all in one. All the three main core muscle groups are activated (figs. 6.15, 6.16, & 6.17).

The Turn on the Forehand asks the horse to master the act of putting his hind foot under his center of gravity and then taking weight on it in a sidestep. To do this he has to do many things at once, such as

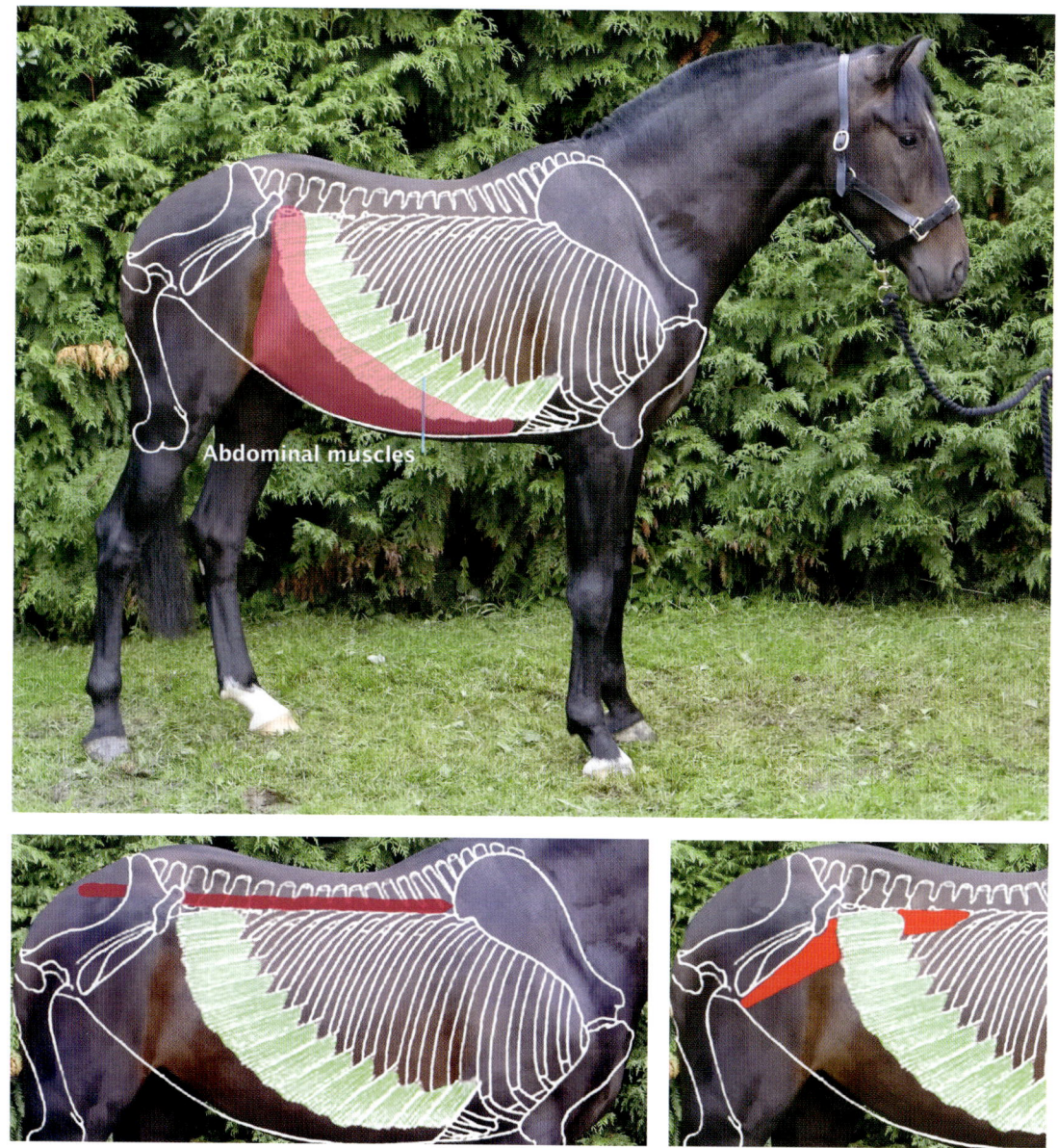

▲ / **6.15** / The abdominal muscles: A taut belly keeps the back supported (top).
/ **6.16** / The *multifidus* muscles: Deep core spinal control muscles (left).
/ **6.17** / The *iliopsoas* muscles: Engage and connect the rear end (right).

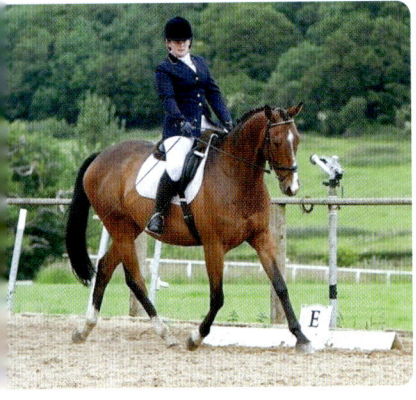

Dana and Ollie

(United Kingdom)

I bought Sudest Island ("Ollie") as a seven-year-old ex-racehorse. He had retired injured, destined for the bullet but saved by his groom because of his exceptional temperament. He came to me having received little in the way of retraining, and had I known how little, he would simply not have been an option for me as my first step into horse ownership!

Nevertheless, I adored him, his quirks, his cheeky side, the unfaltering affection that he showed me. He was a trier, and no matter what I threw at him, he would always give it his all—even when the question probably wasn't clear! We learned and grew together. We overcame tendon and ligament surgery, numerous facial wounds and impressive leg wounds and came back stronger every time!

The summer of 2015 was our season—not much to many, I'm sure, but we were out there competing and even occasionally coming home with a ribbon. In October 2015 we managed to qualify for the Championships of Great Britain (an unaffiliated national championship) at both Preliminary and Novice Level dressage. I had no expectations of winning or even placing as Ollie's movement was never "quality," but I was proud to be there! We had an amazing weekend: seven tests in three days. We even managed to get a ribbon, and Ollie felt as strong and happy on Sunday night as he had when we arrived on Friday morning.

On returning home, Ollie had a couple of well-earned days rest, and on the Wednesday I decided to pop over some jumps as a reward to him for all

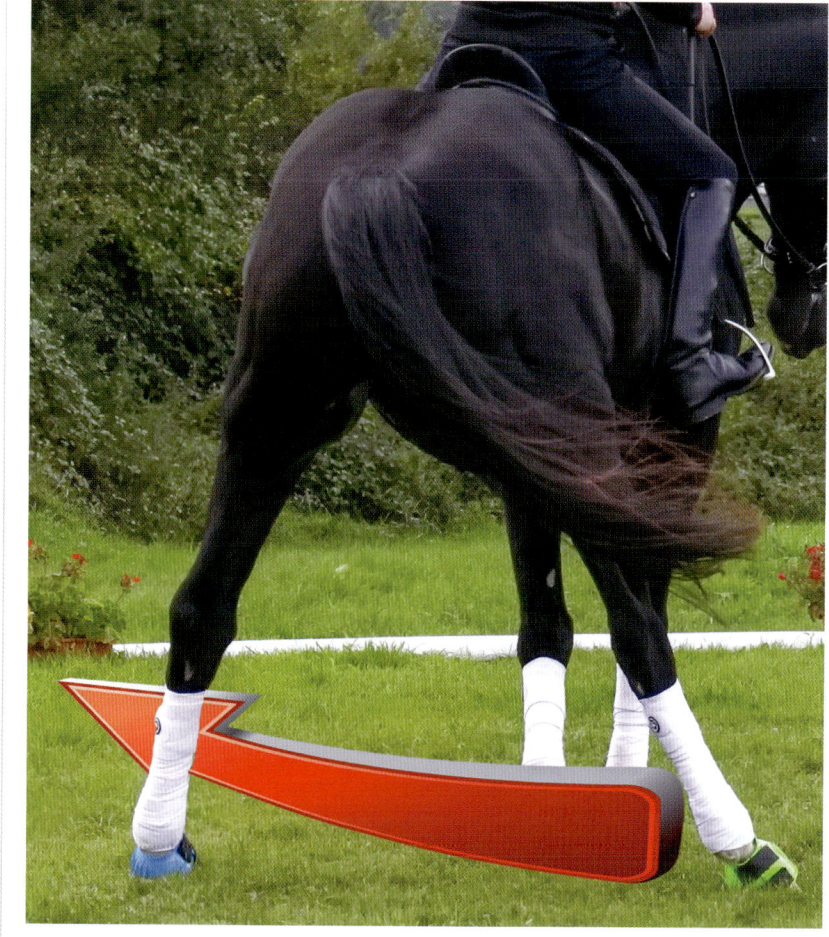

◄ / 6.18 / *Swinging the hind limb across the body builds strength and coordination in the rear end.*

release and rotate through the lumbar back and pelvis while stretching the hind limbs laterally (fig. 6.18). This exercise is done slowly and deliberately for this reason, giving the horse time to bend and release without triggering tension.

"As he turns his hindquarter around the forehand in walk steps, Turn on the Forehand improves coordination and brings about suppleness,"

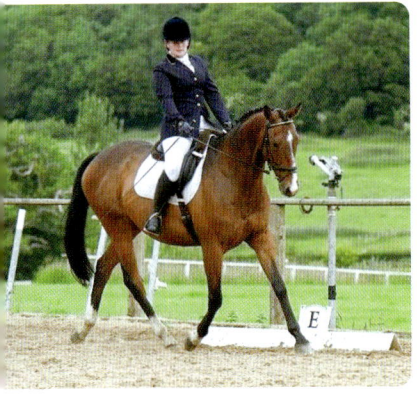

DANA AND OLLIE
CORE STORY

the boring flatwork. As soon as I picked up trot during my warm-up, I instantly knew that something was wrong...he felt "lumpy"! I asked a few others at the barn, and they agreed—something was not right in his back end. I got off and with no obvious heat or swelling, I tucked him in for the night. The next morning I trotted him up, and he looked happy and sound. I gave him the day off anyway and on another clear trot up on the Friday, I hopped back on.... But still "lumpy"!

Over the next few days I tried stall rest, bute, turn out... nothing made a difference. He was sound to trot up and longe but lame under saddle. My vet blocked out the legs and stifles and came to the conclusion that it must be in his back or pelvis somewhere, but there was no sign of any localized pain, and the lameness was bilateral, appearing much more severe on the left rein. Ollie had quarterly physical therapy treatments (as he has never been the strongest), and his saddle was checked and adjusted frequently. The vets were at a loss. The next approach was to bring him into full work to see if the symptoms disappeared, or if it made him worse. We needed him to help us find the problem. He pressed on with his work as asked but was clearly not right. This was probably the hardest part for me—to ride a horse I cared about so much, when I knew I was causing pain, was soul-destroying!

My vet was reluctant to do spinal X-rays as Ollie had always been poor in terms of topline, and his view was that we might see some signs of changes in the vertebrae, but these could have been present for years. He didn't want to jump to conclusions before everything else had been ruled out. Ollie was referred to the hospital for a bone scan. I eagerly awaited the results, only to be told that there was nothing significant to be seen. We were now out of options; X-rays were all we had left.

As soon as the image appeared on the screen, I knew Ollie's bones were not meant to be wrapped around each other as they appeared. The vet recommended that we inject the spine, and if Ollie's pain couldn't be managed with the injections, we could then look to surgery, if necessary. The injections made zero difference. I knew we had to operate. I wasn't ready to give up on my boy. The surgery was textbook, the patient was a star and rehabbed like a pro. He walked in hand well, he turned out without any drama, he longed over poles, and 10 weeks post-surgery his writes the United States Dressage Federation (USDF). "Turn on the Forehand teaches the elementary coordination of the aids essential to the further development of the rider and can be used to provide the rider with effective gymnastic schooling that creates a supple and willing horse."

This is one of the most difficult exercises to perfect at Tone Level because it requires a very deep level of suppleness and connection between horse and rider; but once achieved, it is never forgotten.

Core Score, Level, and Head-and-Neck Position

If your horse has a Core Score of:

- **3–5**, then do this exercise at the **RELEASE LEVEL.**
- **2**, then do this exercise at the **COORDINATION LEVEL.**
- **0–1**, then do this exercise at the **TONE LEVEL.**

Use this exercise in Release Level until Core Release and Long-and-Low HNP is easy for the horse, then progress through the more demanding Levels as the horse improves in Coordination and regularity. Note that the Levels are not adjusted by gait, as in some of the other exercises, but by how many crossing steps you ask for. All Levels perform this exercise from the standstill (fig. 6.19).

As this static exercise focuses on the back, lumbar back, and core, the HNP can be left to wherever your horse feels comfortable. In developing this exercise he has enough to work out inside his body

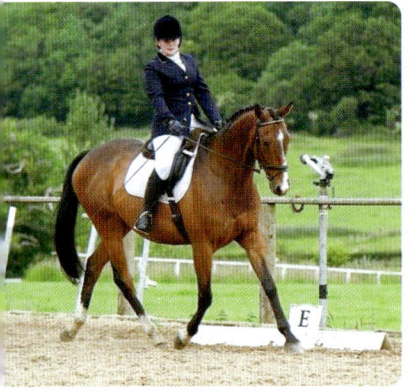

DANA AND OLLIE
CORE STORY

physical therapist and the vet agreed we were ready to get back on. The walk was good… just like I had never been away. He was calm and happy to have me on his back. The trot…was "lumpy" and unchanged. As I fell out of the saddle, hysterical, the vet said the words that everyone dreads: "I don't think he is in any pain; it must be mechanical. He will not be able to do what you want him to do."

I went home that night heartbroken. My world had fallen apart. It couldn't be the end; it just couldn't be. A good friend had reassured me that it was too soon to make the call, that maybe Ollie needed more time. It was around three the next morning, through tired and tearful eyes, that I found an article online by Simon Cocozza called, "Kiss Kissing Spines goodbye." I had not heard of Simon before but read the article and absorbed every word. Could these exercises help my horse to strengthen his spine? Was it really possible to make him stronger than he had been before? I sent Simon an email (not expecting any response), simply thanking him for putting the inspirational words out there. You can't imagine how truly touched I was the next day when a reply landed in my inbox. He reassured me and offered encouragement and support that I could not have dreamed of.

With Ollie's physical therapist's okay, I spent the next few weeks walking under saddle and continuing with the longe work that we had started. We incorporated core strengthening bands: first an abdominal band, and then later we added a hindquarter band to encourage Ollie to engage his core and lift his back. And one day I asked for trot and…the limpy, "lumpy" horse had gone, and an even, balanced stride had returned like magic. Core strengthening was the key!

Ollie and I attended our first clinic with Simon in July 2016, six months post-surgery. Simon had reviewed our progress via photos and videos, and I was overjoyed to meet him in person. Ollie was still being supported by his bands, and I was still reluctant to push him for fear of "breaking" him once again, but Simon gave me the courage to push the boundaries. He made me believe that my horse was indeed sound. The change in Ollie even just within an hour with Simon was unimaginable; it was like someone had flicked the switch.

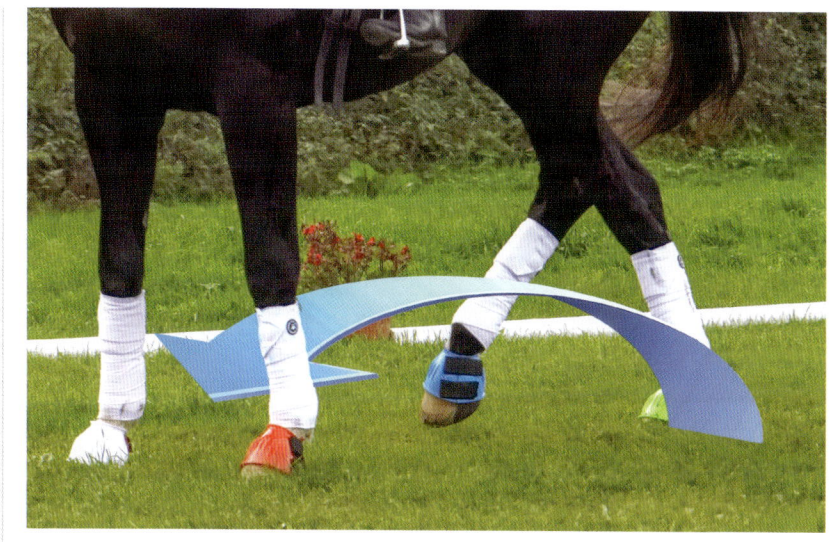

◀ / 6.19 / *Stepping under: The farther the horse steps under the body, the better the exercise will be for his gaits.*

without the distraction of having his head "placed." The exercise itself will gradually and naturally bring the horse "on the bit" by rounding the back first (as it should be done).

- **RELEASE LEVEL** (The Principle of "Stepping Under"): Do one to three steps, then reward. This can be deceptively hard for even very well-conditioned horses that may have a weak core. In the beginning, all you should expect is one or two sideways steps from the hindquarters away from a stimulating inside leg and followed by the Tapping Stick (see p. 146) if needed. One step rewarded quickly and well learned will soon be three, then five, and so on.

- **COORDINATION LEVEL** (Half to One Full Rotation): This is where the horse must learn to coordinate and string multiple steps together in Turn on the Forehand. Encourage, forgive, reward, then try again in the other direction.

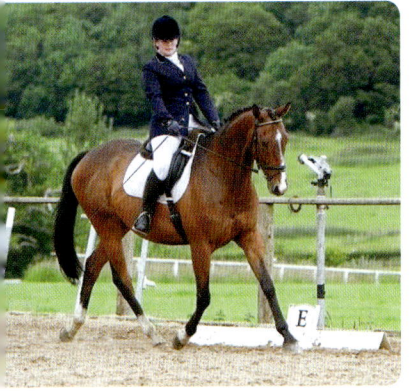

Over the year that followed I worked with exercises that Simon gave us, and the bands were used less and less. By October 2016 we attended a second clinic, band-free, and were competing again—immediately scoring higher than we had in the past. My horse had learned to engage his hindquarters, to stretch through his entire back. I could feel when his spine was lifted beneath me and when he reverted to his old hollow frame and needed encouragement. The exercises and the knowledge had not only made Ollie a better horse, but they had made me a better rider. As the winter season drew to a close in early 2017, Ollie and I were named Winter Champions in the Retrained Racehorse Section at Abbey Dressage.

We clinic with Simon regularly. The learning process will never stop: We learn new exercises and every one unlocks a new door in terms of performance and health. There have been hiccups along the way, and I don't doubt they will continue to arise, but we are armed now, Ollie and I. We have Simon's techniques to bring relief to tight muscles after stall rest, to calm and loosen him in the warm-up ring, to break up a week of disciplined schooling and jumping, just to warm up before any ride and stretch out after. I don't even have to ask the questions anymore: Ollie will look for the stretch and loves his work more than ever. ■

....
Dana and Ollie

DANA AND OLLIE
CORE STORY

- **TONE LEVEL** (Continuous Rotation while Framing): This is where the movement is perfected. Developing the ability to rotate smoothly in Turn on the Forehand is a skill every horse should learn. Establishing rhythm, balance, and fluidity, the mobility of the hindquarters will improve every step of every movement the horse makes. At this Level, create a Framing outside rein (see p. 142) during the Turn on the Forehand rotation and the horse should align enough to drop naturally into Forward, Down, and Out HNP (fig. 6.20). Another good day.

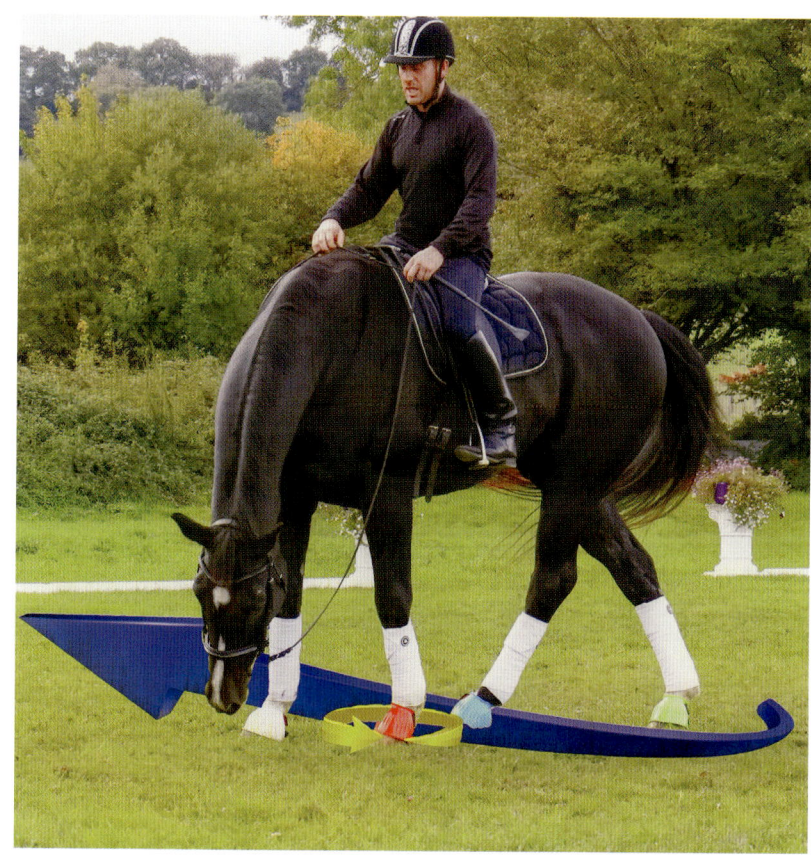

◄ / 6.20 / Turn on the Forehand in Tone Level: When the horse becomes very coordinated and toned in this exercise, the spine aligns so well the horse will be happy to stretch all the way into Forward, Down, and Out.

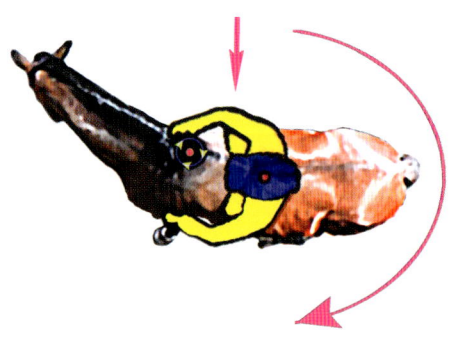

/ 6.21 / *Stretching Flexion: Asking the horse to move away from the inside leg.* ▶

How to Do It

OVERVIEW: The *Turn on the Forehand* is done from a standstill with an inside Stretching Flexion (see p. 139) in the neck (fig. 6.21). Your goal is for the horse to move his bottom in a circle around the shoulders, which stay over the same spot. The hind legs cross to make the turn, with the inside hind crossing in front of the outside hind.

- **STEP /1/** Halt with plenty of room (fig. 6.22). Create a Stretching Flexion in the neck and Hold the inside rein (see p. 141). Using the inside leg at the girth, stimulate the horse to move away from the aid. If the horse doesn't respond to the leg aid, commence the Tapping Stick until the first step is made, then reward.
- **STEP /2/** Initially the horse may be sticky and unsure. Encourage and reward any deliberate crossing steps—however slow or clumsy—as he is just learning them. Build more rotation step by step, releasing to a Long-and-Low HNP, giving a treat if he really invests himself.

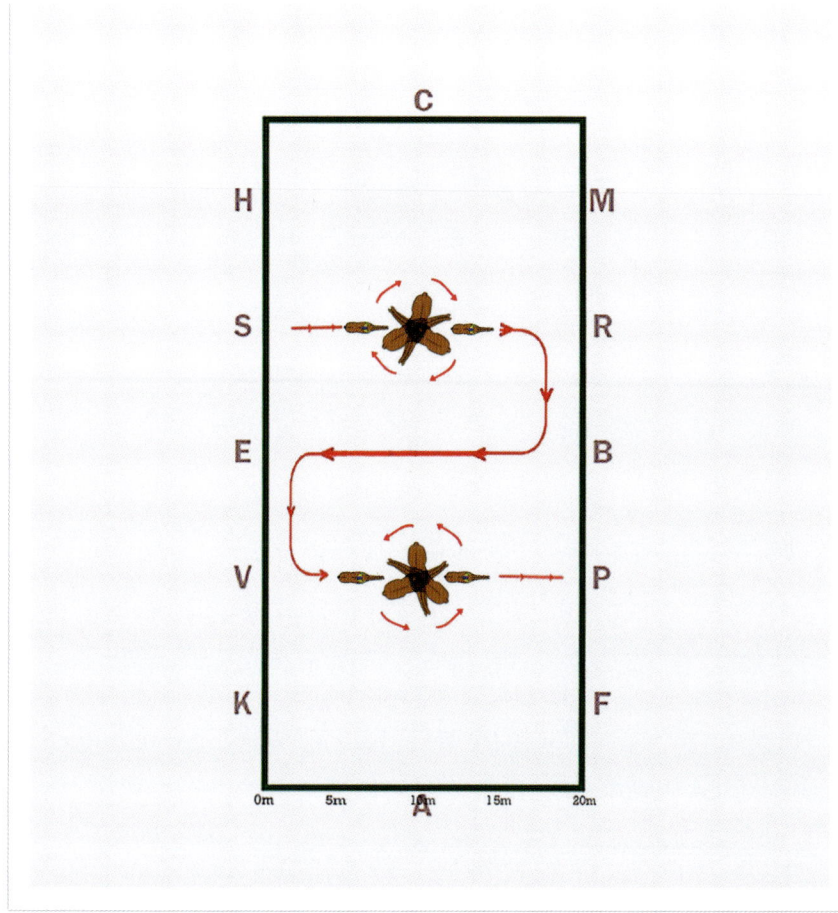

◀ / 6.22 / *Choosing a floor plan: Riding a particular shape for exercise takes care of both directions and helps the horse understand what is needed "next time." Here, the centerline is an excellent place for both Turn on the Forehand left and right with a change of bend at X.*

- **STEP /3/** As it becomes easier for your horse to rotate smoothly and without stopping, keep rotating for two or three full rotations, solving any directional issues as you go. This is both the Tone Level and the exercise's final goal. It cannot be done too elegantly!

When it has become easy, this exercise can be performed in Forward, Down, and Out HNP for an incredible core workout.

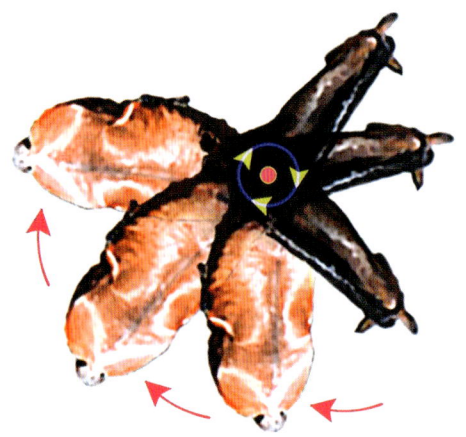

/ **6.23** / *Tone Level: By consecutively repeating the Turn on the Forehand steps, the horse will become smoother, more coordinated, and stronger.* ▶

Common Problems and Solutions

- ***The hind legs will not cross.*** Just to get the ball rolling, attempt the exercise from walk, and "drift" into the first Turn on the Forehand by way of a leg-yield step, before rewarding your horse.
- ***Walking out and walking backward.*** A horse with a sensitive back will try to avoid bending in this exercise. He must try, though, if he is going to get better. If he backs up or walks "through" his shoulder, the best solution is to re-establish the Stretching Flexion and the inside leg response rather than try to correct the evasion itself. It is a just a knack, but a useful one.

The crucial tool in this exercise is practice. It can be very sticky in the beginning, indicating a deep-down lack of flexibility in the area of the horse's back behind the saddle. Gradually, the horse will discover that coordinating a smooth crossing of the hind limbs is the easiest way to turn, and this is a breakthrough moment worth practicing. Making mistakes and being clumsy are all part of the learning process, so particularly with this exercise, I encourage the use of boots and wraps as leg protection.

Core Score Zero Goal

This exercise can be profound. The rotational engagement of the pelvis is unlike any other movement and really hits the mark and brings resolution to some of the stiffening traits of a compromised lower back. When perfected to the point where the horse can bend and engage his body easily, the horse will be automatically wrapped around the inside leg, aligned through the core, and ready for anything.

"The impulsion and elasticity of the gaits depends on the suppleness and especially the springy power of the hind legs. They can be improved a great deal by developing the haunches," wrote Alois Podhajsky. "One of the main training goals of any riding horse must be to strengthen and to supple the haunches and to use them to support the weight of horse and rider." ■

END OF EXERCISE 2
The Yoga Half-Split / The Turn on the Forehand

/ **6.24** / Forward, Down, and Out allows the back to find its full unrestricted freedom. ▶

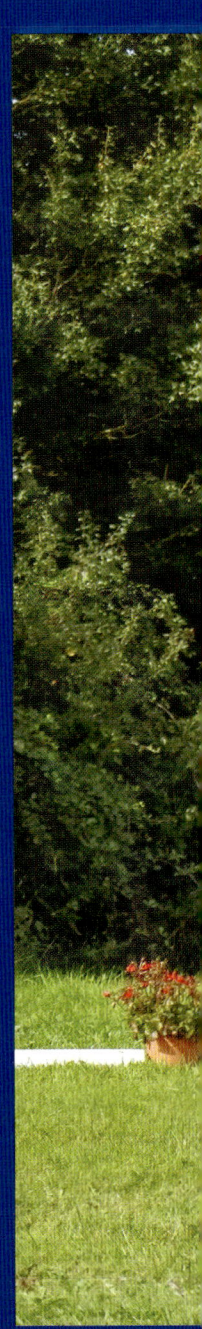

Exercise 3

/ The Cat Pose
/ Forward, Down, and Out (FDO)

The *Cat Pose* is a wonderful, natural, full-spine stretch for humans, of course inspired by our purring house guests. It gives complete liberation through the whole length of your back and luckily proves just as beneficial for our equine friends as it does for us. This exercise for horses—called *Forward, Down, and Out*—takes the longitudinal stretching of the back to its most comfortable position for the horse—that of grazing—and aims to complete the release started by Exercise 1: Core Release Volte in Long-and-Low (fig. 6.24).

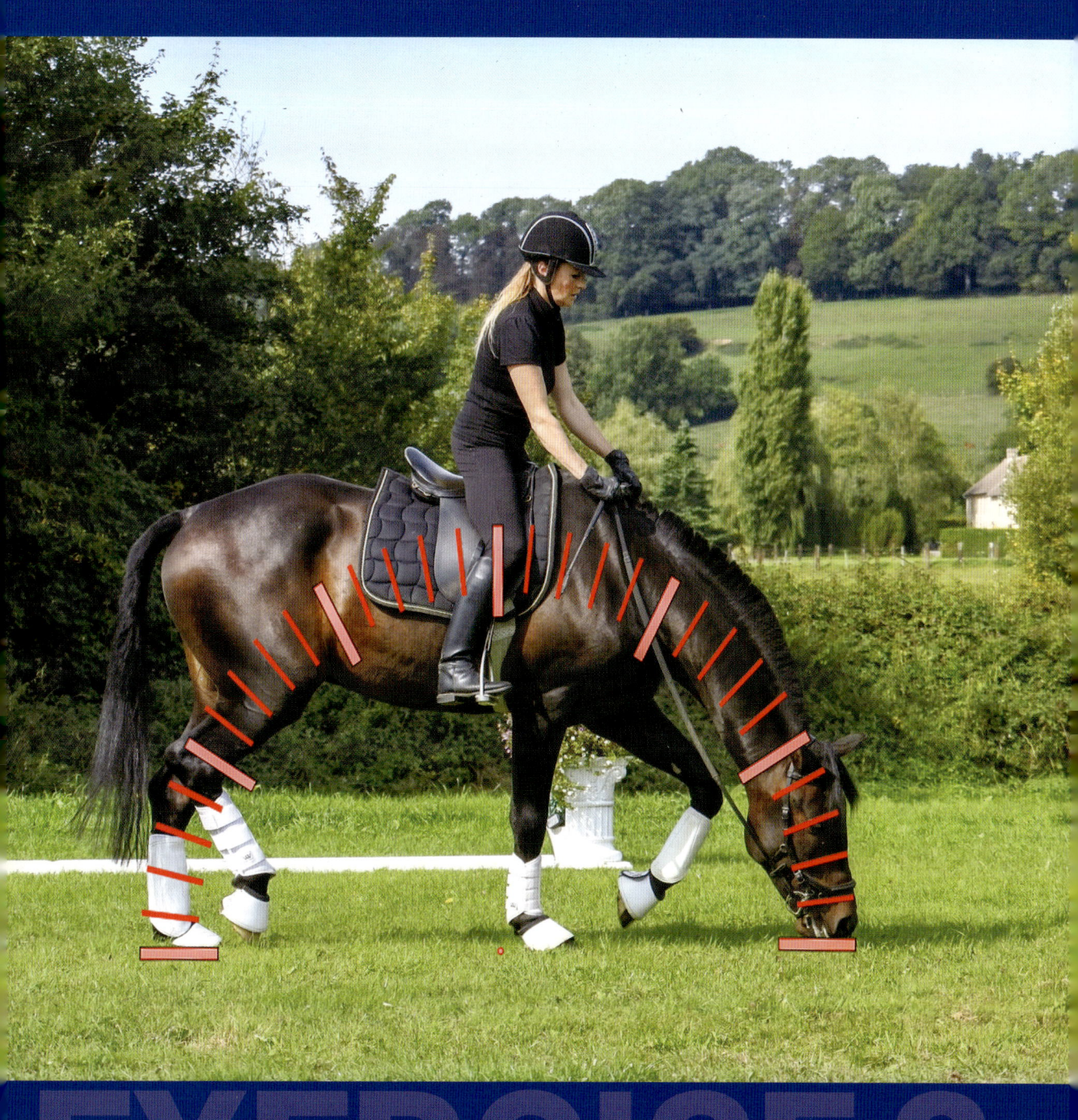

EXERCISE 3

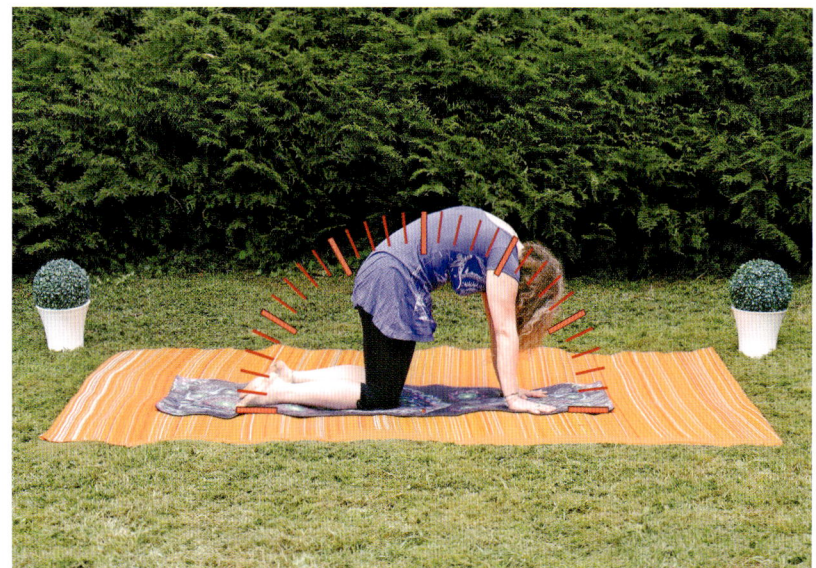

/ **6.25** / *The yoga Cat Pose stretches the human back in a way that gently releases tight muscle and stiff areas.* ▶

🧘 / The Cat Pose

The *Cat Pose* is performed on all fours and involves arching your back and lowering your head, just like a cat stretches. This vertical rounding of the back helps realign, release, and mobilize the human back from the pelvis to neck (fig. 6.25).

This pose helps a human to:

- Gain flexibility in the spine.
- Strengthen wrists and shoulders.
- Tone the abdomen.
- Improve digestion.
- Relax the mind and relieve stress.
- Improve blood circulation to the brain and organs.

The Cat Pose promotes overall durability of the spinal column. It can play a significant role in correcting an individual's posture while relieving tension in the lower back. "The yoga Cat Pose is a movement that combines forward bends with back arches, giving your back the complete movement it needs," explains Indian yoga teacher Shirin Mehdi. "Your vertebrae become mobile, releasing all the tension trapped in the cervical, thoracic, and lumbar areas."

/ Forward, Down, and Out

Forward, Down, and Out is so natural, it happens on its own. This stretching exercise is so named because of its relationship to the Head-and-Neck position we discussed on p. 132—it is the horse's grazing position, after all.

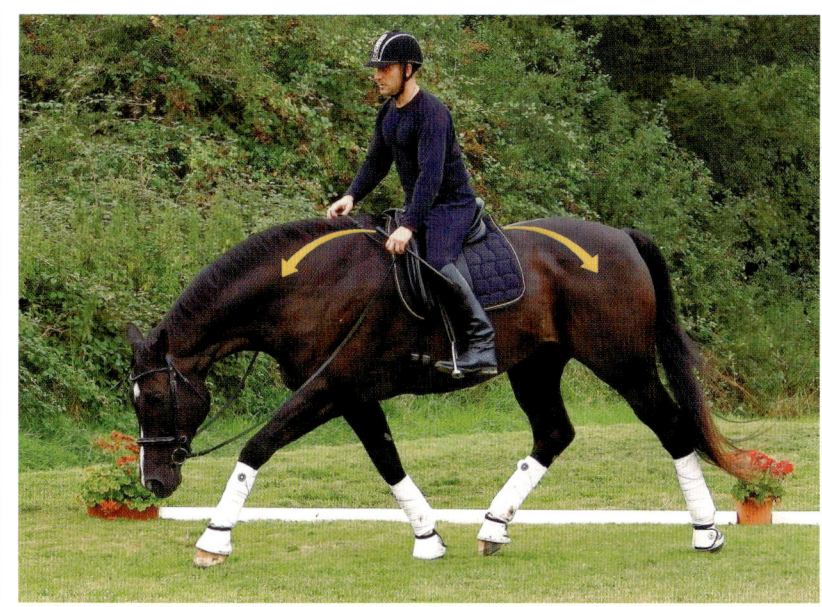

◄ / 6.26 / By gradually allowing Wardance to stretch down in trot d'école, his back is put under a natural traction, lifting and separating the thoracic vertebrae.

"Because of its multiple advantages, the work with the low neck constitutes one of the basic exercises of the physical preparation of the horse," wrote Dr. Jean-Marie Denoix in *Biomechanics and Physical Training of the Horse.*

With our help the horse gradually discovers that he can move and stretch at the same time (fig. 6.26). Nothing engages the core quite like it, and it is so natural that once we have shown a horse he can do it, he quickly adopts it as a preferred way to self-balance in all gaits (fig. 6.27). This exercise begins with the Long-and-Low Outline from Exercise 1: Core Release Voltes (see p. 159),

This exercise helps the horse to:

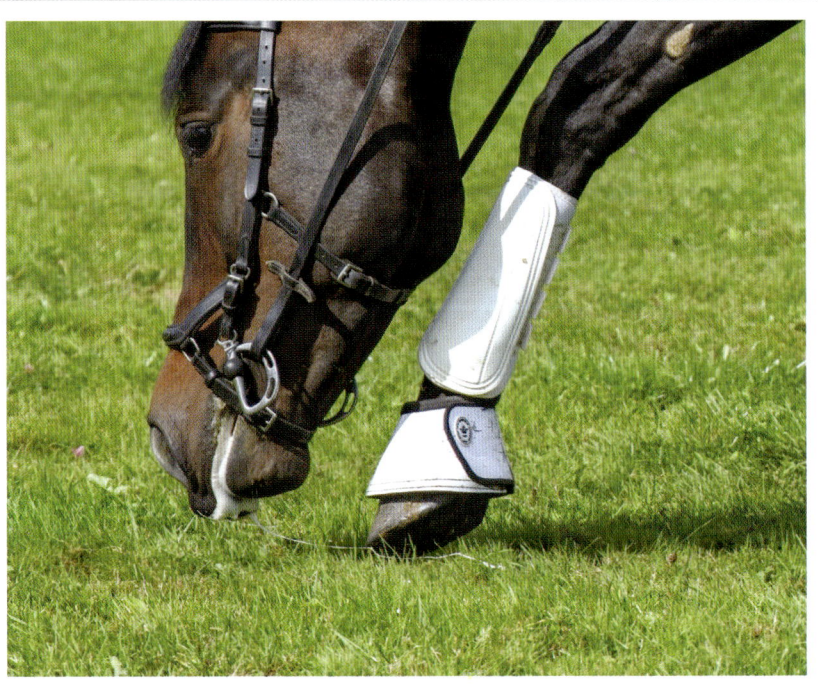

/ 6.27 / *The most natural posture of all: The horse's body is designed to keep his nose in the grass for the majority of the day. Learning to move slowly like this is a natural skill.* ▶

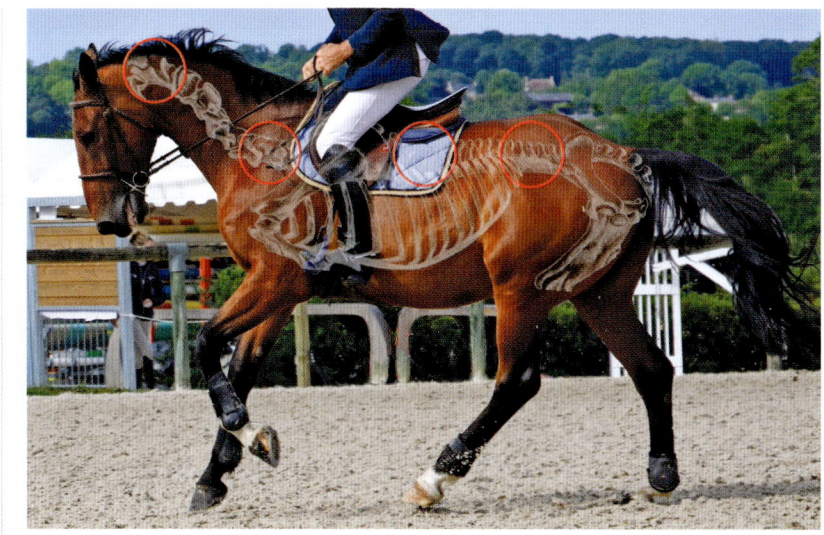

◀ / 6.28 / The full spinal stretch of the Forward, Down, and Out HNP can release all the usual compression points, immediately helping the horse.

- Have a fully supple spine.
- Activate the Thoracic Lift, the Nuchal Lift and the Pelvic Tilt (see the Three Core Powers, p. 44).
- Improve suppleness in all locomotory structures attached to the spine.
- Improve body confidence.
- Reverse dipping in the back.
- Create a smooth and comfortable gait.
- Release all tightness in the back.

The Nuchal and Thoracic Lift actions become noticeable as the horse learns to round his back. The exercise gradually melts tightness at deeper and deeper levels, rounding and stretching the horse a little more in each session (fig. 6.28). "One of the most valuable early lessons in dressage is teaching your horse to stretch down," agrees FEI dressage trainer Jerry Schwartz. "Not only does it confirm and improve his contact on the bit, it also provides you with a valuable tool for

rewarding and relaxing him. It's something you'll use every day in your training no matter what level you're riding so it's all the more important that you don't take any shortcuts teaching your horse to do it."
This exercise helps solve these issues under saddle:

- Hard or unstable mouth.
- Uncomfortable gaits/hollow back.
- High head.
- Stuffy paces.
- Stiff gaits.
- Unhappiness; lack of enthusiasm.

Forward, Down, and Out is also an excellent reward and release between exercises or as a warm-down exercise in itself (see p. 186).

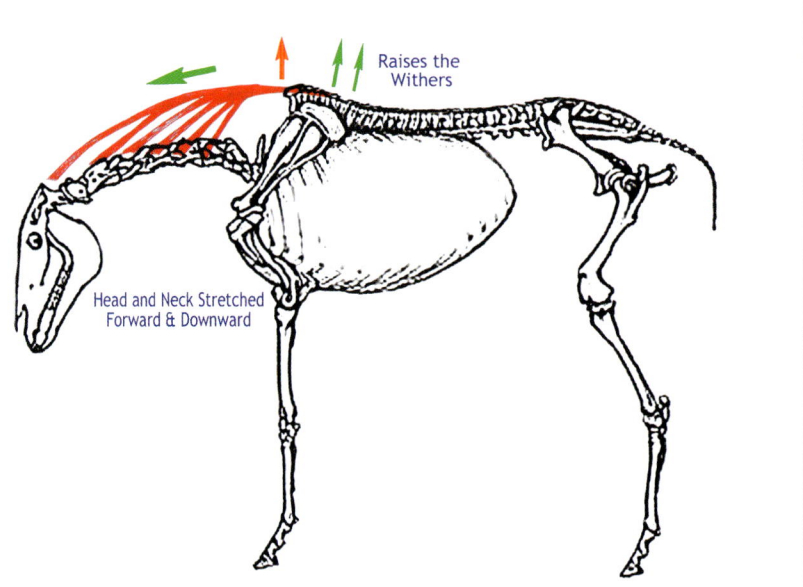

/ 6.29 / *The Nuchal Lift under saddle: By activating this Core Power, the horse's body brings itself into balance without any further help from us.* ▶

What It Does Inside the Horse

Releasing the spine fully allows all of Mother Nature's physical miracles to come to life, whatever the species. As the horse's body gets longer and the nose can stretch lower, this activates all the horse's most powerful internal geometry in such a way that the core pushes the horse's back upward (fig. 6.29). Once the horse learns that by stretching his topline he can then shorten the "lowline," progress can be made in all gaits and movements because this postural improvement lets him keep himself round. In this way a once uncomfortable horse can be retrained into a very pleasant ride.

Core Score, Level, and Head-and-Neck Position

If your horse has a Core Score of:

- **4–5**, then do this exercise at the **RELEASE LEVEL.**
- **3**, then do this exercise at the **COORDINATION LEVEL.**
- **0–2**, then do this exercise at the **TONE LEVEL.**

- **RELEASE LEVEL** (Free-Walk, Long-and-Low to Forward, Down, and Out HNP): A free-walk on a long rein in Long-and-Low (Exercise 1—see p. 130), with the horse's head left alone to "bob" lower, into Forward, Down, and Out.

- **COORDINATION LEVEL** (*Trot d'École*, Long-and-Low, to Forward, Down, and Out HNP): In a light and unhurried rising (posting) *trot d'école* in Long-and-Low, simply offer a more downward hand to invite Forward, Down, and Out.

- **TONE LEVEL** (*Petit Galop*, Forward, Down, and Out HNP): After feeling the Core Release in Tone Level of Exercise 1 (p. 163), allow the horse's head to lower itself from Long-and-Low downward into Forward, Down, and Out.

How to Do It

OVERVIEW: For this exercise you set the horse up well, then let him stretch into it (fig. 6.30). Speed and progress are entirely the choice of the horse. You are there to help him discover how free and balanced he can be (because *you* read a book about it!)

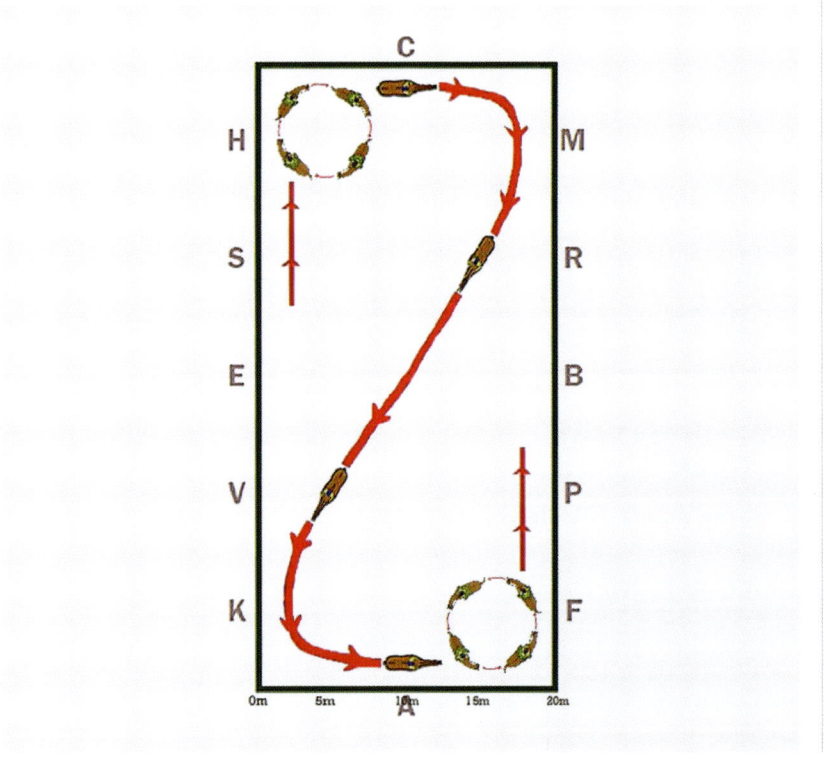

/ **6.30** / *Forward, Down, and Out floor plan: After releasing the core, use the whole arena to allow the horse to discover how to use his body without too many distractions.* ▶

Core Conditioning for Horses

- **STEP /1/** After achieving a Long-and-Low HNP in a Core Release Volte (Exercise 1, p. 156), ride straight away from the volte and allow the reins to slip through your fingers to offer room for the horse's head to stretch as far Forward, Down, and Out as the horse wishes. Steer with a light, guiding contact and always keep a slight inside bend, giving you the option of returning to a volte if the horse loses balance, speeds up, or raises his head too high.
- **STEP /2/** As the horse becomes more balanced while in Forward, Down, and Out HNP, begin to ask for other exercises in your Warm-Up Plan while remaining in FDO (as low as the horse feels comfortable) for very deep core suppling.

Common Problems and Solutions

- ***No Core Release into Forward, Down, and Out and the horse won't stretch down.***

Practice Core Release Voltes until the horse releases in the core and drops into Long-and-Low. While learning to stretch in this way, it is normal for the horse to raise and lower his head frequently between Long-and-Low, Forward, Down, and Out, and perhaps others. This is normal and is indicative of the horse "trying out" different stretches to find his balance. As long as the trend is mostly lowering, stretching, and sticking out the nose—however stiffly—the exercise is working.

"Through stretching the muscles of [the horse's] neck, it will elongate and his back will lift as much as anatomically possible," explains FEI dressage judge and author Christoph Hess. "This process will do your

\\\ Rosie Hope ///

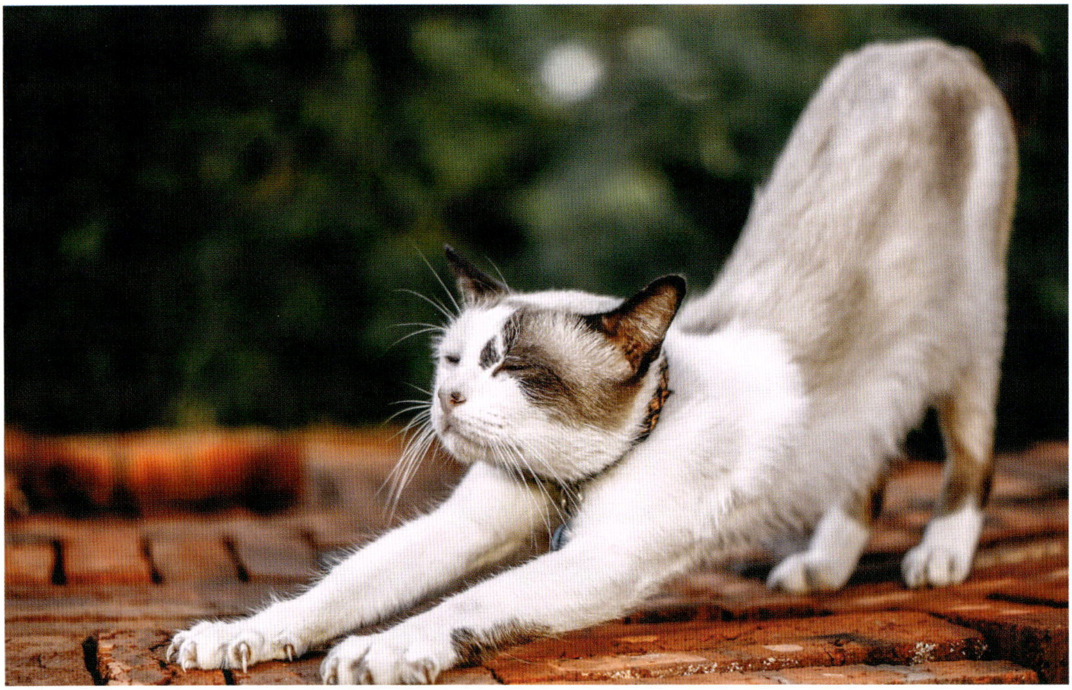

Rosie Hope

"Stretching the back allows the body the space it needs to explore its full range of motion, increasing its functionality to perform and enhance movement patterns."

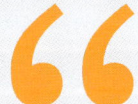

horse good and he will enjoy it. This is his natural position, which you can observe while watching him graze. With consistent practice you create the opportunity for your horse to seek for himself this 'wellness frame' more and more."

Core Score Zero Goal

A 0 Core Score horse in Forward, Down, and Out gives the rider an incredible feeling. When developed to the Tone Level, a horse will be able to walk, trot, canter, and make all the transitions in between with his nose staying voluntarily at coronet level and in front of the vertical. It will look and feel effortless. Then, bringing the head and neck into a Competition Outline HNP is easy. This is the foundation of a sublime ride. ■

END OF EXERCISE 3
The Cat Pose / Forward, Down, and Out (FDO)

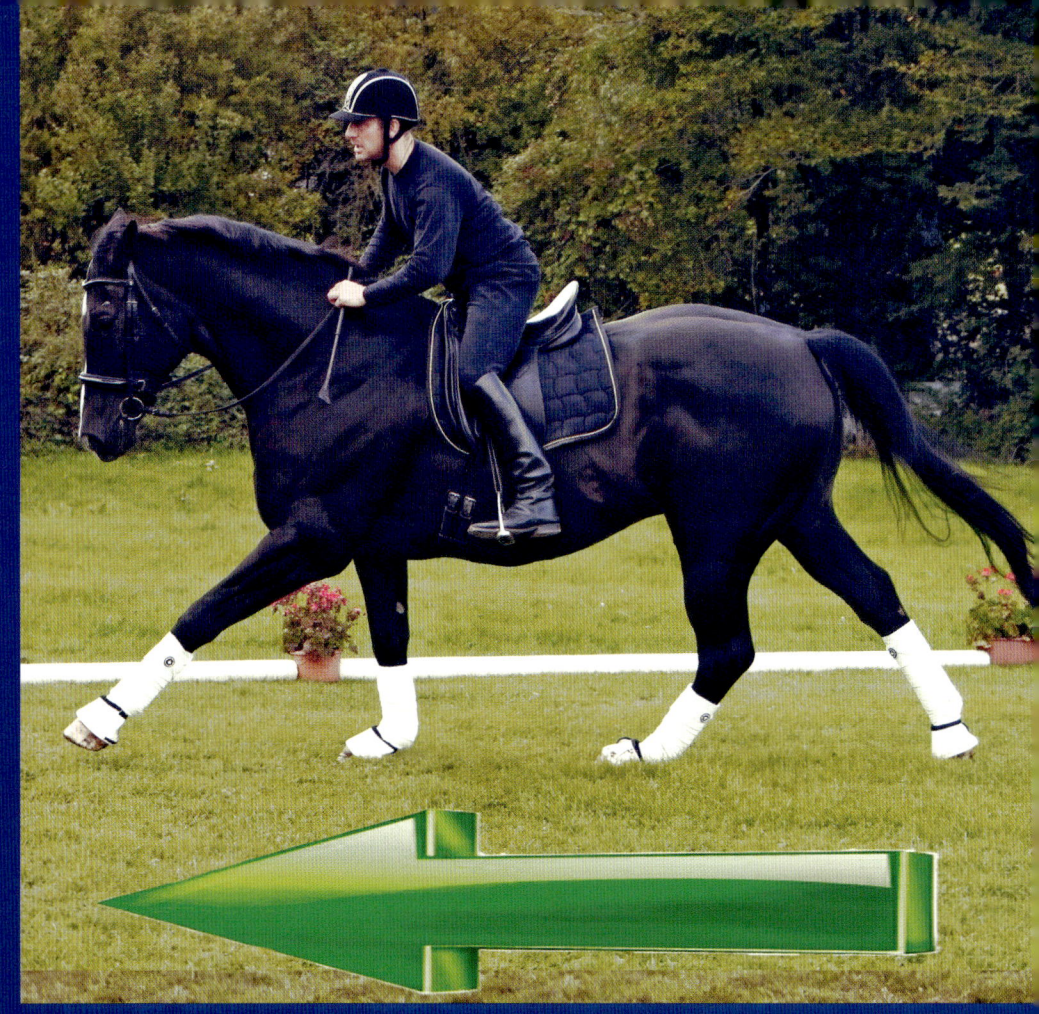

▲ / **6.31** / Forward and Back: As simple as it sounds, lengthening and shortening the stride develops great balance

Exercise 4

/ The Balancing Table to Tiptoe Chair Poses
/ Forward and Back

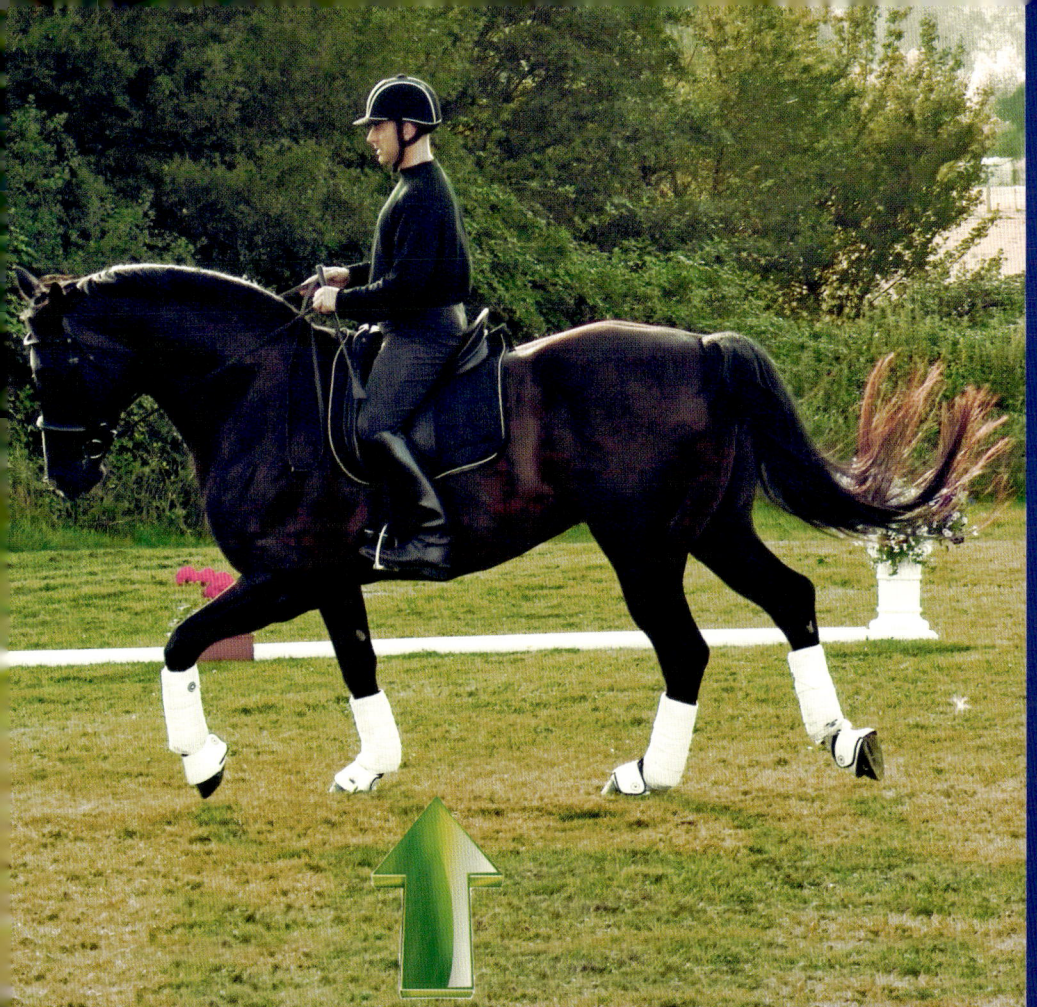

and a stronger connection to your horse.

In this super-simple combination exercise you will show your horse how to stretch and then collect his body, bringing natural athleticism to the stride (fig. 6.31). You do this by alternating between an exercise that mirrors yoga's *Balancing Table Pose* and one like the *Tiptoe Chair Pose*, then back again. This is simply going *forward* and *back* in his different gaits. Nothing could be more useful, natural, and fun.

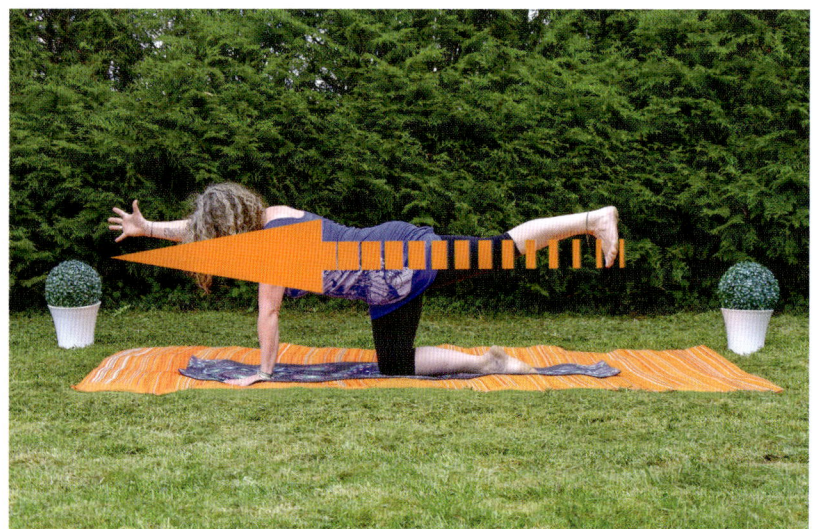

/ **6.32** / *The Balancing Table is the forward stretching phase of the exercise. It challenges your balance and coordination.* ▶

♨ / The Balancing Table Pose

This yoga exercise is a stretching exercise in a forward and active posture (fig. 6.32). As well as warming your body, it primarily brings flexibility to the spine, although this pose also helps to improve focus, coordination, and overall physical equilibrium. Regular practice of the pose will help you build grace and poise.

The Balancing Table Pose helps humans to:

- Strengthen the core and lower back.
- Warm up the body.
- Strengthen shoulders and hips.
- Improve balance and stability.
- Strengthen and realign the spine.
- Improve focus.

"The Balancing Table is a great pose to improve balance!" says British yoga teacher Veronique Gaulthier. "It teaches us to pay attention to our alignment, breath, and our core, and to focus!"

While the Balancing Table Pose stretches, the Tiptoe Chair Pose brings things back into balance.

🙏 / Tiptoe Chair Pose

The second element in this exercise is a shortening, energizing pose called the Tiptoe Chair Pose. It helps develop balance throughout your body from a supple, sitting posture (fig. 6.33). This stance lowers your center of gravity, which cultivates stability and a sharp mental focus. It is as much a mind game as it is a physical challenge.

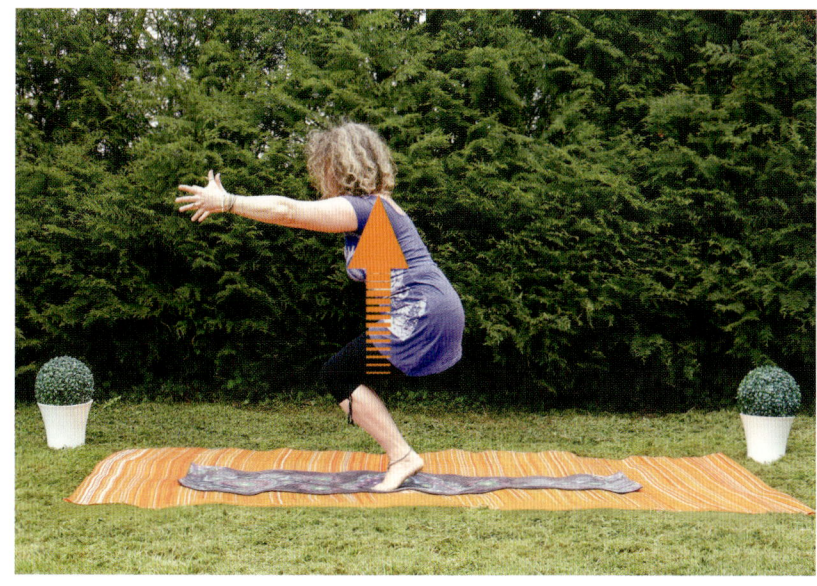

◀ / 6.33 / *The Tiptoe Chair Pose: After stretching forward for the Balancing Table Pose, the Tiptoe Chair Pose brings the body into a near perfect balance.*

This pose helps people to:

- Strengthen the lower back and torso.
- Improve reflexes.
- Exercise the spine, hips, and chest muscles.
- Tone the thigh, ankle, leg, and knee muscles.
- Activate the diaphragm, chest, and upper abdomen.

"Utkatasana (Tiptoe Chair Pose) on toes is packed with huge benefits for your entire body," says Barbora Simek, Canadian Bikram yoga teacher, "and just a little attention and applying yourself to the posture can go a long way."

/ Forward and Back

Forward and Back is the most natural exercise in the world (fig. 6.34). It is packed with goodness for both horse and rider, if you are sensible!

/ 6.34 / *Lengthening and shortening the walk while maintaining rhythm is an excellent way to refine communication.* ▼

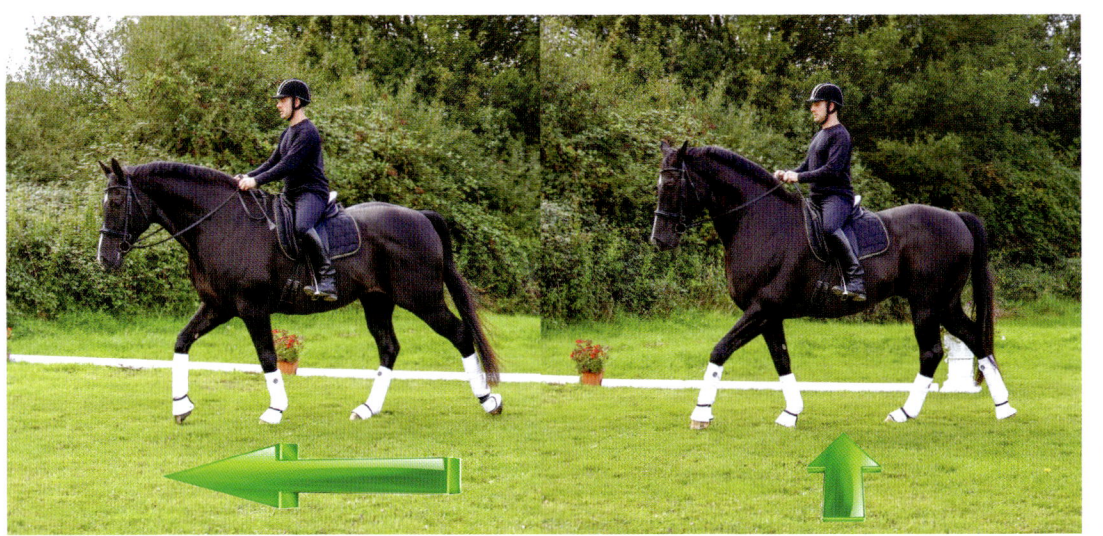

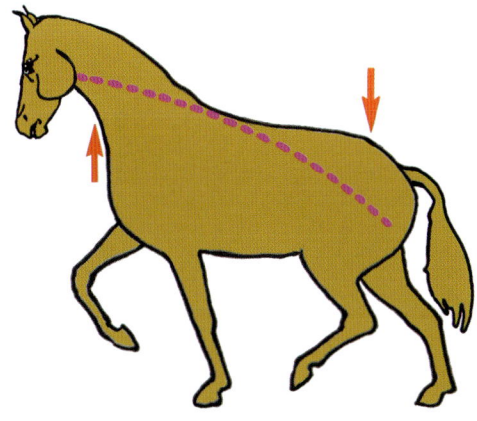

◀ / 6.35 / Bringing the body into balance: The "Back" phase of Forward and Back encourages the horse to sit, lower the hindquarters, and lighten the forehand.

Whatever the breed, horses are dynamic athletes who must do athletic things to remain in good form. This exercise uses the horse's own enthusiasm and energy to improve posture by simply calling it into action.

You are going to teach the horse to go forward and come back using his Core Powers (see p. 44). This will help develop the right reflexes, agility, and deepen your partnership.

This exercise helps the horse by:

- Improving balance.
- Improving enthusiasm.
- Developing the cardiovascular system.
- Increasing agility and reflexes.
- Engaging the three Core Powers.

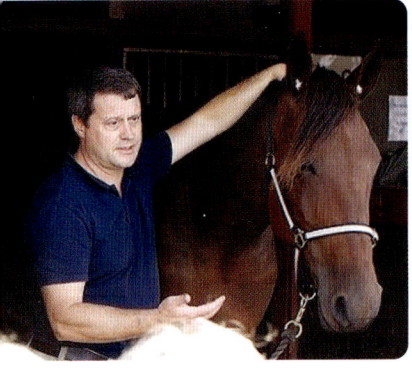

Doychin Lyudov, DVM

(Finland)

My name is Dr. Doychin Lyudov, and I am a veterinary surgeon and specializing in veterinary chiropractic in Europe. In my long practice with horses I have had to treat many patients with back pain and asymmetric or uneven gaits.

Three years ago I met a horse named "Pena" diagnosed with "kissing spine." He was the typical patient with back pain: He had stiff and painful muscles, a poor topline, was difficult to ride, prone to head-shaking, and showed serious changes to the dorsal spinal processes in X-rays. After treatments with chiropractic, acupuncture, and Chinese herbal medicine, Pena improved a lot, but there was always something still "not right" with him.

I recommended the owner use a system of exercises to help Pena improve his balance, muscle condition, and flexibility. That is how we discovered Simon Cocozza's "yoga" for horses. That was the "finish line" for Pena. After one year using these techniques, everything came into place, and my treatments were fully received by his body. This success with Pena encouraged me to start recommending Simon's exercises to all my patients with similar problems. It turned out to be very helpful and useful for all kind of horses: dressage, jumpers, driving horses. I consider his exercises a significant part of my treatment plan for all of my patients with orthopedic and behavior problems nowadays. ■

....
Dr. Doychin Lyudov

A balanced gait is a result of good posture. By encouraging the horse's body to be able to lengthen and shorten itself, the horse can learn to adjust his balance from the core all on his own. This exercise encourages him to place weight only on those structures designed for it, gradually giving him more body confidence (fig. 6.35). The physical involvement of this exercise will bring a new attitude to the horse. A little bit of excitement can hold his concentration better than any aid, yet be sure it is only a little!

This exercise helps solve these issues under saddle:

- Bored or sleepy attitude.
- Slow to go, no to slow.
- Gaits on the forehand.
- Distracted mind.
- Lack of natural engagement.

The horse will be able to give you shorter, bouncier strides and better forward reflexes from smaller and smaller aids. This effect is particularly important for jumpers needing an elastic and supple stride that can shorten and lengthen easily and instantly.

Core Score, Level, and Head-and-Neck Position

If your horse has a Core Score of:

- **0–1**, do the exercise in **TONE LEVEL.**
- **2–3**, do the exercise in **COORDINATION LEVEL.**
- **4–5**, do the exercise in **RELEASE LEVEL.**

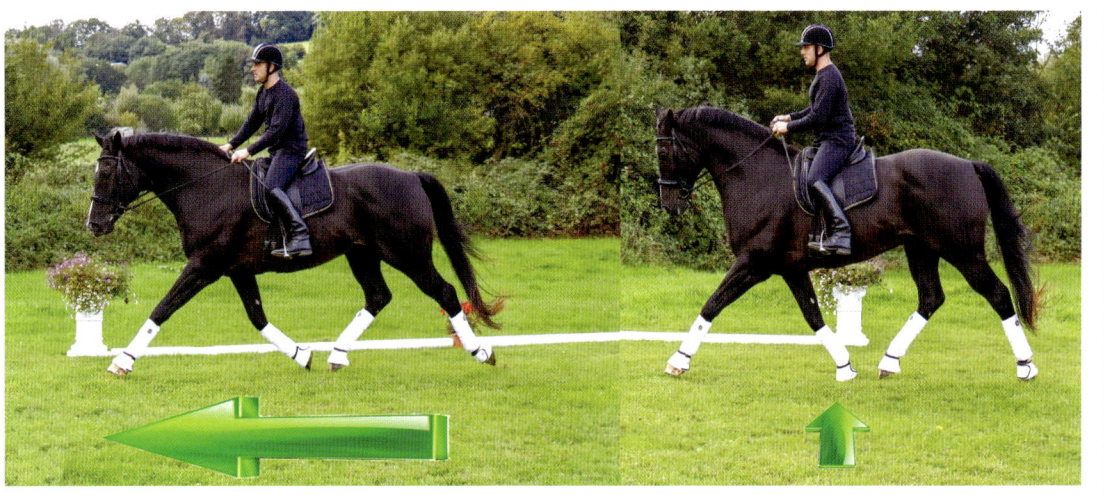

/ 6.36 / *An example of Forward and Back in the trot. Stretching and then connecting the horse's body has many benefits—for both the body and rideability.* ▲

- **RELEASE LEVEL** (Free-Walk, Allowing Horse Freedom in His HNP): Lengthening and then shortening within the free-walk—easy-peasy. Simply shorten for a few strides, then lengthen for a few. If Core Release is experienced regularly in this level, it is an indicator to move up to the *trot d'école*.

- **COORDINATION LEVEL** (*Trot d'École* to Working Trot and Back Again in a Long-and-Low HNP): Simply ride forward from a short, balanced, and easy rising or sitting *trot d'école* into a working trot for five to ten strides, then gently ask the horse to shorten and return to the *trot d'école* (fig. 6.36). The trick is to try to help the horse keep the same rhythm in both the short *trot d'école* steps and long steps. If perfected, this exercise can end up being the transition between the piaffe and passage, if you are that way inclined.

- **TONE LEVEL** (*Petit Galop* to Working Canter and Back Again, in a Long-and-Low HNP): This is where all horses and their riders

■■ Core Conditioning for Horses

start to have fun. The natural swing and energy of Forward and Back in the canter gait is a superb warm-up for any discipline. When perfected, this Level gives you ultimate sporting stride control.

How to Do It

OVERVIEW: You will simply be stretching and gathering the horse in each gait (figs. 6.37 & 6.38), What is vital are communicative, measured hands and a following seat as you want the horse to stretch forward into a Long-and-Low HNP eventually in both the "Forward" and "Back" parts of the exercise at all Levels. "Riding your horse 'on and back' involves asking him for a few lengthened strides before

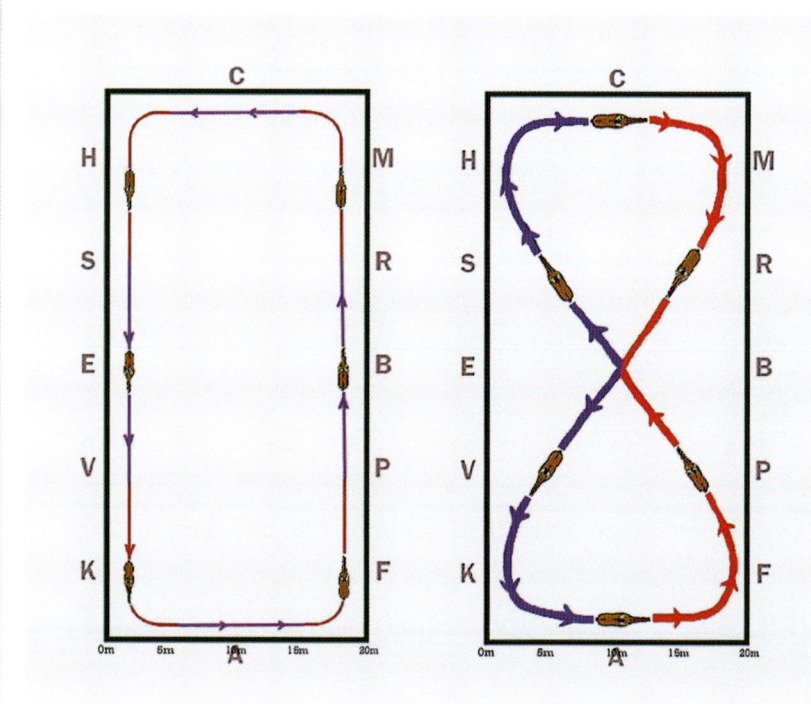

◄ / 6.37 / The Forward and Back floor plan for walk and trot uses the track, allowing you to concentrate on lengthening and shortening the strides while maintaining rhythm and energy (left).

◄ / 6.38 / The Forward and Back floor plan for the canter has you turn the arena into a very large figure of eight that gives you space to move into and also an opportunity to change canter leads at X either through walk or with a flying change (right).

asking him to come back to his working pace, then repeating it several times," notes five-time Olympian Carl Hester. "This will help you to get him to carry his head and neck, and achieve self-carriage."

- **STEP /1/** Shorten the reins and adopt a slight half-seat with your heels well down, appropriately ready for action.
- **STEP /2/** Pick up the appropriate gait for the horse's Level, then begin, gradually at first, pushing the stride forward with your seat (see Exercise 5: The Driving Seat—p. 211). Ride at this length for two or three strides, then gradually bring the stride length back to where you started, making sure to lighten the aids the very moment the horse responds. Even when bringing the horse back, be sure your seat follows the movement of the horse's back.
- **STEP /3/** Repeat the forward-and-back transitions, making the extremes longer and shorter, and trying to be even lighter and more encouraging with each repetition. The exercise itself creates the improvement with enough practice; you just have to remember that the horse has to get it wrong before he can learn to get it right. Let him, then try again, always ready to reward a good attempt.

Common Problems and Solutions

- ***Overheated horse.*** Steady there! Simply stop and do something else to dissipate the hysteria. This exercise can pique the interest of every horse, so be careful and use preventive judgment, as always.
- ***Horse raises the head while shortening his stride.*** This happens sometimes as an evasion, even when the rider does everything right.

Firstly, be sure to not lean back or be heavy in the stirrups or with the hands. Consider establishing a Long-and-Low HNP in a lower Level, as well as using Exercise 1: Core Release Volte (p. 156) to help begin this exercise well.

Core Score Zero Goal

When the horse has developed good core condition from the other yoga-inspired exercises in your plan, this one becomes smooth, easy, and very, very useful. The ability to lengthen and shorten easily is a dynamic skill that changes what you can do with your horse. It improves everything, from the flexibility of dressage gaits to show-jumping stride placement, as well as being invaluable if you are one of those riders who likes to gallop at one of those "bear traps" deceptively labeled as a cross-country jump! ∎

END OF EXERCISE 4
The Balancing Table to Tiptoe Chair Poses / Forward and Back

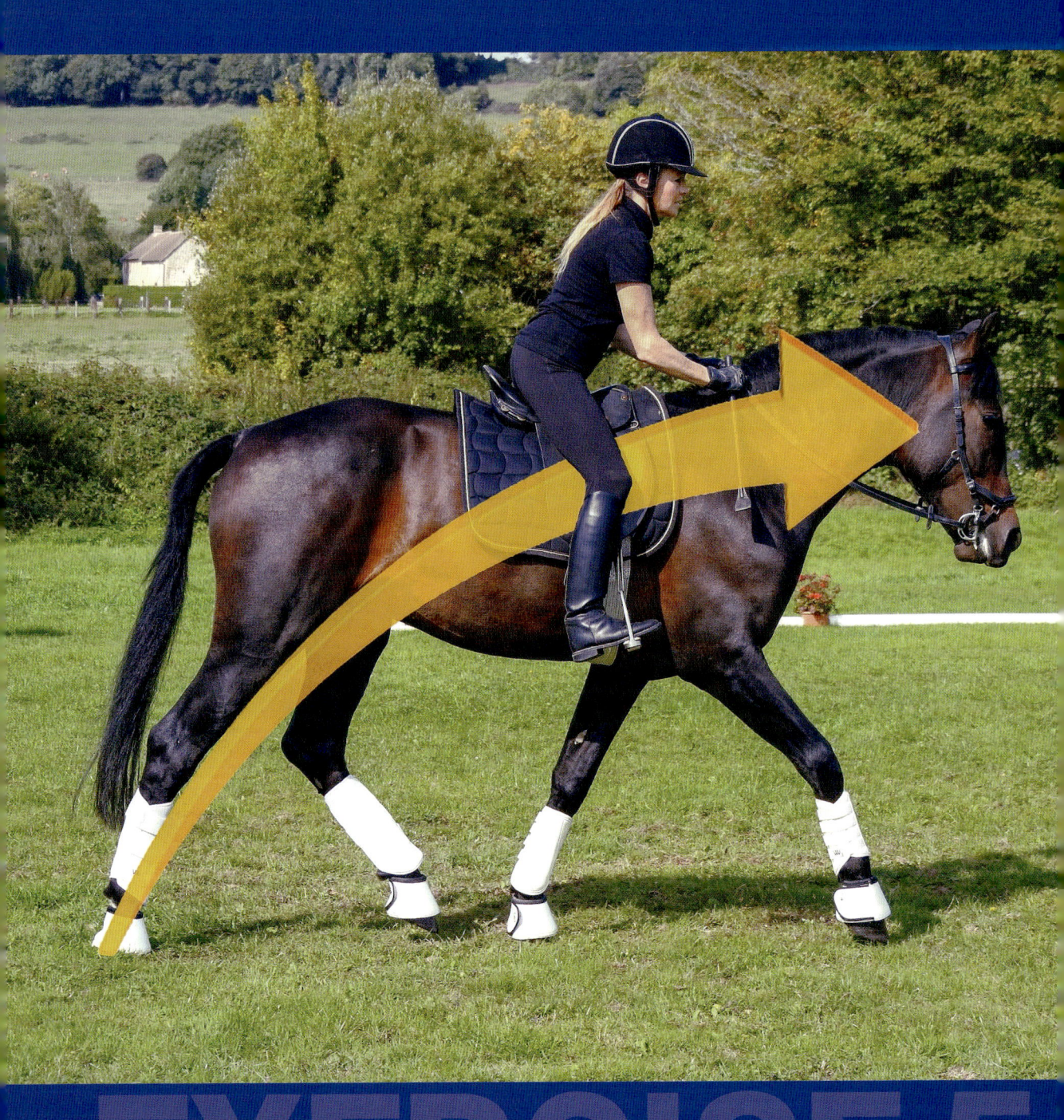

EXERCISE 5

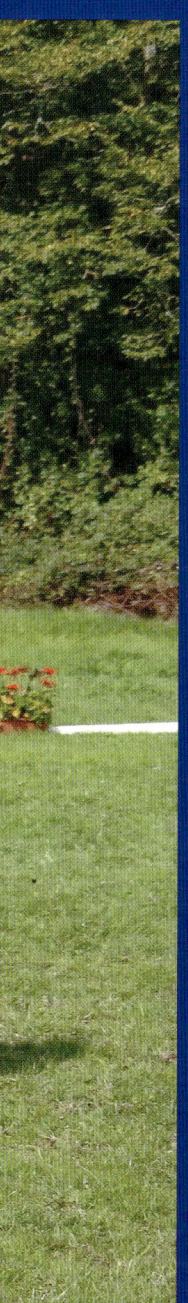

◀ / **6.39** / *The Driving Seat: Going forward from the seat makes transitions smoother and more harmonious than from the leg.*

Exercise 5

♠ / **The Chair Pose**
♞ / **The Driving Seat**

A "readiness" posture is the foundation of agility. The exact way in which you stand before you even begin to move is critical to both the mastery of your center of gravity and to bring balance to whatever comes next. Only then can your body be agile, quick, and useful. The yoga *Chair Pose* and core conditioning's *Driving Seat* (fig. 6.39) are as simple as they are effective in bringing mind and posture to be ready for action.

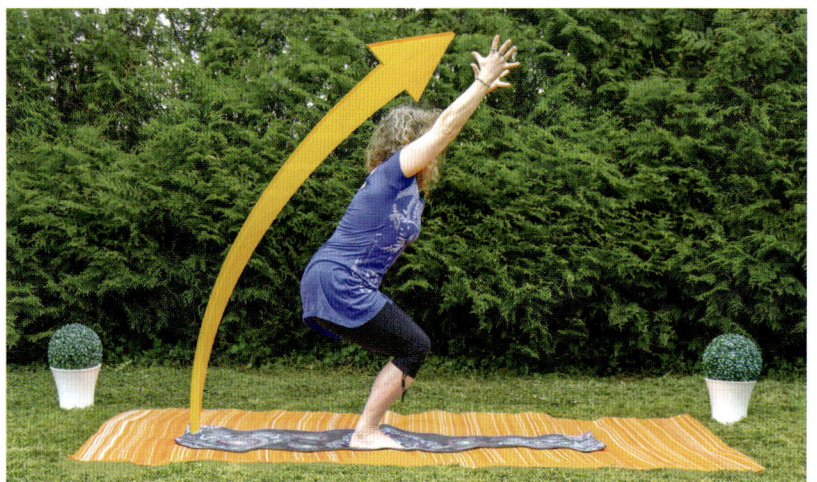

/ **6.40** / *There is a fine balance to be found in the yoga Chair Pose. It stretches your muscles, tones your core, and focuses your mind.* ▶

🙏 / The Chair Pose

The *Chair Pose* is a centering movement. Performed regularly, it tones most of the human body while honing balance and core stability (fig. 6.40). Holding this pose for several breaths increases the heart rate, stimulating the circulatory, metabolic, and balancing systems.

This exercise helps a human to:

- Strengthen the spine, hips, and chest muscles.
- Strengthen the lower back and torso.
- Tone the thigh, ankle, leg, and knee muscles.
- Balance the body and bring determination to the mind.
- Activate the diaphragm, chest, and upper abdomen.

"Sitting in a chair may sound very easy and comfortable," said yoga guru Sri Sri Ravi Shankar. "But sitting in an imaginary chair might be a little challenging! And this is exactly what we do in *Utkatasana* or Chair Pose. The literal meaning of *Utkatasana* is intense posture or powerful posture."

/ The Driving Seat

This is an exercise that, much like an airplane, doesn't sound like it will work until you see it. The *Driving Seat* gets both horse and rider to rethink the driving aids and clarify them, as a team. The connection you share with a horse through the seat is the most profound of them all, and in real terms, your seat is the most efficient driving aid you have. It is not used much by adults for reasons that will become clear, yet it is super effective, and if you are a child rider, it makes all the sense in the world.

The Driving Seat is a driving aid that replaces the leg as the signal for the horse to go forward. This teaches the horse to go at the slightest inclination of your seat aid, which makes riding easier from one important angle, because it makes more sense to the horse than using the leg as the driving aid.

This exercise helps the horse to:

• Engage the lower back.
• Naturally activate all core muscles.
• Understand your driving aid.

Our leg aids are, more often than not, terrible communicators. They already have their "hands full," so to speak. Wobbling about and almost falling off near the letter K erodes the horse's faith in the subtlety of our gentle leg aids. All too easily our communications become lost in a sea of white noise on the horse's sides.

Our seat, though, jiggles far less. It may not be perfect, but it is much closer to the horse's core, making it a much clearer aid than a flapping leg could ever be. For this reason the Driving Seat shows you how to complement your leg aids with a clear, voluntary confirmation from your seat. This does many good things. Most importantly, it frees up your legs to relax, become softer, and give clearer lateral aids that appear to the horse as signals, rather than pressures. Secondly, it teaches the horse to go forward from the suggestion of your seat, making it invisible, and lastly, it focuses, engages, and excites your horse's inner dancer.

This exercise helps solve these issues under saddle:

- Distracted mind.
- Resistance or lack of reaction to the leg aids.
- Slow moving.
- Nervousness and indecision.
- Sloppy posture.

It is the horse's own mindset that brings a better posture (fig. 6.41). When he understands this exercise he "wakes up" and readies himself to go from the seat instead of the leg. The energy created by you and transmitted through your seat instinctively encourages the horse to "listen" and prepare to act, improving your connection and partnership a great deal.

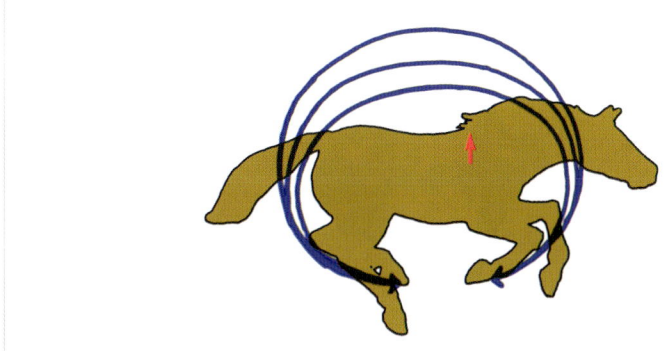

◄ / 6.41 / *Upward energy: By improving his own posture, the horse's core makes him rounder and more balanced.*

What It Does Inside the Horse

- Makes him alert and physically ready.
- Tightens the core and improves posture.
- Focuses his mind on you.
- Quickens reaction time.

As the exercise evolves and your horse begins to key into your smaller and smaller seat aids, creating movement—and even increasing it—with the seat becomes instinctive for both you and the horse, improving extensions and jumping stride-placement with instant responses. This works excellently in conjunction with Exercise 4: Forward and Back (see p. 198).

Core Score, Level, and Head-and-Neck Placement

If your horse has a Core Score of:

- **4–5**, do this exercise in **RELEASE LEVEL.**
- **3**, do this exercise in **COORDINATION LEVEL.**
- **0–2**, do this exercise in **TONE LEVEL.**

\\\ Bertil Voss ///

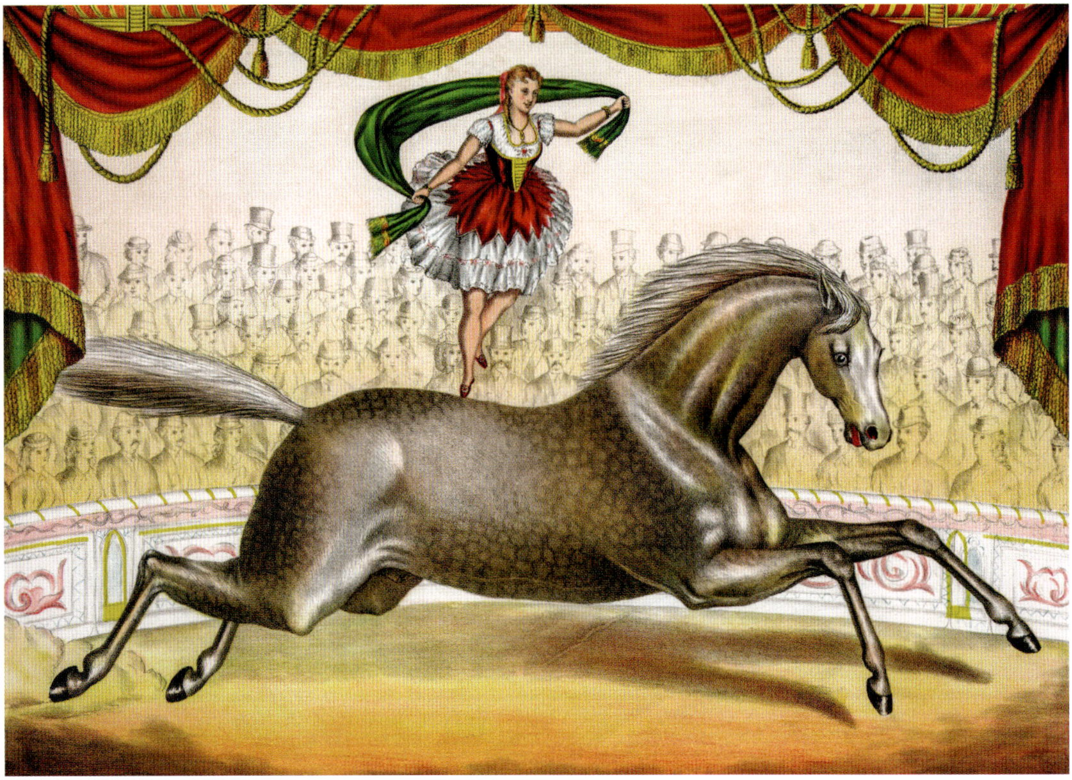

"You must never rush a horse out of his natural balance."

- **RELEASE LEVEL** (Free-Walk into Trot Steps): From a free-walk, begin the Driving Seat and Tapping Stick aid until a trot is achieved. The type of trot or head carriage does not matter as it is the horse's decision you are focusing on. Too much information will dilute the message, so keep it simple to start with.

- **COORDINATION LEVEL** (Halt to Trot Steps, Allowing a Long-and-Low HNP): This is identical to the Release Level, yet from the halt. Be sure the horse is ready and listening as quick reactions are part of this lesson. If the horse is soft in the contact and has released in the core from previous exercises, a Long-and-Low HNP will help maintain roundness in the transition.

- **TONE LEVEL** (Free-Walk to Canter): Go from the free-walk directly into any kind of canter. Gather into a *petit galop* in Long-and-Low HNP after the exercise becomes well understood and fluid. As with the Coordination Level, if the horse is soft enough to the contact to remain easily Long-and-Low from the beginning of the exercise, this will work all the right parts of the core and immediately bring a depth of roundness to his way of going.

How to Do It

OVERVIEW: You will synchronize your core with your horse's to get a smooth, new, and clear driving aid. Remember, the transition is the horse's decision to make; it is his body. All you are trying to do is ask him to make the decision to go forward immediately, but not from whip, spur, or leg (fig. 6.42).

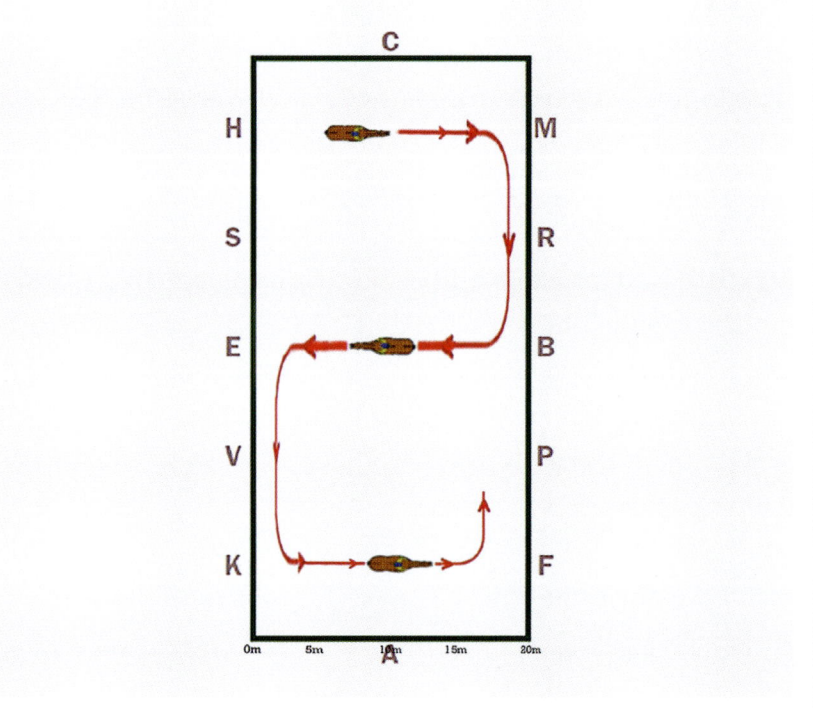

/ **6.42** / *The Driving Seat floor plan: Using the centerline as a target, you can get many Driving Seat transitions into a short time, multiplying the effects.* ▶

- **STEP /1/** Find a clear area with nothing in front of the horse and preferably with no one watching. It may look silly for a minute or two, but remember, you are doing this for the horse!
- **STEP /2/** For the Release Level, you want the horse to understand and deliver a free-walk to trot transition from the seat only. From the walk, begin by pushing your pelvis forward in the saddle, urging the horse to go faster, just and exactly like a nine-year-old kid in Pony Club (fig. 6.43). This is the Driving Seat aid. Do not give in to the temptation to use your legs. If the horse does not give you a trot transition (which would be unlikely), begin and continue using the Tapping Stick (see p. 146) behind one of your

legs while continuing to push the seat forward (fig. 6.44). At some point the horse will decide to move forward in the hope you will stop driving and tapping, and you should. Release, reward, and repeat.

- **STEP /3/** Each time the horse should react a little more quickly, so your reactions need to be kind and quick (fig. 6.45). Repeat the exercise until the horse trots away from walk easily from the first Driving Seat aid and with no need for the Tapping Stick.

Bravo, you now have a means to refine the seat aid into something very subtle in the Coordination and Tone Levels, giving a reliable and invisible driving aid while allowing your leg to relax completely and lengthen effortlessly, just like a pro. "FORWARD—straight away,"

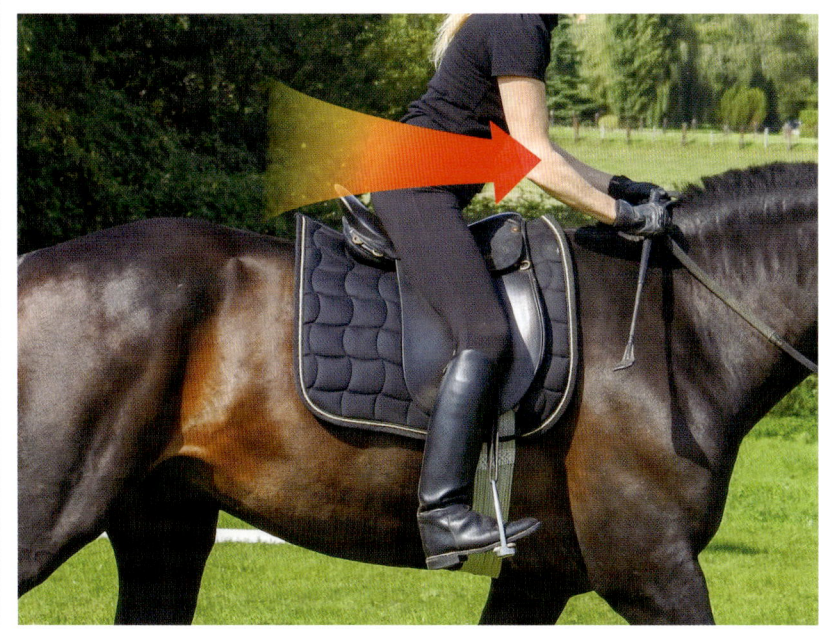

◂ / 6.43 / *The Driving Seat aid: Your center of gravity can connect with the horse's, making the "go" signal both intuitive and immediate.*

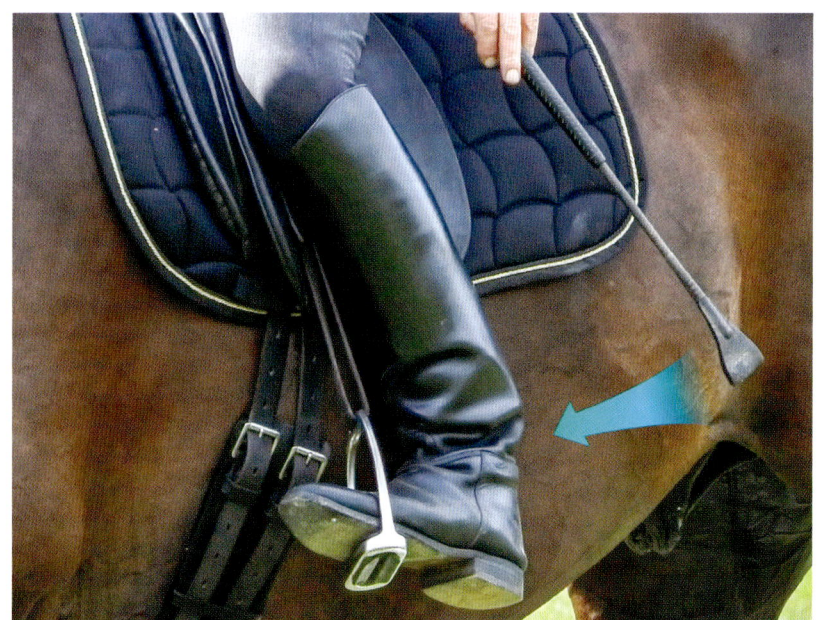

/ **6.44** / *The Tapping Stick aid: Tapping will help the horse connect your Driving Seat aid with the act of moving.* ▶

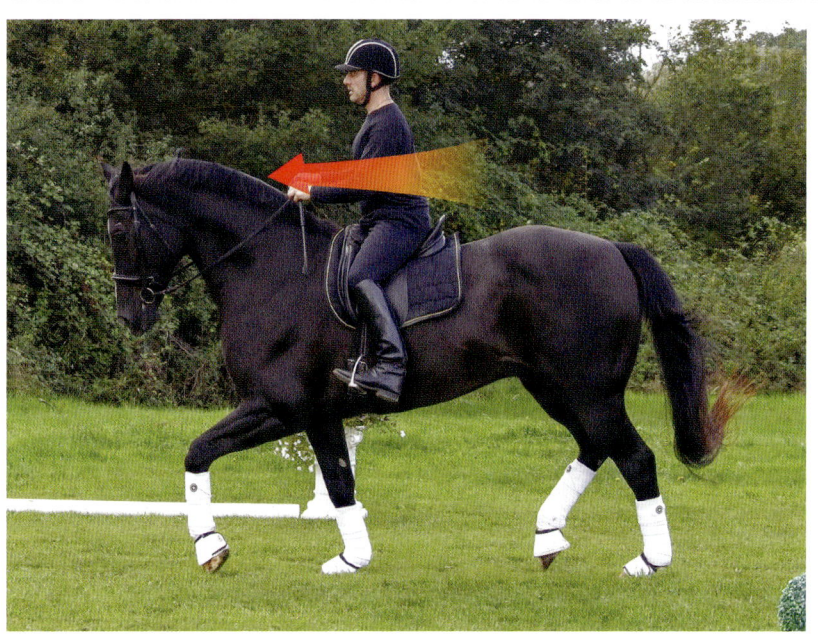

/ **6.45** / *For the horse to trust your request to go forward, you have to prove to him that you are ready to "go with him." A proactive seat is always ready to follow the horse's back.* ▶

insists Olympic gold medalist Charlotte Dujardin. "[Horses] have to react from the smallest aid; when you get to Grand Prix, you just want to steer."

Common Problems and Solutions

- **The horse isn't reacting quickly enough.** Sometimes our horses doze off, and who can blame them. Just before doing this exercise at any of the Levels, be sure to have him ready and waiting, as surprise aids never get a good reaction.
- **Exercise makes the horse a little crazy.** A fiery horse will pick this up and run with it like he is, well, on fire. When Mr. or Mrs. Bonkers makes an appearance, change the exercise to one that calms your horse's instincts. After a few minutes (or when reason has returned), the lesson can be continued and will give an easy, effortless impulsion to your ride.

Core Score Zero Goal

A Core Score 0 horse has great posture and instant reactions to your Driving Seat, so moving in any direction feels Bentley-like smooth. When this aid is refined, you get superb feedback through your seat, opening new levels of refinement for your lateral leg aids and collection.

Happy days. ■

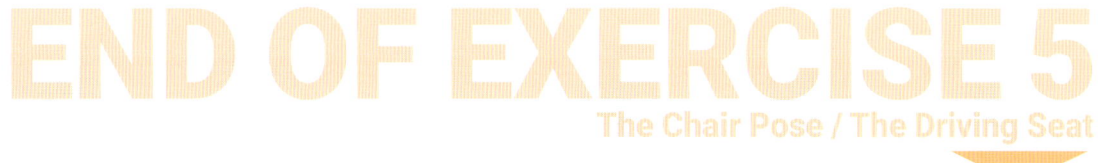

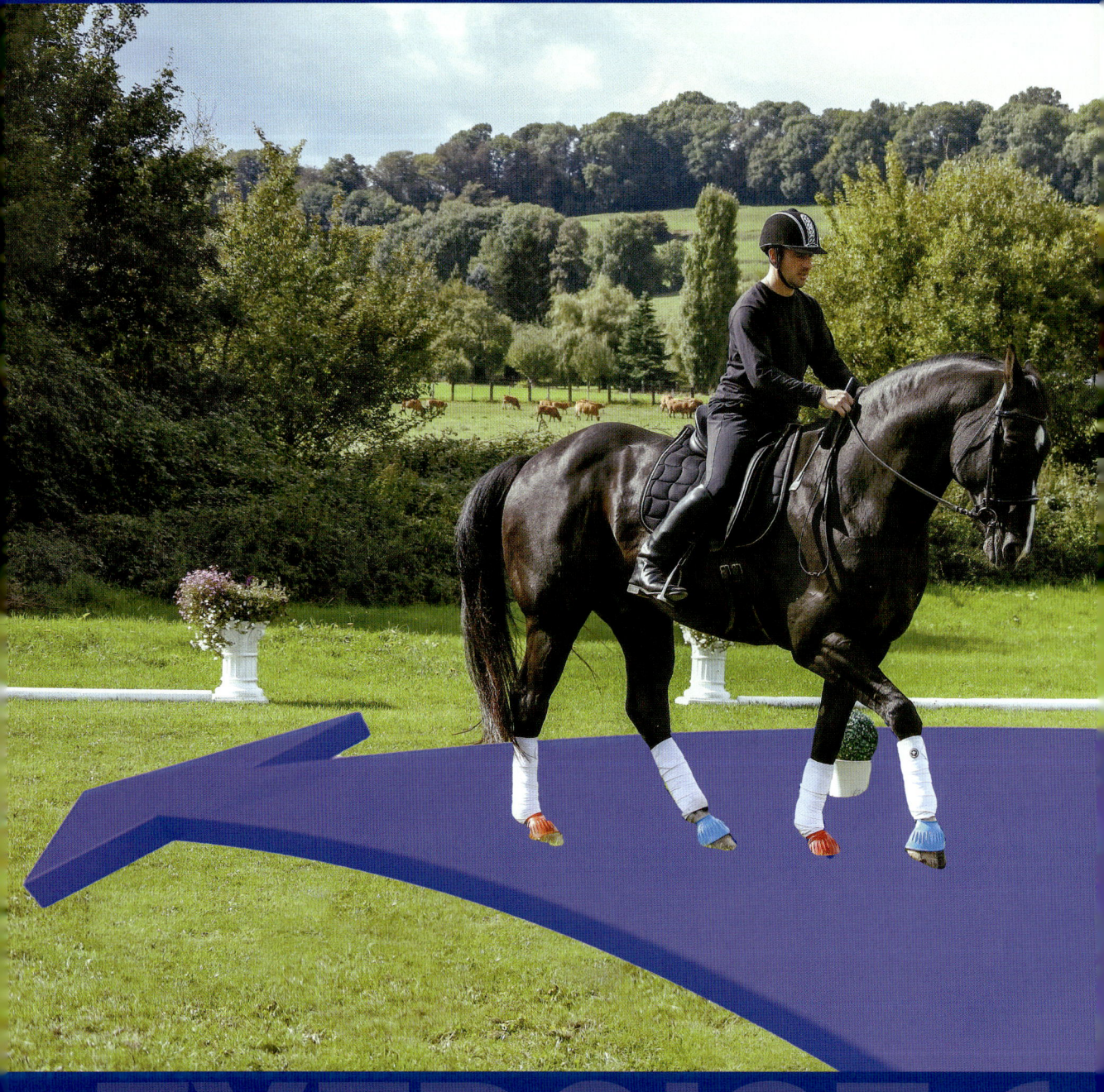

EXERCISE 6

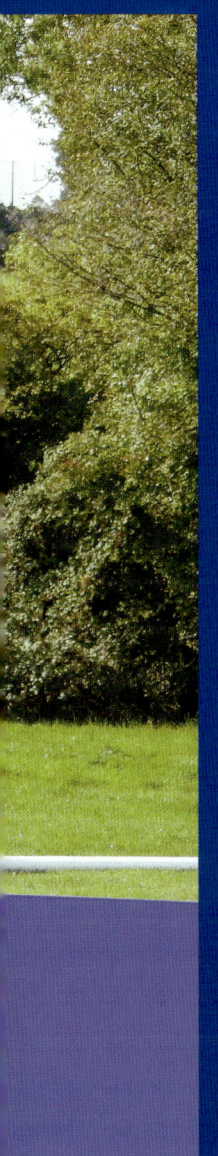

◄ / **6.46** / *The Rounding Rein-Back: Going backward really, really well helps a horse go forward really, really well.*

Exercise 6

♣ / The Garland Pose
♞ / The Rounding Rein-Back

An easy yet very powerful movement, the *Garland Pose* is an instant posture improver. As a sitting and lowering pose, it is a natural way of rebalancing the human body. The *Rounding Rein-Back* is the equine equivalent (fig. 6.46).

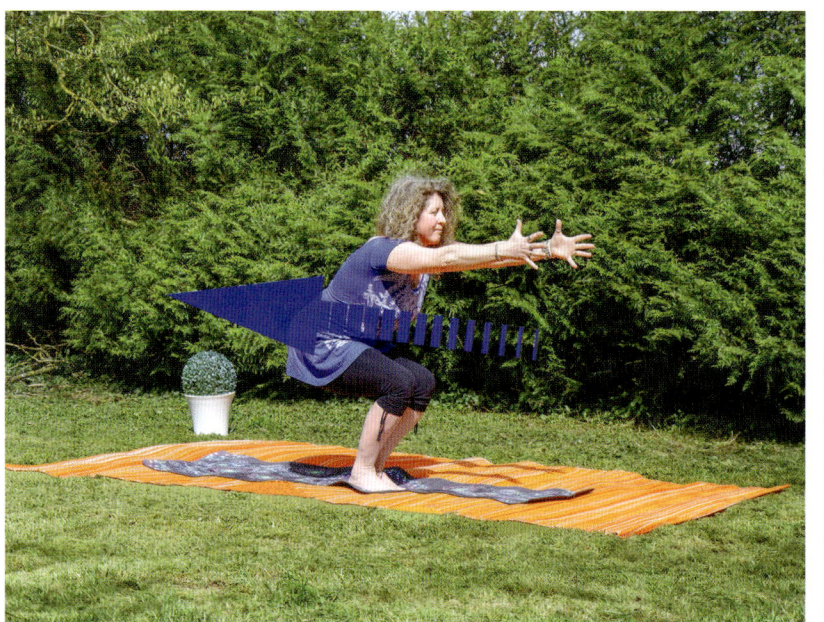

/ **6.47** / *The Garland Pose: Bringing your point of balance over your heels will center your body and engage your core muscles.* ▶

🙏 / Garland Pose

The low, strong, and solid foundation of the *Garland Pose* flexes all the angles and muscles in your thighs and back, establishing a more centered and agile posture (fig. 6.47).

This pose helps people to:

- Stretch the back and pelvis.
- Improve hip mobility.
- Relieve backache.
- Learn better posture.
- Strengthen the core.
- Improve balance.

"The Garland Pose can improve your posture, stretch your back, elasticize your knees and ankles, and help improve your digestive function," says Iyengar yoga teacher Marla Apt. "It is a forward bend—the back softens and releases from head to tail as the ankles, knees, and hips flex. The heels root the hips back, and the spine lengthens as it rounds."

/ The Rounding Rein-Back

As General Albert Decarpentry, one-time President of FEI Dressage, said: "The goal is not to raise the [horse's] neck; it is to lower the hips."

Backing up is a two-time movement and is technically a reverse trot. This makes it ideal for getting into a rhythm while you encourage this exercise's party piece: a powerful, rounding effect on the horse's body, just by going backward (fig. 6.48). How easy is that?

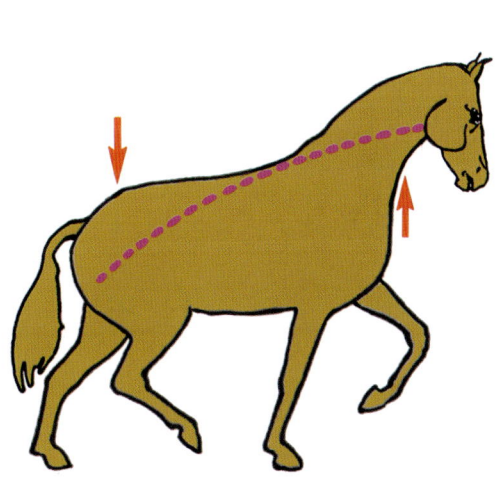

◀ / 6.48 / When the horse moves backward confidently he lowers his rear end naturally.

The Rounding Rein-Back helps the horse by:

- Creating a Core Release.
- Engaging the three Core Powers (see p. 44).
- Improving trust.
- Coordinating front to back and side to side.
- Engaging the hindquarters fully at low impulsion.

At Coordination and Tone Levels, the horse naturally rounds into Core Release, which gives an immediate improvement in posture and weight distribution. As the horse's hocks can then reach easily under his center of gravity, you walk away with a more balanced and much rounder horse (fig. 6.49). This effect is immediate. FEI 5* judge Anne Gribbons attests, "In the ring, the rein-back is either a testament to the suppleness and throughness of the horse or just the opposite!"

This exercise helps solve these issues under saddle:

- Hollow back.
- High head.
- Hard contact.
- Unbalanced body.

There is an interesting psychological aspect to this exercise. As the horse obviously can't see where he is going while in rein-back, he must develop trust in you that the path is clear. For an equine, this is an important step toward your credibility as his leader. This exercise gradually helps the horse believe in you. Just make sure the path is indeed clear or the horse will remember that, too (probably forever).

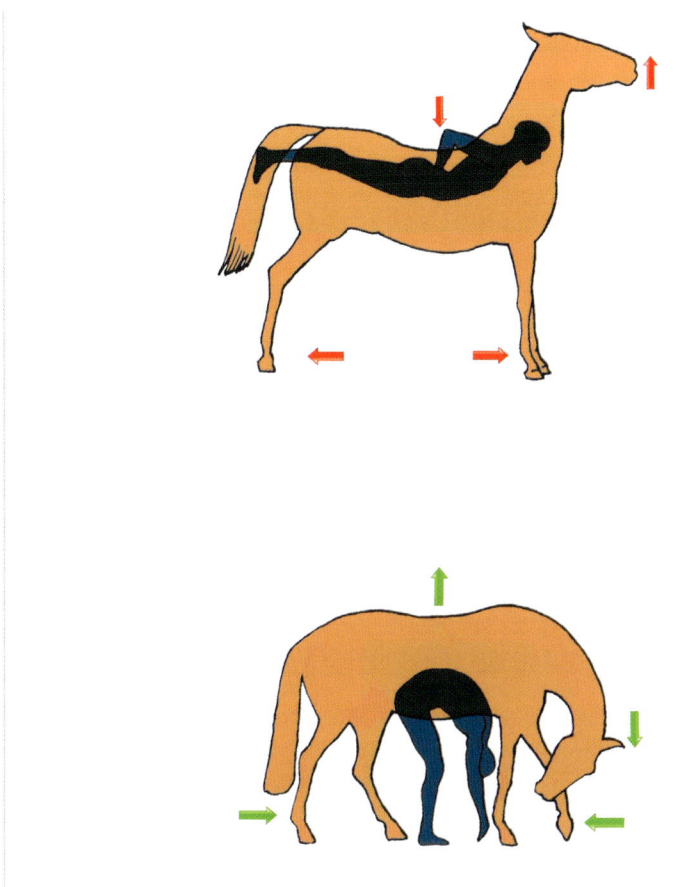

◀ / 6.49 / *This exercise creates a posture in the horse that pushes upward, under the back, by contracting his core.*

What It Does Inside the Horse

The rearward motion of multiple rein-back steps gives the horse a strong incentive to take the central mass of body weight over his hocks, making reversing much more stable for him. Once he has learned how easy this is and begins offering it regularly, sitting a little more on the hocks has several profound and immediate effects upon the horse's body:

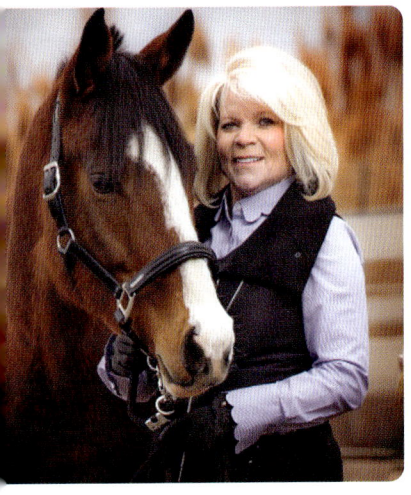

Debbie and Chaussette

(United States)

In mid-March of 2017, my six-year-old Appendix mare Chaussette began to show significant resistance in her dressage work. Her trainer suggested that she was showing signs of kissing spine and that we should have some X-rays completed. Her X-rays confirmed the presence of three mild kissing spine. My veterinarian recommended steroid injections down her back to alleviate the inflammation, and I was advised by trainers with some experience with this condition that nothing could be done that would help her, and that it would be best to put my horse to pasture. I was heartbroken!

I relayed this advice to my vet, who strongly disagreed. He asked me, "When you fell from your horse and hurt your back, did you feel best just sitting or was it better to keep moving?" There was no question to my answer. Without a doubt, I knew I had to follow my veterinarian's advice, as well as my own instincts, to do all I could to help Chaussette heal and move comfortably. We proceeded with the injections.

I began researching her condition to learn as much as I could. To my disappointment, I was not able to find many experts who gave a positive outlook on recovering from kissing spine. Feeling defeated, I came upon an article online entitled, "Kiss Goodbye to Kissing Spine" by Visconte Simon Cocozza. He suggested that working the horse in exercises that

- It pushes the chest upward in the Thoracic Sling, activating Thoracic Lift.
- It rounds the lumbar back to engage Pelvic Tilt.
- Weight taken willingly to the rear immediately lightens the forehand.

Core Score, Level, and Head-and-Neck Position

If your horse has a Core Score of:

- **0–2**, do this exercise at **TONE LEVEL.**
- **3**, do this exercise at **COORDINATION LEVEL.**
- **4–5**, do this exercise at **RELEASE LEVEL.**

We back up in the same pace, so the difference between Levels is simply how many steps we ask for.

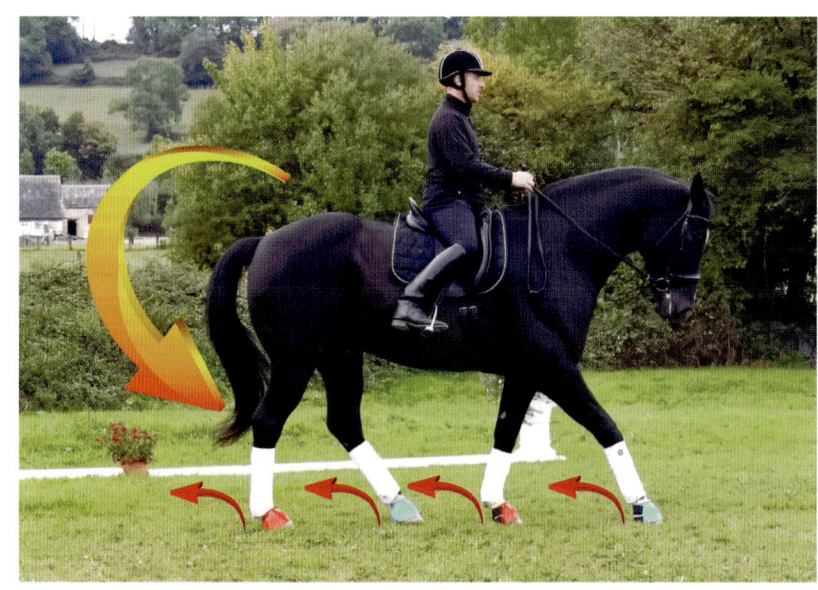

◄ / **6.50** / *Going backward activates the Pelvic Tilt—While the horse reverses he naturally rounds through the back behind the saddle and pelvis to "sit" with more stability.*

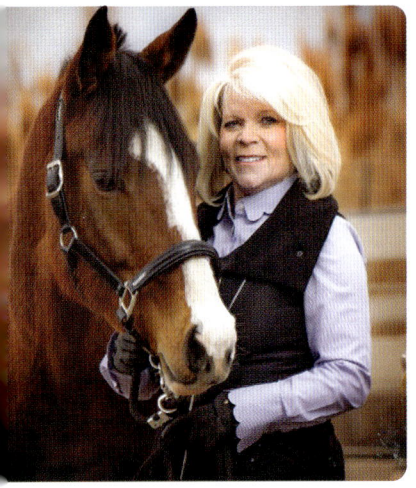

DEBBIE AND CHAUSSETTE — CORE STORY

strengthen core muscles would alleviate the defensive tension and pain that come with kissing spine. Everything he expressed made complete sense to me and prompted me to take a wild chance and contact him. Although I never expected a response, one came quickly... I was elated! I told him Chaussette's story and expressed that, while she was not a Grand Prix horse, she was my horse, and I loved her and wanted to do whatever I could to help heal her and keep her moving forward. Visconte Cocozza was completely encouraging and reminded me that Chaussette had a whole life ahead of her. It would take time, he said, and it would be a long process—12 to 18 months to completely heal her. However, he said I sounded like I was up to the task and, if I was, he would help me. I was thrilled!

Our program started on April 1, 2017, just two weeks from Chaussette's initial diagnosis. As we began, I was quite concerned that by asking her to move I would be causing her more pain. The Visconte reassured me that I knew far more about Chaussette's injury than she did. He predicted an even stronger bond between the two of us as she would come to understand that I was taking away her pain. And that is exactly what I saw happen! The respect, obedience, and willing submission that I started to receive almost immediately from Chaussette was unbelievable. I knew that just wishing for her to heal would not happen without me putting in my time. I decided then that I would not and did not miss a day of working with her, knowing that inconsistency would be the enemy of any hoped-for success.

In July 2017 I had a chiropractor check Chaussette to be sure that we were not dealing with any underlying injuries. As he examined her he was impressed by her suppleness, not expecting her to be so, given her diagnosis. He inquired as to what I was doing and I told him of the program by Visconte Cocozza. At that time, he could tell where the kissing spine was as the vertebrae were fixated. He encouraged me to keep the course and was excited to see her progress as time went on. In December 2017 the chiropractor returned and she was even more supple and relaxed. Chaussette was pain-free upon palpating, and her vertebrae were no longer fixated. With a smile on his face, he showed me how he could move every vertebra! Tears welled up in my eyes as I looked into the eyes of my beautiful, happy horse. We both had received a wonderful gift!

- **RELEASE LEVEL** (Short Rein-Back): Just 1 to 3 backward steps, then release and reward. The principle is the only consideration at this Level (fig. 6.50). Allow the horse to question throughout and gently continue to explain the aids, quickly rewarding the first step attempted. Throughout this beginning Level, allow the horse's head to express itself and the horse to concentrate on his legs. Once three steps are coming fairly easily, don't hesitate to move on to the next Level, even if it is far from perfect. This exercise is learned on the go.

- **COORDINATION LEVEL** (Add Steps Backward): Now ask for 5 to 10 reverse steps in Long-and-Low HNP. Keep the horse straight with your legs and soft in the hand. The horse will now offer to keep a contact, so gentle guidance toward Long-and-Low will come naturally.

- **TONE LEVEL** (Increase the Challenge): At this Level, 15 to 20 steps down the centerline or quarterline is the goal. At this Level the horse should be on the bit or in a Long-and-Low HNP from the beginning and for most of the 15 to 20 rein-back steps. Smoothness, softness, and harmony are the goals here. You will know when you feel it, then ride forward, and enjoy an instant balance upgrade.

How to Do It

OVERVIEW: Patience and gentle aids will be required throughout this exercise as the decision is, as ever, the horse's to make (fig. 6.51). So, there is no need for any strength to be used; repetition is enough to get the point across. When the horse understands, longer smoother step sequences will come naturally. The aids should be light, yet

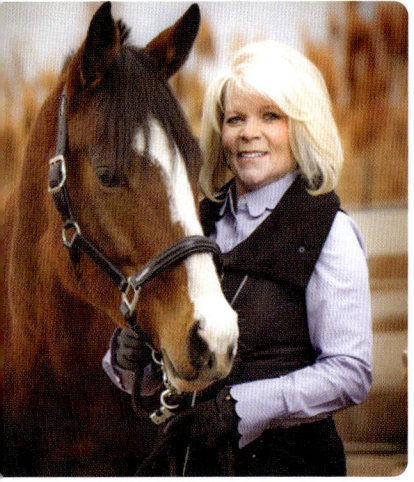

Our journey is not finished, nor will it ever be! We will continue, always with the advice and wisdom from Visconte Cocozza and his program. There is still so much to do to get Chausette where she fully deserves to be. But what a joy it is to be along for the ride!

My gratitude to Visconte Cocozza is immeasurable. Although I have not had the pleasure of meeting him personally, I am so grateful to one who is so prominent in the horse world, taking his precious time to patiently guide and instruct me in the recovery of my beautiful horse. He is a true "horseman" in every sense of the word. The Visconte's support, along with my barnmates who fully backed me in this effort, have sustained me during a time when I was otherwise feeling abandoned and alone in this task. I can only hope that by Visconte Simon Cocozza's selfless example, I too may be able to return the favor to another owner who is being told that having a horse with kissing spine is a hopeless situation. It definitely is not and my beautiful Chaussette is living proof of that! ■

....
Debbie and Chaussette

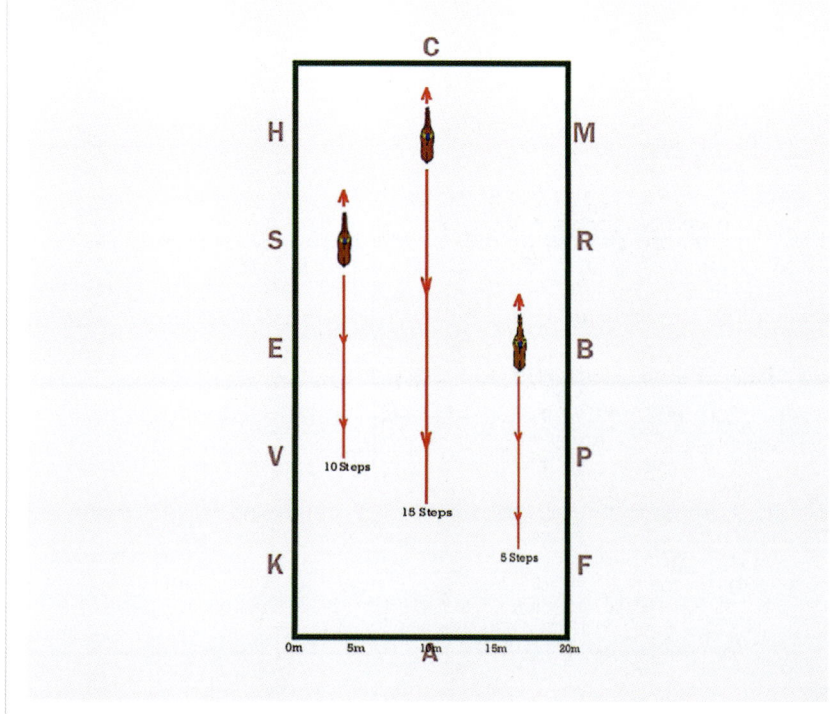

◀ / 6.51 / *The Rounding Rein-Back floor plan: The Levels of difficulty are the length of the rein-back. It is best practiced away from the track to develop independence and line control.*

communicative at all times—even if the horse has not yet understood, he is surely considering it.

- **STEP /1/** Release Level requires only the reflex to go backward from your aids. One step is enough for a reward. Halt as squarely as convenient; then sit quietly for a moment.
- **STEP /2/** Lean forward just a little and bring both legs behind the girth, stimulating the horse's sides gently while pulsing the rein connection in both hands onto the horse's tongue in a gentle but clear rearward "pulse-then-give" contact. Be sure not to pull or hold, which may trigger tension and make the horse feel trapped. After some repetition,

the horse will decide to try a rearward step. Immediately reward with a treat. When 1 to 3 steps are achieved with no tension, move on to the Coordination Level with 5 to 10 steps.

- **STEP /3/** As the horse becomes more fluid in the movement and trusting of you, he will round his back to make the exercise easier. This triggers a natural Core Release and a soft Long-and-Low HNP.
- **STEP /4/** Tone Level should feel smooth, easy, and natural for 15 to 20 steps with Long-and-Low HNP. Tone Level is where practicing backing up is honed to become as smooth and controllable as going forward. The horse will learn how to use his three Core Powers to sit more, round his back, and lighten the forehand, bringing more magic to his posture in everything he does (fig. 6.53).

/ 6.52 / *The aids must be clear. A lightening of the seat and a lower leg aid behind the girth should be the primary aids for the rein-back, with only a light, communicative contact on the horse's tongue.* ▶

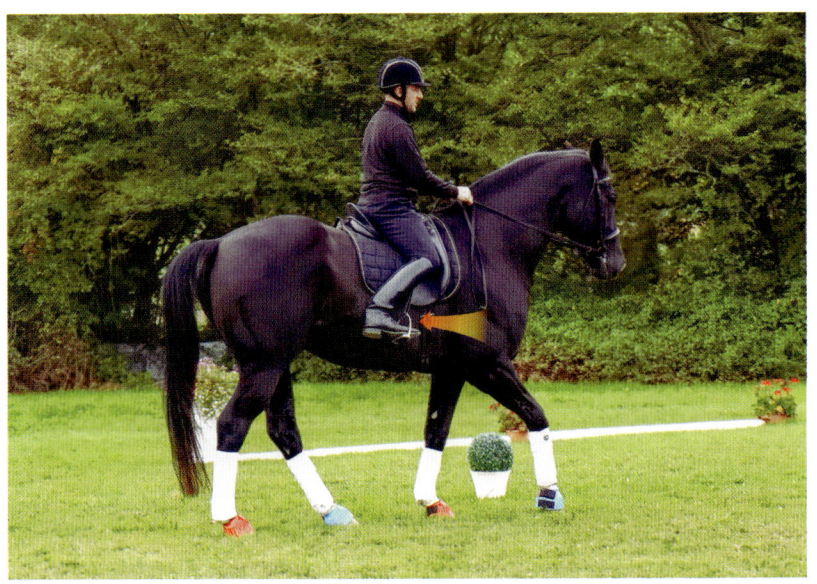

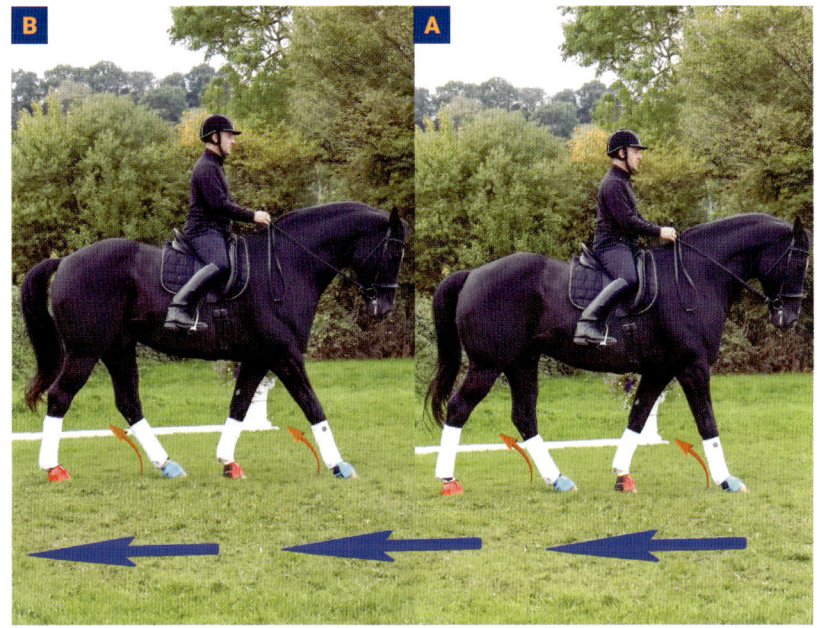

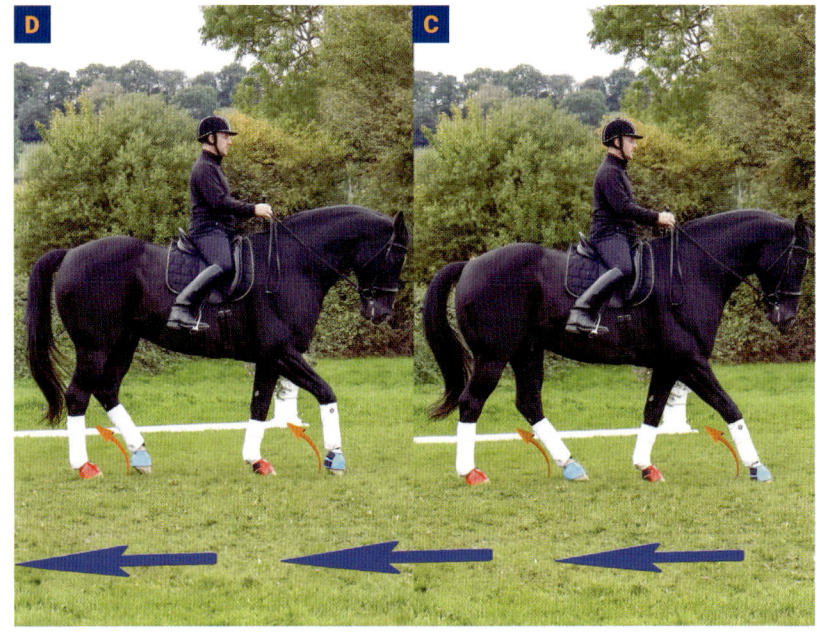

◄ / **6.53** / *Like its forward-pointing brother, the trot, the rein-back needs a rhythm, a good contact with the horse's mouth, and a seat that encourages the next step.*

Common Problems and Solutions

- ***Lifting the head. Be light with the hands.*** This is all about communication, and the horse's mouth should only be "talked to" gently. It will lower with nonconfrontational daily practice. It may be helpful to do Exercise 1 (see p. 156) beforehand to help relax and round the horse's back prior to the exercise.
- ***Wiggling left and right.*** Practice this exercise away from the wall or fence of the arena, using your left and right leg aids to channel the horse backward on a straight line. Practice makes perfect.
- ***Going too fast; taking it personally.*** If the horse feels unsafe or upset, as with all exercises, you should stop and do something easier. If the horse will not respond well to gentle aids in the Rounding Rein-Back, there may be a secondary reason that needs addressing before the horse will be able to build confidence in this exercise or simply, as with all things equestrian, tomorrow is a new day and another chance to talk things over.

Core Score Zero Goal

After some months of practice, almost all horses become very smooth at this movement. It becomes easy, fluid, and rhythmical, complementing the other exercises and serving as a wonderful way to easily create a more naturally engaged posture at any point in the ride and with no real effort from either of you.

The Core Score 0 horse will flow backward confidently and with pin-sharp coordination. At this point, adding challenges, such as rein-back to canter or reversing around corners, are great fun and deepen your connection even more. "The rein-back will be the proof of the degree of the suppleness of the horse, of the action of the rein going through the body," wrote Alois Podhajsky. "Above all, it will be proof of the correct bending of the joints of the hind legs." ■

END OF EXERCISE 6
The Garland Pose / The Rounding Rein-Back

/ **6.54** / *The Limbering Leg-Yield: Crossing the front and hind legs while going sideways supples the horse's spine and back.* ▶

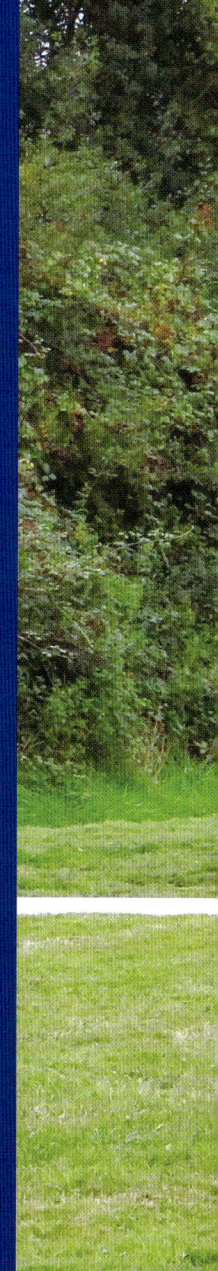

Exercise 7

♞ / The Revolved Triangle Pose
♞ / The Limbering Leg-Yield

This is a tricky exercise to get right, but when done well it can release old stiffness and rejuvenate the spine. The *Revolved Triangle Pose* and its horsey equivalent, the *Limbering Leg-Yield* (fig. 6.54), create a powerful yet natural swirl of movement that has a profound loosening effect upon resistance found throughout the back.

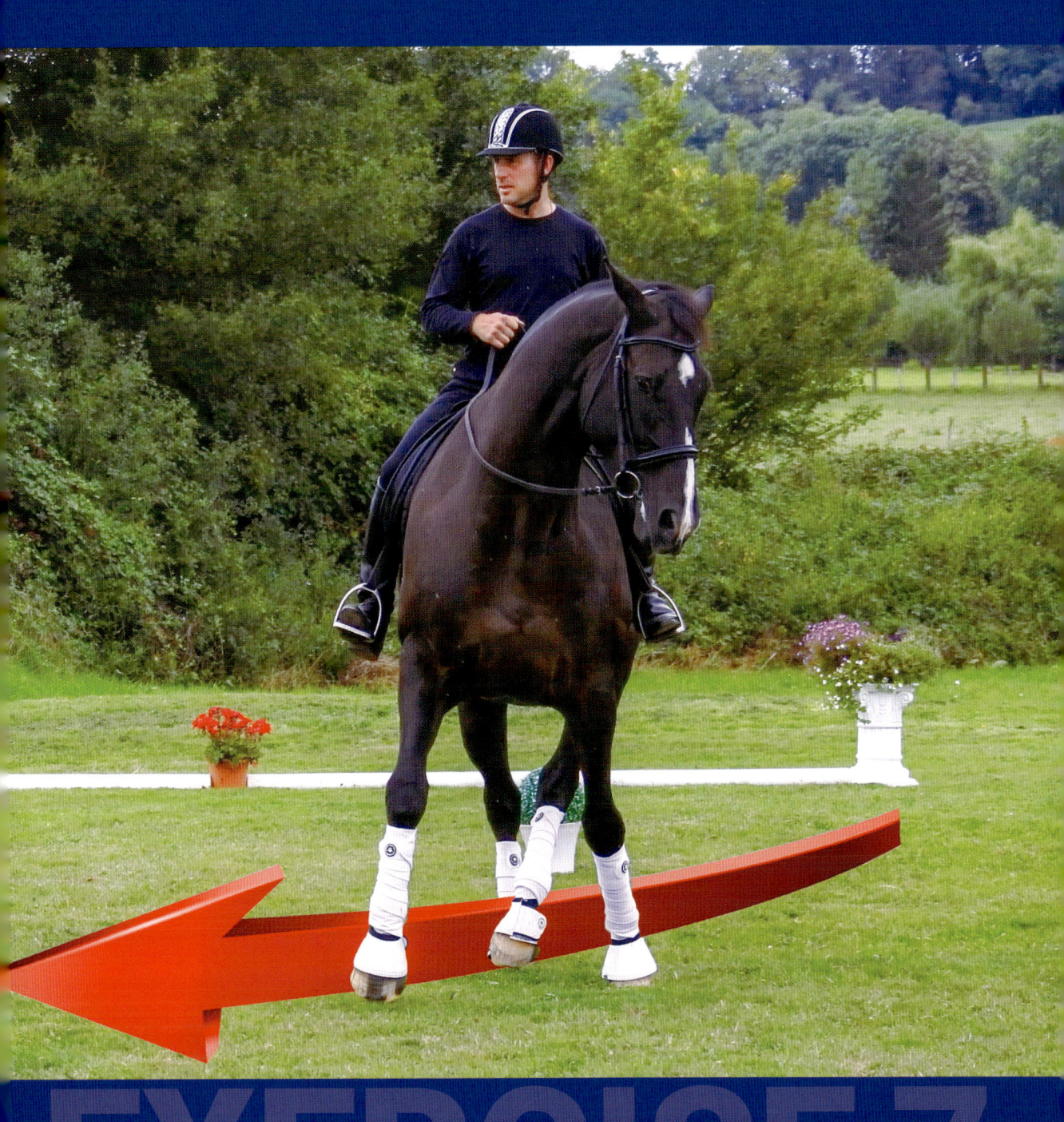

EXERCISE 7

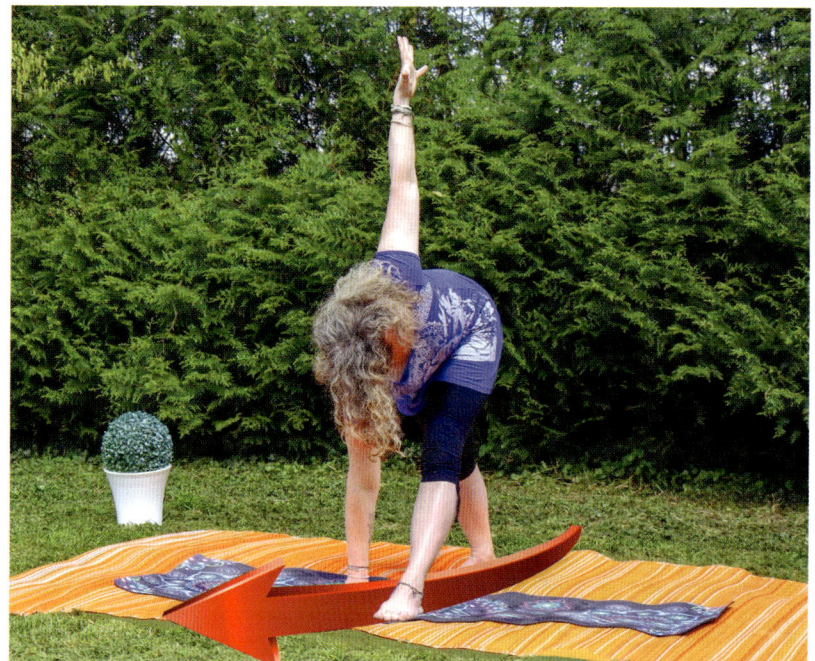

/ 6.55 / *The yoga Revolved Triangle Pose looks easy, but it takes time to master. It involves putting a twist through your lower back and stretching your whole body.* ▶

🧘 / The Revolved Triangle Pose

The *Revolved Triangle Pose* is all about the twist. It is a gentle way to rotate the back, creating a natural suppling action through the different sections of the spine and core (fig. 6.55).

This pose helps people by:

- Increasing rotation through the torso.
- Improving balance.
- Conditioning the legs, feet, ankles, and abdominal muscles.
- Increasing flexibility in the hamstrings, shoulders, and upper back.
- Activating core muscles in the abdomen.

"The Revolved Triangle Pose helps activate the spine with the help of the internal and external obliques," explains American yoga and fitness trainer Jaclyn Nguyen. "It also lengthens and releases any muscle tension in your glutes and hamstrings. This pose is also great for your sense of balance and coordination."

/ The Limbering Leg-Yield

The leg-yield is something we all know. It is often used in a Competition Outline (see Head-and-Neck Positions, p. 130) while schooling. Unfortunately, the Competition Outline HNP has a very high risk of triggering back tension, so often the goodness in the movement is blocked out. To make sure a horse can benefit from this great exercise, this yoga-inspired version is practiced in a Long-and-Low frame and called the Limbering Leg-Yield, because it does exactly that (fig. 6.56).

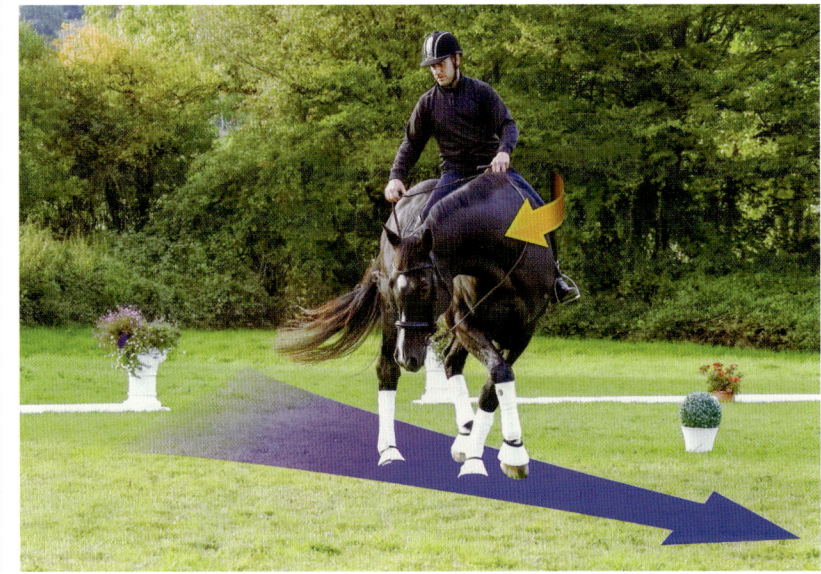

◄ / 6.56 / *To allow the horse's back to supple deeply, ask him to leg-yield in a Long-and-Low HNP with an inside Stretching Flexion (see p. 139) to keep his spine aligned.*

The ability to easily bend the horse around the inside leg in any gait is the best and easiest way of keeping a horse straight and round through the back. The mechanism that manages skeletal straightness is practiced and tuned when you develop the Limbering Leg-Yield.

This exercise helps the horse to:

- Learn to be supple, loose, and aligned through the spine.
- Increase range of motion throughout the core.
- Deepen body balance.
- Tune in to your inside leg.
- Coordinate the limbs.

"Leg-yield helps to shift the weight of the horse from side to side while moving forward," explains Dr. Sheila Schils, dressage rider

/ 6.57 / *The horse gradually relaxes his topline into the lateral movement, and with new freedom in the spine, he can discover how to better coordinate his legs.* ▶

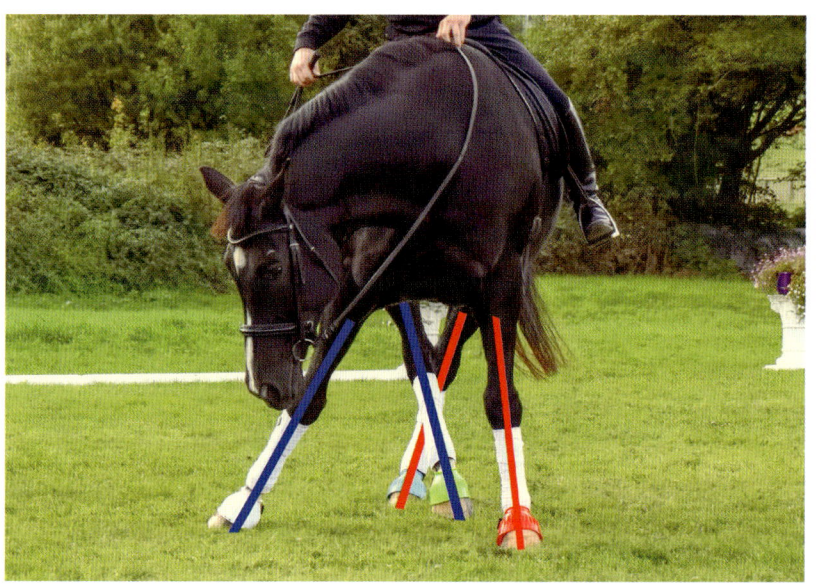

and professor of equine biomechanics. "This is an important skill for horses to learn so that they can carry their weight, and the weight of the rider, evenly distributed between all four legs, not just on the two legs that are the strongest and most coordinated" (fig. 6.57).

This exercise helps solve these issues under saddle:

- Stiff through the legs.
- Nonresponsive to the inside leg aid.
- Poor lateral work.
- Heavy contact.
- Tight neck.
- Stiff back.
- Poor coordination.

What It Does Inside the Horse

The rotational action of the Limbering Leg-Yield has the shoulder and pelvis of the horse twisting in opposite directions, reaching deep into the core's finer control system. The thoracic section of the spine has to flex laterally, while the lumbar section must both round vertically and twist rotationally (fig. 6.58).

Many horses lack confidence in their core and do not allow the spine to rotate in this way while using power as it risks bruising deep and sensitive structures that may hurt already. The Release Level's free-walk develops range of motion along the spine very gradually, giving the horse enough confidence to allow this movement into his overall gaits. Once established through the Levels, the rider will notice that the

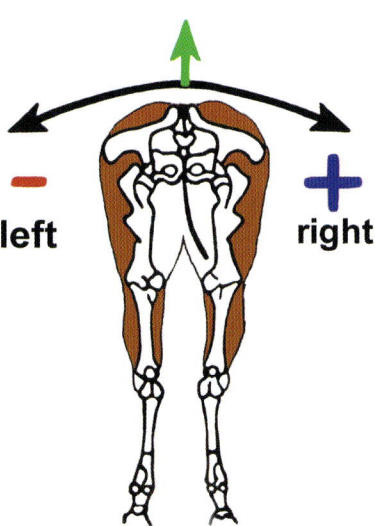

/ 6.58 / The Limbering Leg-Yield encourages rotation in the horse's lumbar spine, liberating the pelvis's full range of motion. ▶

horse's back feels more "still" as the spine's rotational qualities can now absorb more of the movement going on under you. This makes a less complex movement for you to follow.

Core Score, Level, and Head-and-Neck Position

If your horse has a Core Score of:

- **3–5**, do this exercise at **RELEASE LEVEL.**
- **2**, do this exercise at **COORDINATION LEVEL.**
- **0–1**, do this exercise at **TONE LEVEL.**

- **RELEASE LEVEL** (Free-Walk, Long-and-Low HNP): The Long-and-Low frame in leg-yield creates an excellent formula for suppling a horse's back. Set up the horse well for a line of leg-yield steps toward the wall or arena fence. It is important to get this exercise right at Release Level, so practice may be needed.

- **COORDINATE LEVEL** (*Trot d'École*, Long-and-Low HNP): Rising (posting) *trot d'école*, then sit for the lateral section only. Sitting on a lateral movement is easier than when going forward on a line, with the addition that it allows you to be clearer with the inside leg aid—and perhaps a Tapping Stick just to help him take the leg aid as a priority. As with most physical training, if it is "happening" but a little sticky, it is working.

- **TONE LEVEL** (*Petit Galop*, Long-and-Low HNP): In the most *petit galop* we can ask for a smooth and agile leg-yield into a Long-and-Low frame. It will take daily practice to achieve, yet the good steps will quickly outnumber the difficult ones.

How to Do It

OVERVIEW: Here we help the horse into a Long-and-Low outline to release the core *before* asking the horse to cross both his front and hind legs on a diagonal across the school (fig. 6.59). "Riding a leg-yield at the beginning of the warm-up is the perfect exercise for a horse at any level of training to test his reaction to your lateral moving (sideways) aids," notes the United States Dressage Federation (USDF).

- **STEP /1/** Ride into a corner and make one 6-meter Core Release Volte (see p. 156) before coming straight down the school close to the quarterline, parallel to the track and holding a Stretching Flexion (see p. 139) in a Long-and-Low outline.

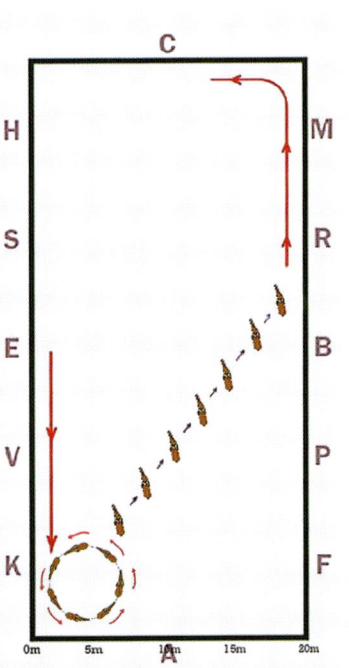

/ **6.59** / *Limbering Leg Yield floor plan: Beginning with a Core Release Volte to obtain a soft Long-and-Low HNP really helps keep the horse's back from tensing during the leg-yield.* ▶

- **STEP /2/** Ride straight for a few strides before stimulating the horse with the inside leg to leg-yield to the track on the other side of the arena. Don't worry about accuracy, beauty, or grace. These will come only with practice. Ride it, encourage the horse a lot, and get good at it while inviting him to stretch down.
- **STEP /3/** Be sure to follow with hand and seat in the lateral stretch. The horse may need more than leg aids to get to the other side of the ring, so encourage, release, and reward his efforts for day-to-day improvement.
- **STEP /4/** To amplify the suppling effect when the exercise has become very smooth, put the hindquarters a touch ahead

of the shoulders so they lead very slightly across the arena (fig. 6.60). This will align the spine for optimal loosening, and you will get a very supple horse as a result.

Common Problems and Solutions

- **The horse leads with the shoulder.** Ride several voltes before the leg-yield until the core releases; this will give more ability to Frame the shoulder (see p. 142) because the horse's back will be a little rounder.

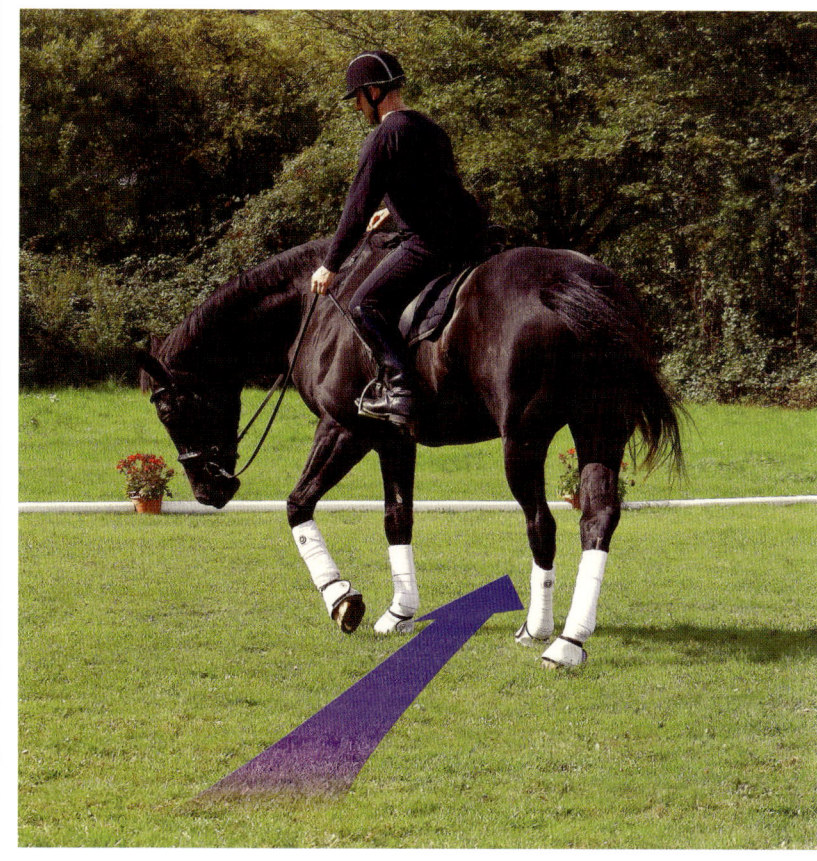

◀ **/ 6.60 /** *When the exercise becomes easier for the horse, the effect of its suppling action can deepen by asking the horse to lead slightly with the hindquarters while Framing the outside shoulder for him.*

\\\ Jason Crandell ///

Jason Crandell

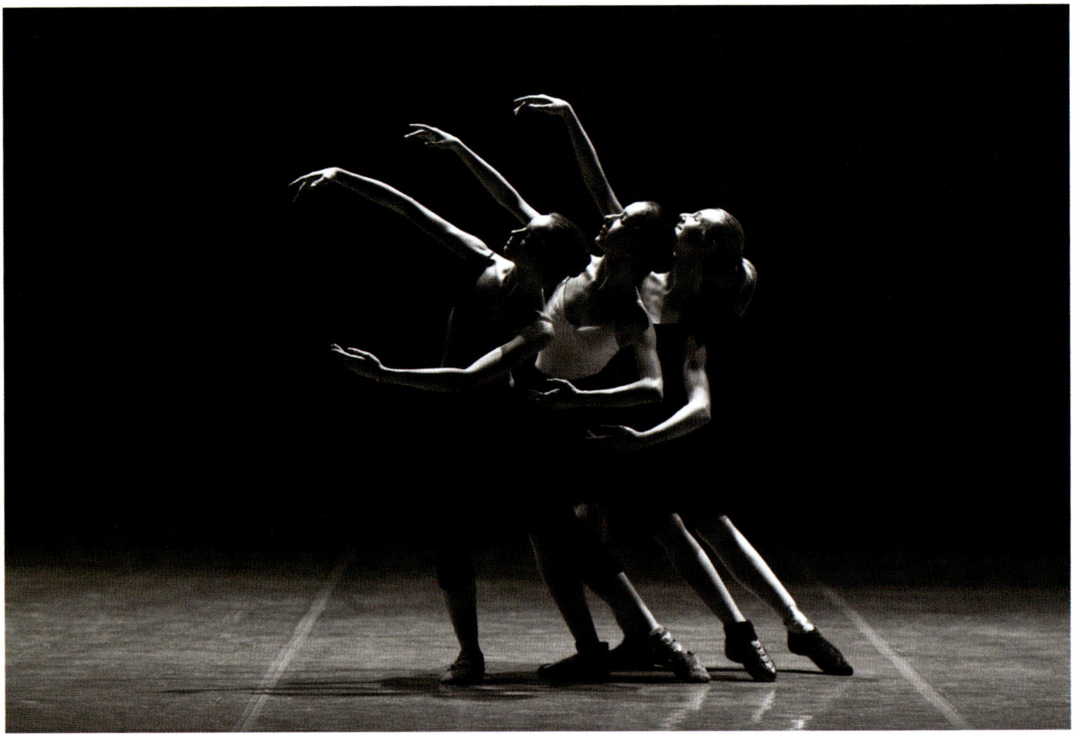

"The Revolved Triangle
is a tricky pose to do well. Remember, though:
you don't need to be flexible to do yoga.
Flexibility is the end result of doing yoga!"

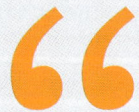

- ***No reaction from the inside leg.*** Practice the Release Level with the Tapping Stick (see p. 146) and reward. All horses can master this one!
- ***The horse resists and raises his head.*** Try using a Core Release Volte to put the horse into a comfortable Long-and-Low HNP before coming down the centerline to leg-yield. This will help to begin with relaxation in the back.

Core Score Zero Goal

The activation of the core to this level will have the horse floating sideways like a ballet dancer. Imagine that. ■

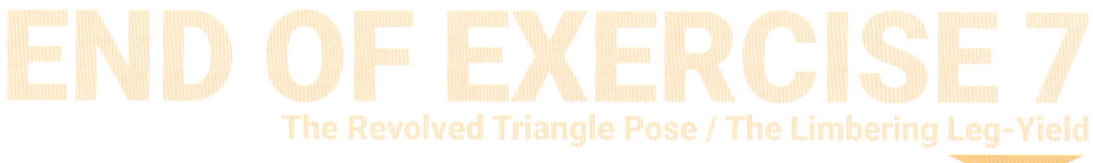

/ 6.61 / *The Perfect Pirouette: Walking slowly and carefully both forward and sideways gives Wardance more range of motion in the shoulders and encourages the Thoracic Lift Core Power.* ▶

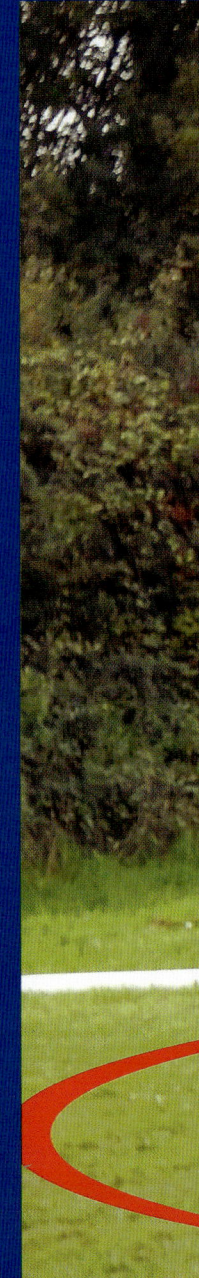

Exercise 8

🔥 / Thread the Needle Pose
🐴 / The Perfect Pirouette

Your upper torso has a lot of complex muscles that can make the limbs express themselves in highly dexterous ways. Lack of use of even the smallest muscle can leave this area less toned than it should be, and this can limit posture and agility when called upon. The *Thread the Needle Pose* helps to gently release a greater range of motion in a person's upper body.

Its horsey counterpart exercise, the *Perfect Pirouette*, can significantly improve the range of motion of your horse's front end (fig. 6.61). This low-impact stretch isolates and awakens that magnificent piece of bioengineering—the Thoracic Sling.

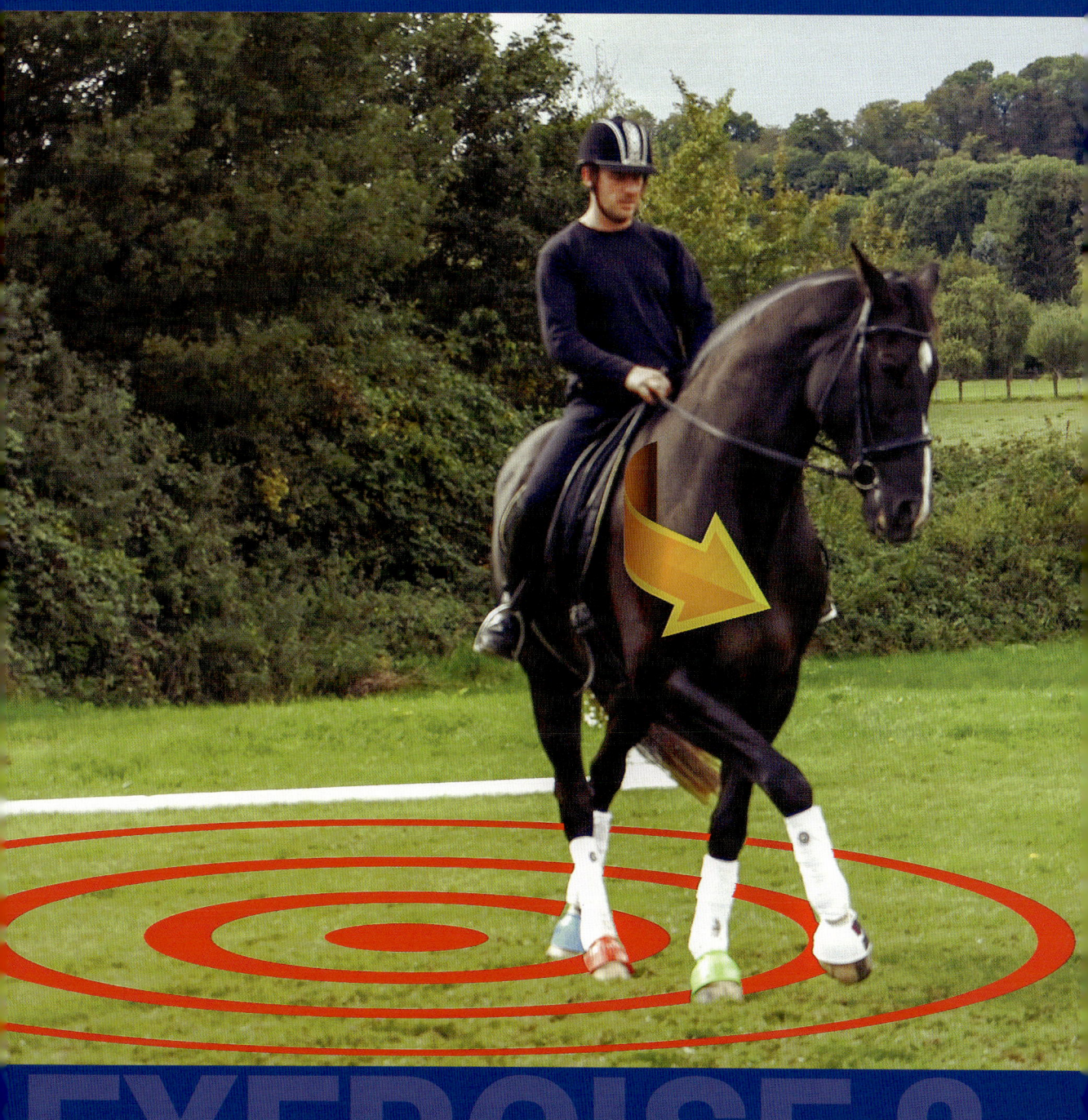

EXERCISE 8

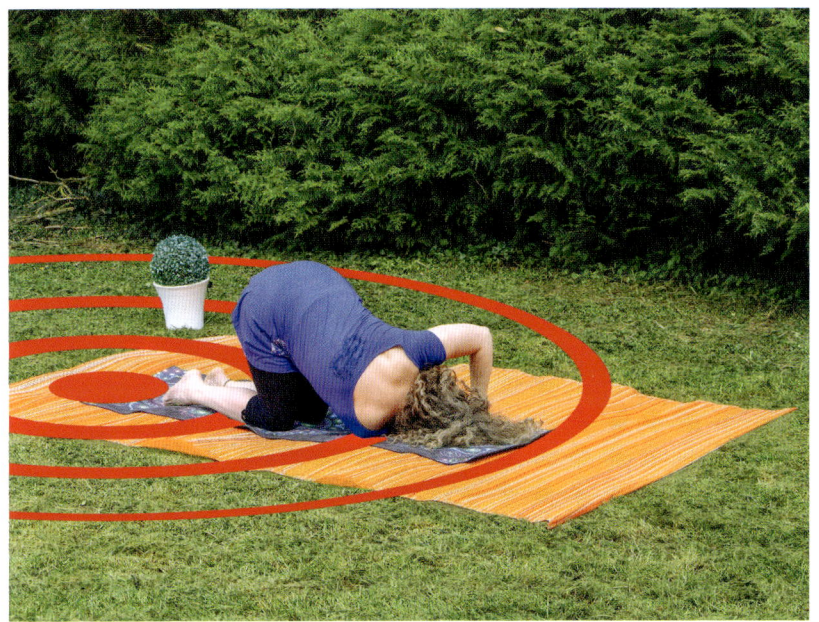

/ 6.62 / The Thread the Needle Pose is an upper body stretching exercise. By stretching the arm across the body, the spine must release and allow itself to gently twist while the shoulder muscles elongate. ▶

🙏 / Thread the Needle Pose

The *Thread the Needle Pose* is a static stretch where you slide your arm across and under your body, rotating and suppling the upper body's components from the head through to the pelvis (fig. 6.62).

This pose helps a human to:

- Stretch the shoulders, chest, arms, upper back, and neck.
- Release tension held in the upper back.
- Stretch the abdominal muscles.
- Increase shoulder range of motion.
- Encourage relaxation.
- Strengthen the arms.

"The Thread the Needle Pose is a great way to open the back and lengthen the muscles around the shoulders and in the neck," agrees Becky Litwicki, mobility and mind-body-awareness teacher.

/ The Perfect Pirouette

The *Perfect Pirouette* will supple and strengthen the front end of your horse (fig. 6.63). Walk is the key to this exercise, so it is very possible for any horse to perfect it.

Collection is not required; you want to keep things very simple to understand and as free-flowing as possible. For its range-of-motion

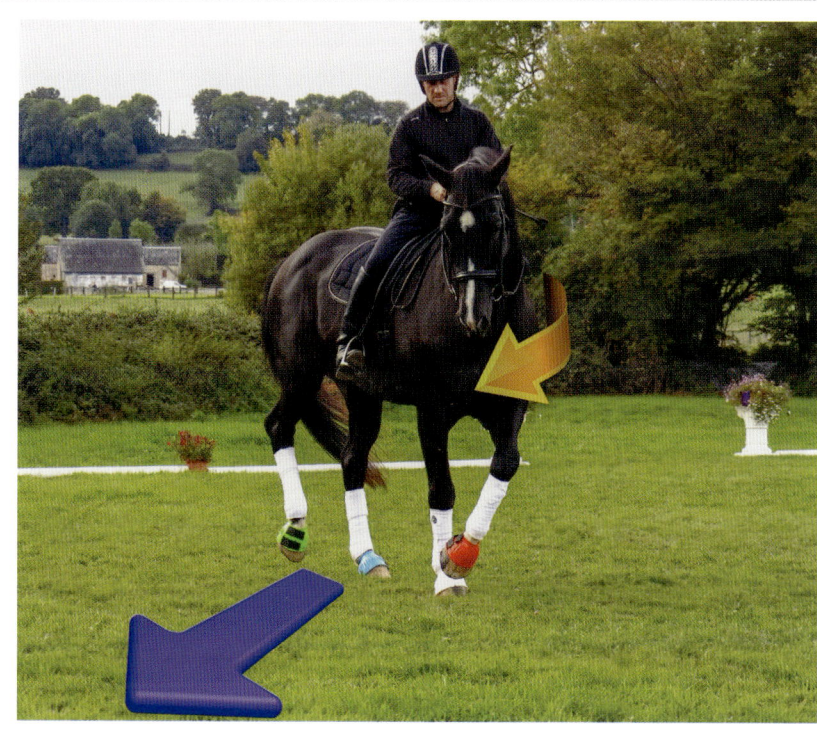

◀ / **6.63** / *Coordination, range of motion, and rider connection are all challenged in the Perfect Pirouette. The horse must be released in the core and light to the inside aids if he is to respond lightly to the outside aids.*

focus, this exercise is done in the same spirit as a turn on the haunches, where good bend and coordinated crossing of legs are the goal, rather than focusing on making a precise shape in the sand.

The *Perfect Pirouette* creates a soft inside flexion while asking the horse to learn to step *into the bend*, as opposed to leg-yield where the horse steps *away from the bend*. This makes it a wonderful, low-impact opportunity to develop clear communication while Framing through the outside rein. It is a wonderful technical challenge. Thankfully, your horse will find it easy to master, and every improvement in technique will bring developments in steering and mobility that advance everything else you do together.

To balance the challenge of this exercise against the benefits, it is best to perform the Perfect Pirouette with the hindquarters allowed to move on a small circle rather than staying on the spot, often called a "working pirouette" (fig. 6.64).

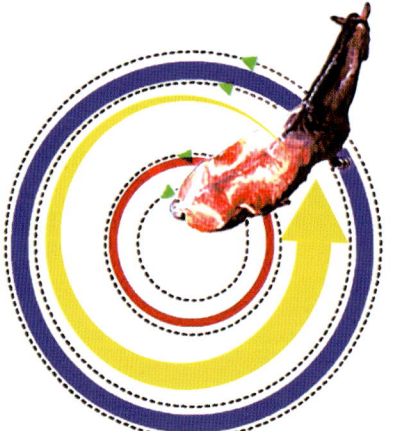

/ 6.64 / *A big circle around a little circle: To maximize the suppling action of the Perfect Pirouette, the horse's front end and rear end must each be walking on a circle.* ▶

This exercise helps the horse:

- Mobilize through the shoulders and neck.
- Awaken elasticity in the Thoracic Sling.
- Widen the stance.
- Stretch the neck.
- Connect the body to the back through the outside aids.
- Remain calm in a slow, deliberate movement.

"It is important for riders to hone their skills perfecting turn on the haunches and walk pirouettes before attempting canter pirouettes," wrote German Grand Prix dressage trainer Gerhard Politz. "In the walk, we have more time to coordinate the aids. I advise seeking many opportunities to practice walk pirouettes to reduce frustration for you and your horse" (fig. 6.65).

This exercise helps solve these issues under saddle:

- Steering problems.
- Stopping problems.
- Lateral work that falls through the outside shoulder (see Framing, p. 242).
- Flat front leg action.

The rider needs to be able to bring the horse's shoulders inward easily. This is the basis of every turn and every lateral movement, and is essential when a particular destination is in mind. If the horse's core is weak in the Thoracic Sling, the rider's position when Framing will resemble the technique used to land a tuna. The Perfect Pirouette will wake this powerful core mechanism, making bulging biceps a thing of the past.

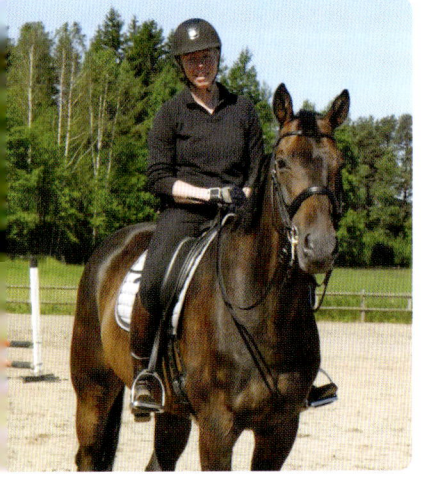

Marina Kallioniemi

(Finland)

My horse was diagnosed with kissing spines in January 2015. He is a big Trakehner gelding, and for me, it was a big setback—for a while I thought our journey was over. He was first treated with acupuncture and I started rehab just by hand-walking. I then tried to find all possible information about how to work with this new challenge and what I should now do differently.

One of my friends forwarded me the article "Kiss Kissing Spine Goodbye" by Visconte Simon Cocozza. I read the article and got really interested in how to do the exercises in a way that could help my horse: How often? How long? In what way? I had many questions and got the courage to contact Simon to ask for more help.

Simon was very kind from the very beginning. He told me to forget everything I had done in the past and start with four basic exercises, riding in walk only, no other gaits, no longeing. I decided to do as he advised. My horse was also regularly checked and treated with acupuncture and chiropractic by our vet. After one week, we started to feel how my horse's back was coming up, especially in a turn on the forehand exercise. Within three weeks of starting the exercises, his pain had abated. From the fourth week onward, we started to trot also for short periods while using the yoga-inspired exercises, and we did lots of

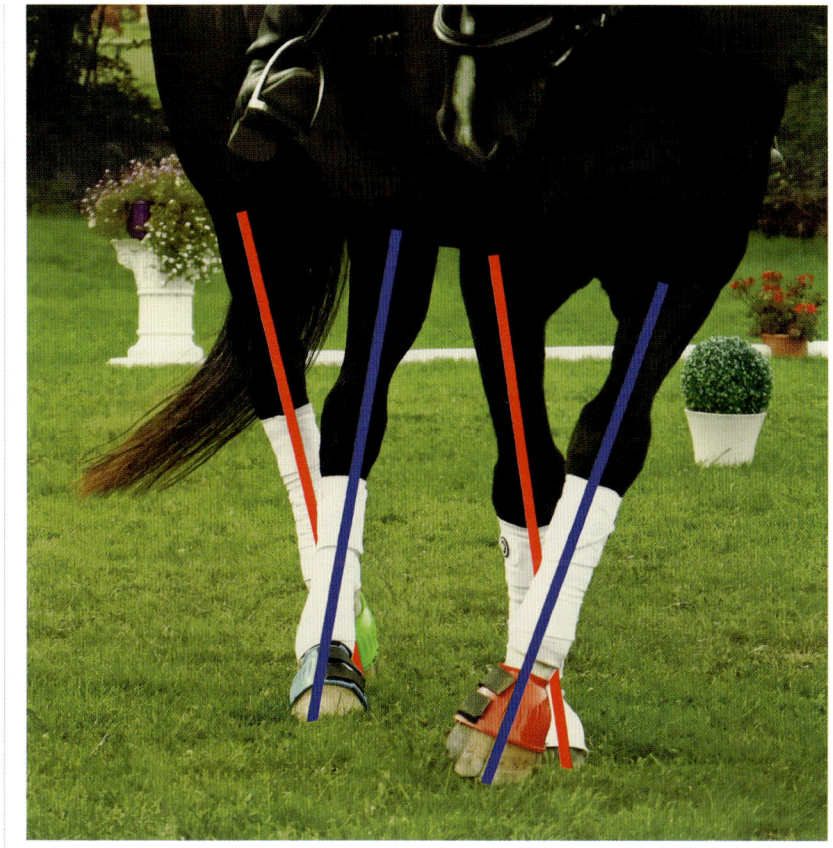

◄ / 6.65 / When it comes to coordinating the legs, the horse needs slow speeds to refine his technique. As his range of motion increases, he can learn to be more coordinated in the limb at higher impulsion levels.

What It Does to the Inside of the Horse

The front legs of a horse can't bend at the knee under weight as ours do, so the horse's front end depends upon this part of the core being in excellent working order (fig. 6.66). The Perfect Pirouette has the horse bend in the back while isolating the shoulder muscles in the Thoracic Sling. This will gradually increase the height at which the horse carries his chest between the shoulders, making the horse "uphill" in motion.

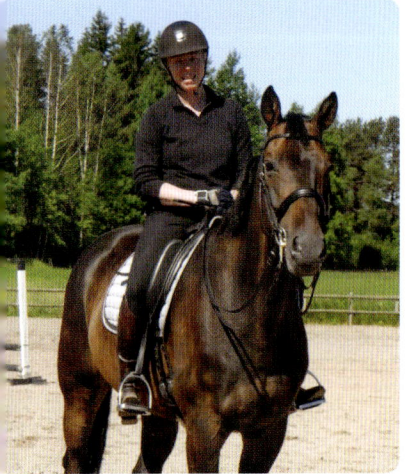

transitions back to walk if my horse started to lower his back. I would use the basic exercises to get his back lifted again before moving back to trot. From week eight onward, Simon advised I introduce canter but no straight lines in the beginning: shoulder-in and leg-yield.

In May 2015 Simon visited Finland for the first time, and my horse and I were already able to practice the exercises in all gaits.

It was amazing to experience how fast my horse adapted to Simon's exercises. When your horse gets stronger and more elastic, you truly find there are no limits in perfecting the movements. During Simon's visit to Finland we reached the next level: getting more fluidity, easiness, and softness, and especially getting my horse's back lifted and his spine aligned to find the natural balance. I now have a toolkit for myself that helps me figure out how to correct my horse if he is crooked, does not bend, or gets tense: always take it one gear down, fix it in the walk—"the queen of gaits"—and then start again.

I recommend this concept and Simon's exercises wholeheartedly—hopefully many can start and feel the difference in their horses without going through challenges like kissing spine first.

These exercises fit all horses, riders, and levels. All horses deserve to be happy in their work. I am ever thankful for Simon's support and coaching during this journey, and also all the riders around us here in Finland who have joined us. It has been amazing to see the transformations in many horses, the easiness and beauty as they move to their own potential. Every horse deserves it.

....
Marina Kallioniemi

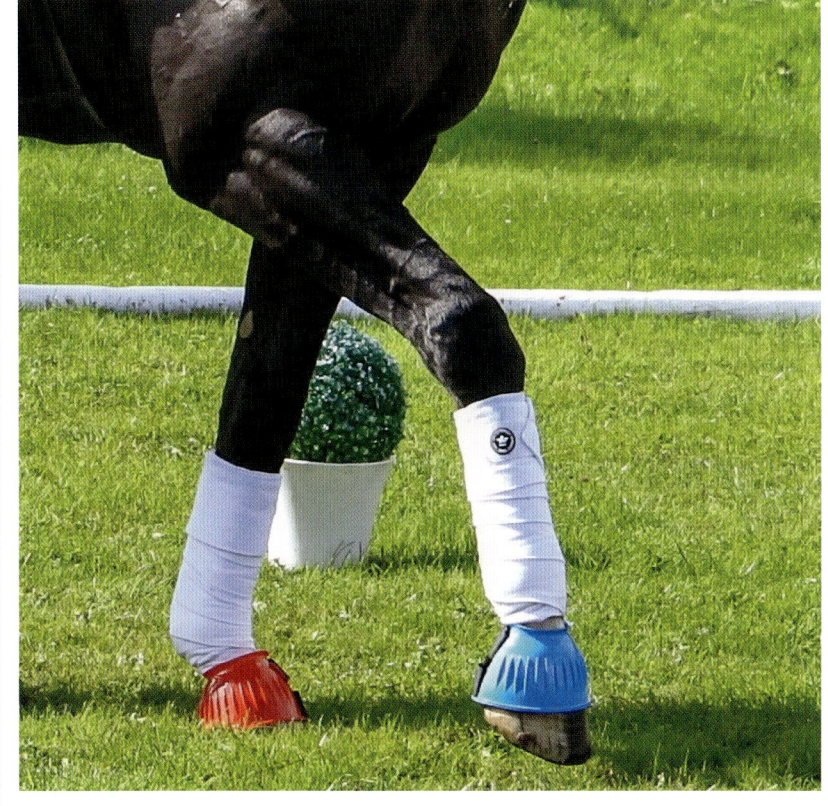

◀ / 6.66 / *The horse has no power in the knee and can only put weight onto a straight front leg. For this reason, full shoulder mobility is the answer to front-end agility.*

Core Score, Level, and Head-and-Neck Position

If your horse has a Core Score of:

- **3–5**, do this exercise at the **RELEASE LEVEL.**
- **2**, do this exercise at the **COORDINATION LEVEL.**
- **0–1**, do this exercise at the **TONE LEVEL.**

In this exercise, Levels are reached by increasing the number of steps and their quality.

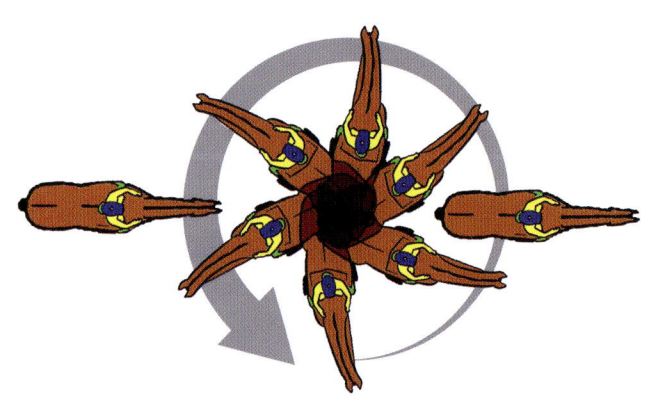

/ 6.67 / *The Perfect Pirouette develops the horse's ability to be light and athletic through the shoulders, as well as allowing us to learn to control them.* ▶

- **RELEASE LEVEL** (1 to 3 Steps into the Flexion): At this level, you should release and reward the very first step sideways by the horse's shoulder that is in the direction of the flexion. All correct responses to your requests, however small, deserve a reward at this point. Acorns build oaks. Allow the horse to carry his own head and feel free to express his own questions.

- **COORDINATION LEVEL** (180-Degree Half-Turn, Long-and-Low HNP): Once Release Level gives three steps with ease and the horse understands the exercise, simply keep going round in an a rough semi-circle while Framing his shoulders in a continuous conversation through your aids.

- **TONE LEVEL** (One Full Rotation): Aim for a smooth and rhythmic crossing of the front and hind legs that is reliable, soft, and light while steadily resting on a light Framing outside rein (fig. 6.67). It should be possible to maintain a Long-and-Low HNP from beginning to end.

How to Do It

OVERVIEW: It is useful to begin by halting on the centerline, giving you space all around (fig. 6.68). The horse is allowed to get it wrong a lot before getting it right once. Simply reward on the first right attempt, and the exercise will begin to take shape.

- **STEP /1/** Begin at the halt in Long-and-Low with a Held Stretching Flexion (see p. 139). Stimulate with the outside leg and outside rein only. Begin Tapping the horse sensitively on the outside shoulder to instigate that first, inward step with the front end. When this happens, release and reward.

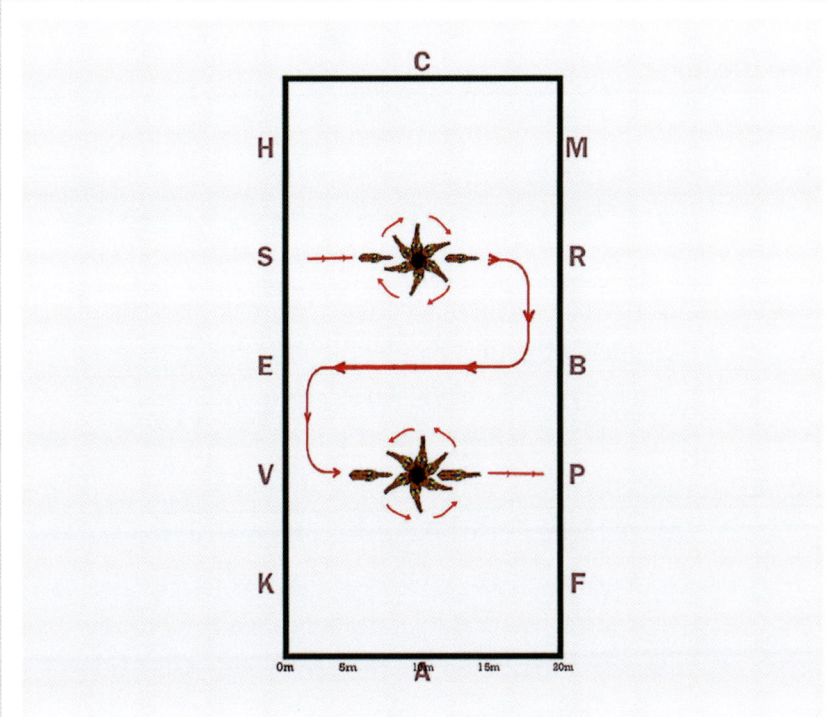

◀ / **6.68** / The Perfect Pirouette floor plan: With a simple pattern, this exercise can be done on the centerline in both directions with a tidy change of direction at X.

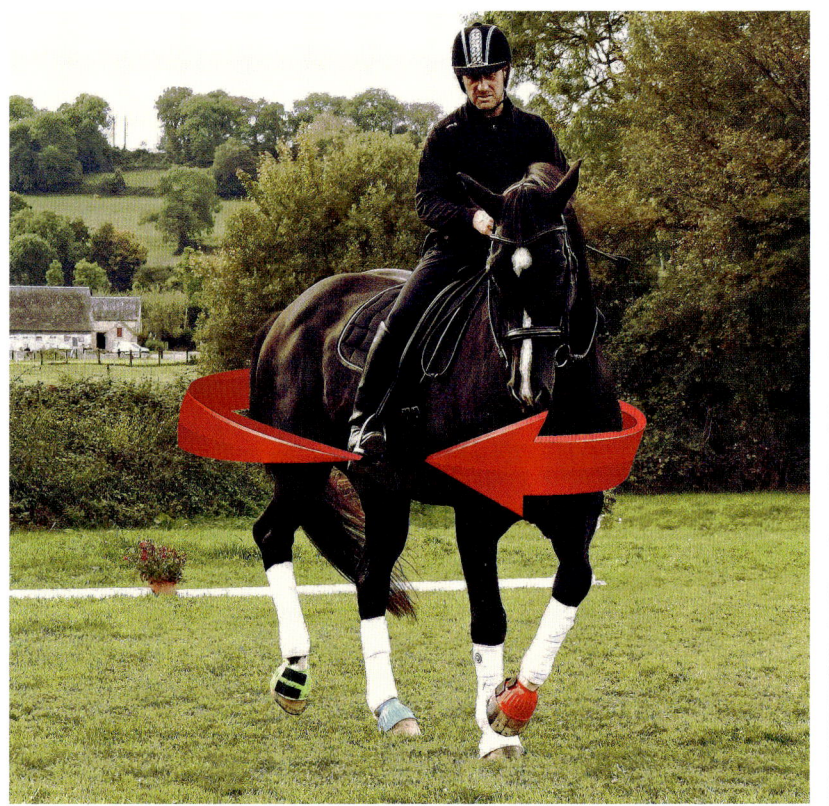

/ 6.69 / Coordination in motion: When the horse has learned the Perfect Pirouette at Tone Level, he will have a soft inside bend throughout his body. ▶

- **STEP /2/** After much repetition, the steps will begin chaining themselves together. Balance the aids to guide both the shoulders *and* the hindquarters onto a medium-sized semi-circle by riding forward and sideways at the same time.
- **STEP /3/** Tone Level is one full rotation around in Long-and-Low HNP (fig. 6.69). This is a deceptively challenging exercise. It will involve very subtle aids that will be needed to guide your horse into a light and smooth ballet. Once the exercise is understood to the Tone Level, a seat aid will often replace the leg completely.

Common Problems and Solutions

- ***The horse is not turning inward.*** Reestablish the hold in the Stretching Flexion (see p. 139), making sure the horse's core is already released. If not, Exercise 1: *Core Release Volte* and Exercise 3: *Forward, Down, and Out* need more practice.

Make sure your inside leg is not on your horse. Sometimes the problem is us! "The important point to remember in executing the pirouette is that it is the forehand which is being asked to come around the hindquarters; therefore the outside leg should address the forehand," emphasizes British eventer Christopher Bartle.

Core Score Zero Goal

You will gradually need less and less rein contact and leg pressure to bring the horse's shoulders inward, and all the aids will become more intuitive. This will make it easy to precisely help the horse place his shoulders well for the next challenge.

This exercise naturally leads to an effortless half-pass and intuitive canter pirouettes—as they should be. ∎

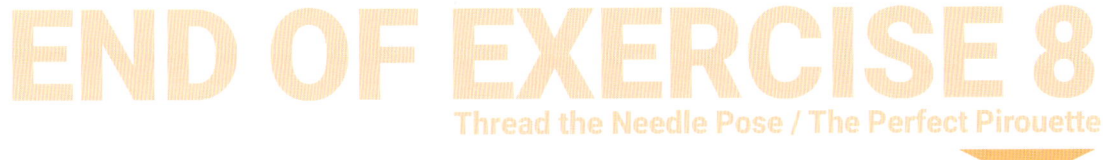

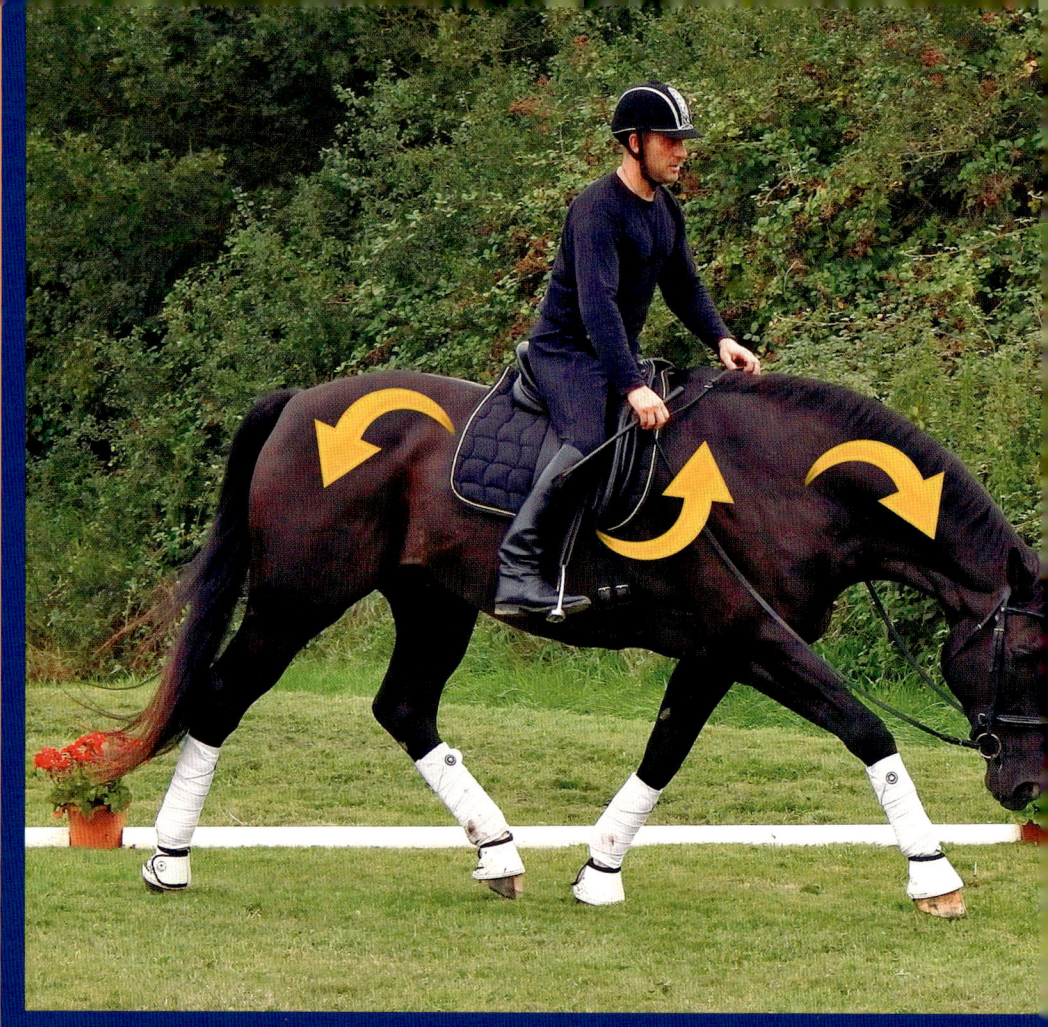

▲ / 6.70 / This range-of-motion exercise takes the horse's body from a full back stretch, all the way up to an engaged,

Exercise 9

♞ / **The Cat to Cow Pose**
♞ / **Forward, Down, and Out to Competition Outline**

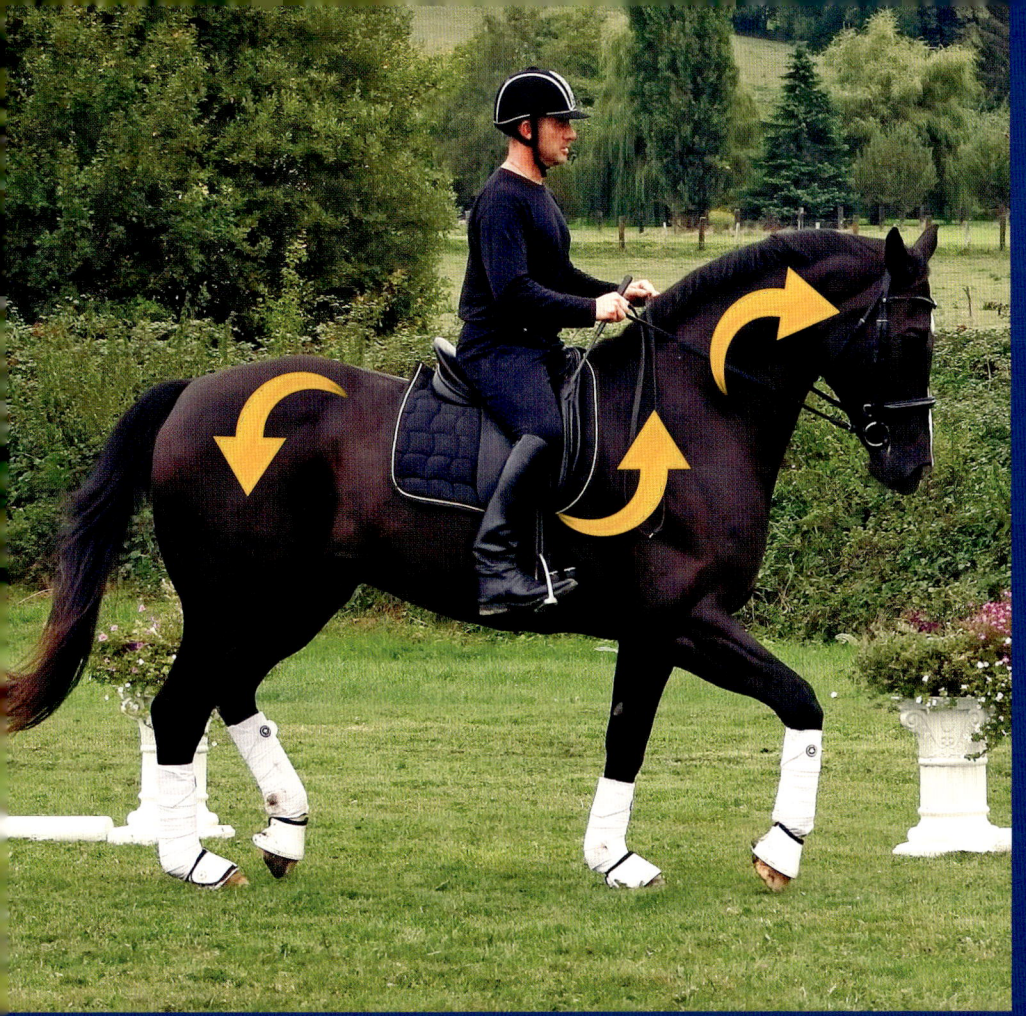

yet soft, classical posture.

The *Cat to Cow Pose* is an essential yoga stretch for humans and with good reason. It's *the* foundation "range-of-motion exercise." Adapted for our horses, moving the horse's outline from *Forward, Down, and Out* all the way through to *Competition Outline* is the key to maintaining healthy back tension while under higher energy—a valuable skill indeed (fig. 6.70).

🙏 / The Cat to Cow Pose

For details of the Cat Pose, see Exercise 3 on page 186 (fig. 6.71).

The Cow Pose introduces tension to the human back under controlled, soft, and temporary circumstances (fig. 6.72). It is very useful to bring the back muscles into play while maintaining correct core posture obtained in the Cat Pose stretch.

Cycling from Cat to Cow Poses helps a human to:

- Learn to introduce strength without tension.
- Improve posture and balance.
- Strengthen the spine and neck.
- Stretch the hips.
- Massage the organs.
- Relieve stress.

Cat to Cow Pose is best seen as a gentle flow between the two poses. This warms the body and brings flexibility to your spine and the core. The engage-release sequence also helps develop postural awareness and balance throughout the body.

"Cat-Cow back stretch and extension is a wonderful, balanced exercise for the back because it is both a stretch (Cat) and an extension (Cow) exercise," explains Marguerite Ogle, American wellness and fitness instructor. "Cat-Cow develops flexibility in the spine and is one of the exercises often recommended for back pain."

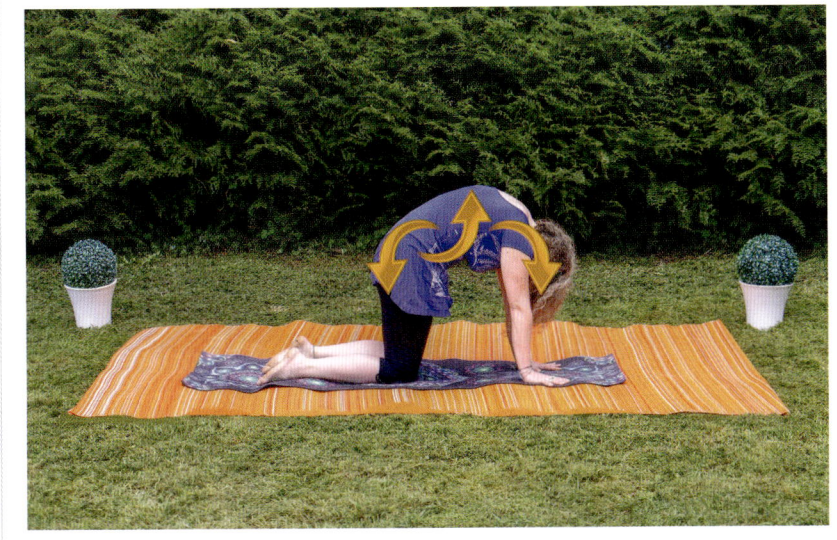

◄ / 6.71 / *The Cat Pose raises and stretches the length of your neck, back, and lower back.*

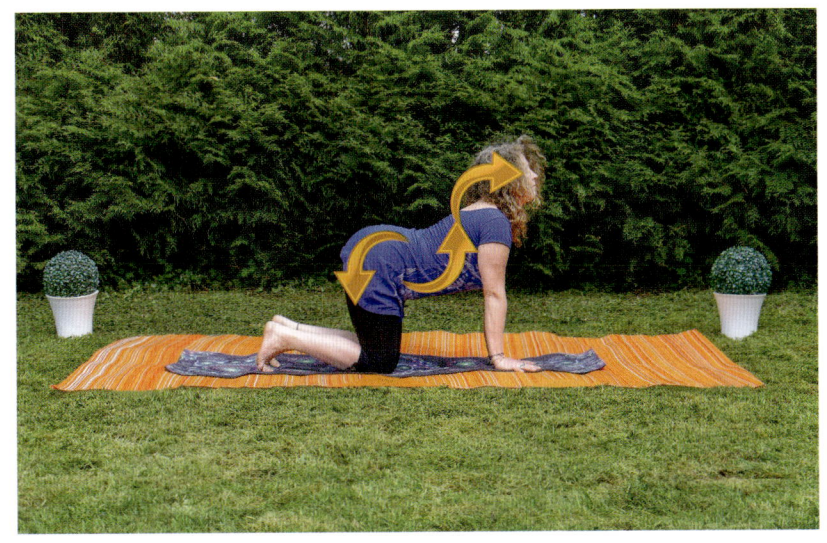

◄ / 6.72 / *The Cow Pose brings the big muscles into play while retaining the Core Release and suppleness from the Cat Pose. Gradually, your body learns to balance the use of both the lifting and pushing muscles.*

🐴 / Forward, Down, and Out to Competition Outline

This exercise will create a weightless head and neck in the horse that can effortlessly and easily be placed in a Competition Outline (see p. 264) while maintaining roundness through the horse's core (fig. 6.73).

This exercise helps the horse to:

- Gain body confidence to fully release, then employ the spine.
- Improve balance and stability.
- Transfer relaxation into connection.
- Easily perform with the weight of the rider in sitting trot.

This full spinal range-of-motion exercise both connects the horse's core to his limbs and creates the horse's all-important trust in our aids to help rather than hinder him. Forward, Down, and Out to

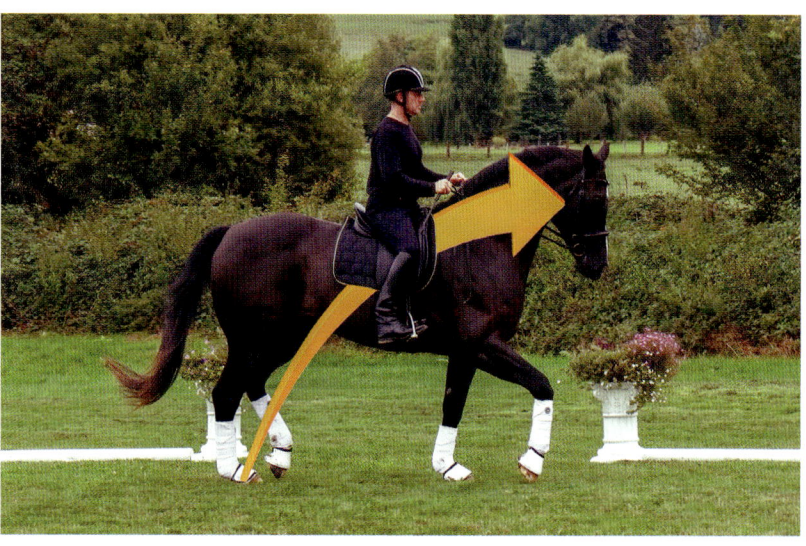

/ 6.73 / The Competition Outline is only harmonious if completely light and free. Using this exercise, you can gradually raise the horse's HNP into a both easy and anatomically correct outline for sport. ▶

Competition Outline performed well represents a milestone in training, and the horse will be very rideable as a result.

This exercise helps solve these issues under saddle:

• Tense or hard contact.
• Running onto the forehand.
• Head too low/high.
• Tense back when on the bit.

What It Does to the Inside of the Horse

Forward, Down, and Out to Competition Outline asks the many areas of the core conditioned by the other exercises to do their part now as an orchestra. These will be the effects:

• Core Release.
• Nuchal Lift, Thoracic Lift, and Pelvic engagement (Three Core Powers).
• *Abdominals, iliopsoas,* and *multifidus* activation.
• Relaxed mind.
• An easy, soft, and forward Competition Outline.

Core Score, Level, and Head-and-Neck Position

If your horse has a Core Score of:

• **4–5**, do this exercise at **RELEASE LEVEL**.
• **2–3**, do this exercise at **COORDINATION LEVEL**.
• **0–1**, do this exercise at **TONE LEVEL**.

- **RELEASE LEVEL** (Free-Walk): Release the head and neck into Forward, Down, and Out HNP, then bring the head up to the Competition Outline, while maintaining the same rhythm and energy. Establish for a few strides before returning to Forward, Down, and Out. Repeat until smooth as silk and light as a feather.

- **COORDINATION LEVEL** (*Trot d'École*): Alternate between Forward, Down, and Out and a Competition Outline in this light, rising trot. When the horse feels very round under your seat, it is time to introduce sitting trot.

- **TONE LEVEL** (*Petit Galop*): Alternate between Forward, Down, and Out and a Competition Outline in a balanced and easy *petit galop.* Your horse will love it.

How to Do It

OVERVIEW: While riding simple figures such as circles, figures of eight, and serpentines, repeatedly practice fully lowering and raising your horse's head carriage, guided by the horse's signs of what is comfortable. When the horse eventually feels strong enough, holding the Competition Outline will become easier and easier for longer and longer.

- **STEP /1/** Ride a Core Release Volte (see p. 156) followed by Forward, Down, and Out (see p. 186), and when there are very light and balanced moments, raise the horse's head into an even, straight Competition Outline without changing the gait (fig. 6.74). Allow the horse to self-adjust. Be sure to follow with your seat while you bring the horse onto the bit.

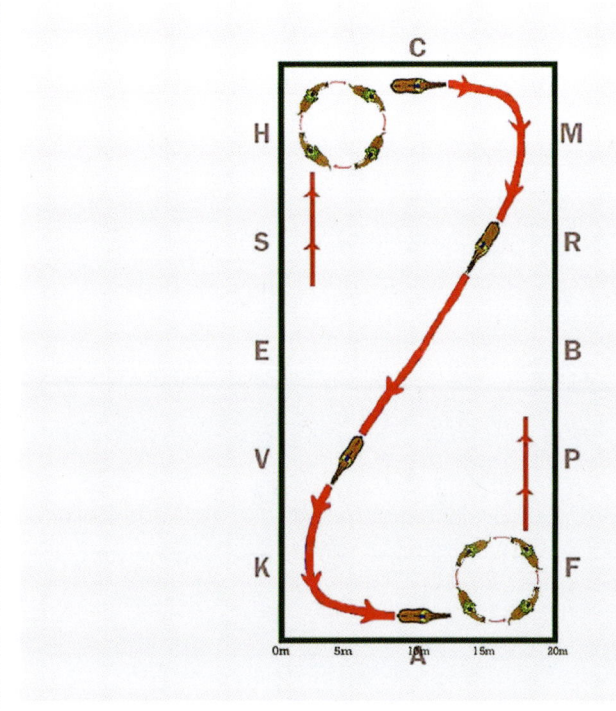

◀ / 6.74 / *Forward, Down, and Out to a Competition Outline floor plan: By incorporating Core Release Voltes to first find a soft Long-and-Low HNP, we can then use the arena in long lines to stretch or raise the HNP when the horse feels ready.*

· **STEP /2/** After a few seconds in a Competition Outline, tension may begin to build through one or both reins. Simply return to a Forward, Down, and Out HNP in a softer gait for a while before repeating the exercise. This is a gradual process that takes practice to build the required muscles and reflexes (fig. 6.75).

· **STEP /3/** When the free-walk is soft and rhythmical in a Competition Outline, it is time to begin introducing the Coordination Level, rising to the *trot d'école*. Over time it will feel possible to spend more time in the Competition Outline than Forward, Down, and Out without resistance or tension. When this happens, it is time to introduce Tone Level.

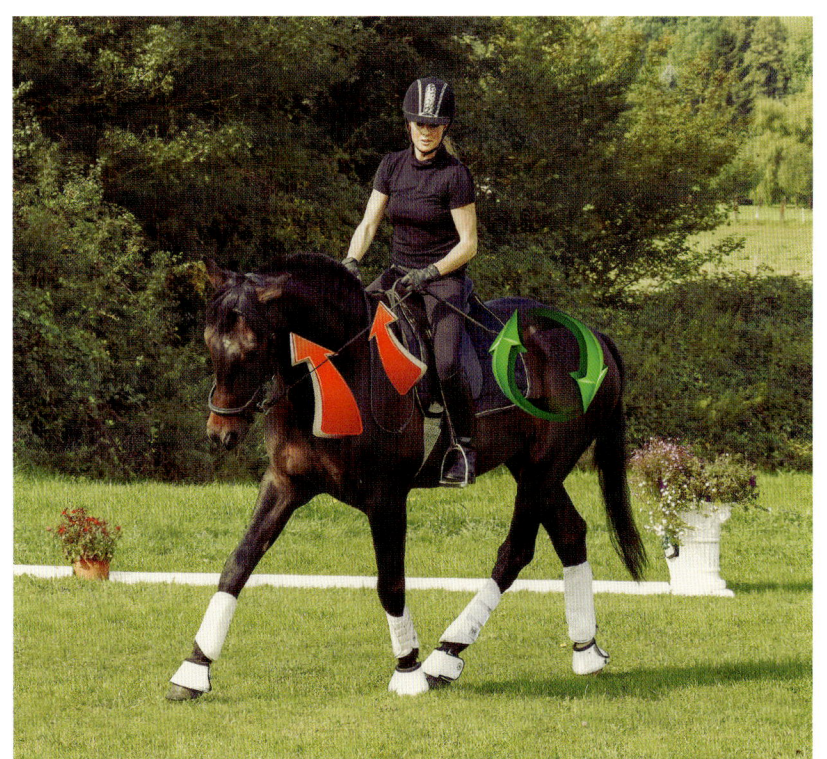

/ 6.75 / *This exercise improves the horse's full range of spine activity. As it gradually restores the core and back functions, the three Core Powers begin to improve the horse's paces.* ▶

- **STEP /4/** Gradually increase the length of time spent in the Competition Outline at Tone Level *(petit galop)* until the horse's back remains as supple in Competition Outline as it is in Forward, Down, and Out. At this point the back will feel very round, supple, and stable.

Common Problems and Solutions

- ***The horse is over-bent.*** It sometimes takes time for the horse's back to fully "unfurl." As long as you are "giving" with the rein contact and not holding his nose in, this will correct itself in time.

- ***The nose is not stretching down in Forward, Down, and Out.*** Practice Exercise 1: Core Release Volte to show the horse how to stretch into Long-and-Low HNP before trying again.
- ***Tension creeps into the Competition Outline.*** Muscle takes time to build. Keep practicing this exercise with longer periods in Forward, Down, and Out. The body's adaptation is not linear and there will be better days than others. If tension is unusually present on a particular day, choose a "softer" exercise for a few warm-ups.

Core Score Zero Goal

A horse that is supple enough to lower the nose to the grazing position of Forward, Down, and Out, smoothly followed by an "on the bit" frame without tension in the mouth, contact, or back, is a success of core conditioning. Your horse will be extremely intuitive and comfortable to ride after mastering this challenging exercise, as it will make different outlines, transitions, and lateral movements feel smoother, more predictable, and always in great balance. ∎

END OF EXERCISE 9
The Cat to Cow Pose / Forward, Down, and Out to Competition Outline

/ **6.76** / La Giravolta Longe: Giving the horse every chance to learn how to align, release, and round his own body, in his own time. ▶

Exercise 10

🧘 / The Revolved Half-Moon Pose
🐎 / La Giravolta Longe

The tenth exercise in this yoga-inspired series is based on the *Revolved Half-Moon Pose.* For the horse, it is known as *La Giravolta Longe* (fig. 6.76). Core alignment just got serious.

There are times when we can't, or shouldn't, ride. When you are experiencing equipment problems, injury, or perhaps a horse that is just impossible to ride well enough to be safe or fun, this is Plan B. La Giravolta Longe is a precise aligning tool that helps the horse improve himself. You are going to use it as a longeing tool, as it will be easier to reverse poor posture without a rider in the way. When the horse develops the skills required to do the Giravolta well, he will be well-aligned, released in the core, and ready for ridden exercises.

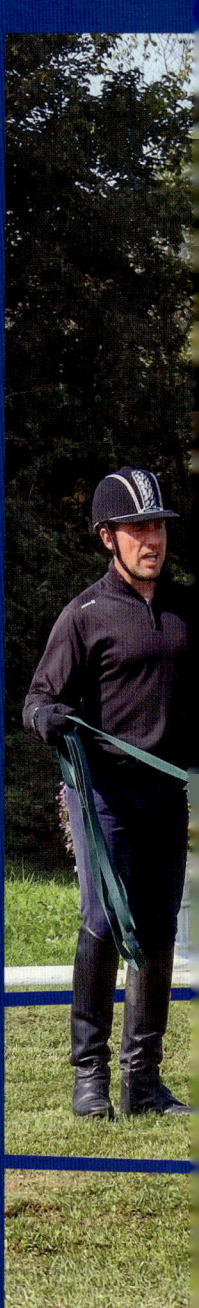

How to Use This Book

In this book I will show you how to assess, evaluate, and then completely condition the horse's core. The pages ahead will explain how to:

• Understand the horse's core.
• Assess the horse's core condition.
• Create a 20-minute, yoga-inspired, Core Warm-Up *exactly* for your horse.
• Ride your Core Warm-Up exercises safely and effectively.

By showing you how to spot what the horse's core needs from you, the rider, in the very subtle language used by your equine friend, you will be able to pinpoint what you can do to help your horse move better. Using "Core Indicators," you will assess the horse's core strength before deciding upon his "Core Score," which helps you then choose just the right Core Warm-Up to help him become connected, agile, and flexible. As your horse's core becomes stronger and the exercises easier, you can choose to develop another Core Warm-Up "plan." Eventually, your horse will become a true "Yoga Master"!

I've organized this book into two parts: You will begin with introductory material that will help you understand the horse's core and how to "score" it. In Part Two, you will learn the key exercises to improve your horse's core condition.

/1/ **The Back: Where All Movement Begins**
/2/ **The Source of the Force in the Horse: The Core**
/3/ **Horses Are People, Too**
/4/ **Assessing the Horse's Core and Choosing a Warm-Up Plan**

UNDERSTAND THE HORSE'S CORE

PART ONE: UNDERSTANDING THE HORSE'S CORE

\\\ Leonardo Da Vinci ///

Leonardo Da Vinci

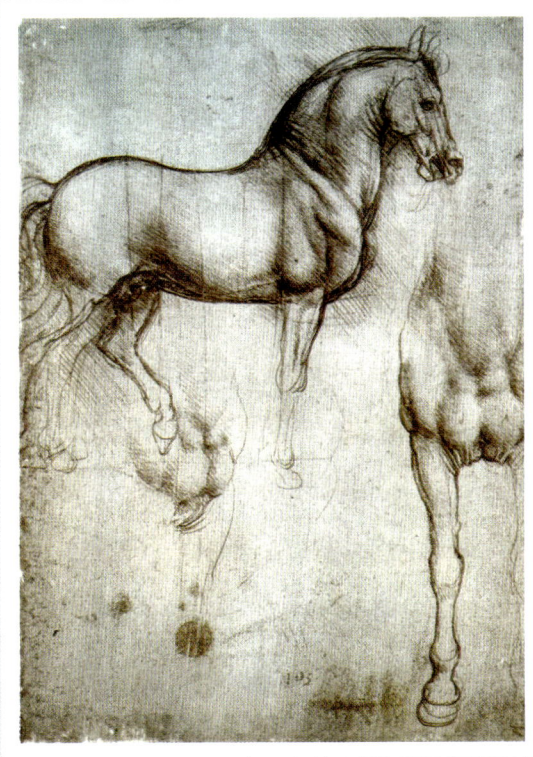

*"Once you have tasted flight,
you will forever walk the Earth
with your eyes turned skyward."*

❝

1

The Back: Where All Movement Begins

The Magic Inside Every Horse

Leonardo da Vinci was fascinated by the mechanical complexity inside the horse's body. He was looking for the "magic" behind the muscle.

Most serious riders have felt that magic that lives inside a horse. In that breathtaking moment when a horse is physically and mentally "free" under the saddle, you get to become part of a true wonder of the world: the equine athlete's magic in motion. Once experienced, this sensation is something you never forget. This is perhaps why the search for this deep connection between human and horse has been an obsession of our many cultures for millennia.

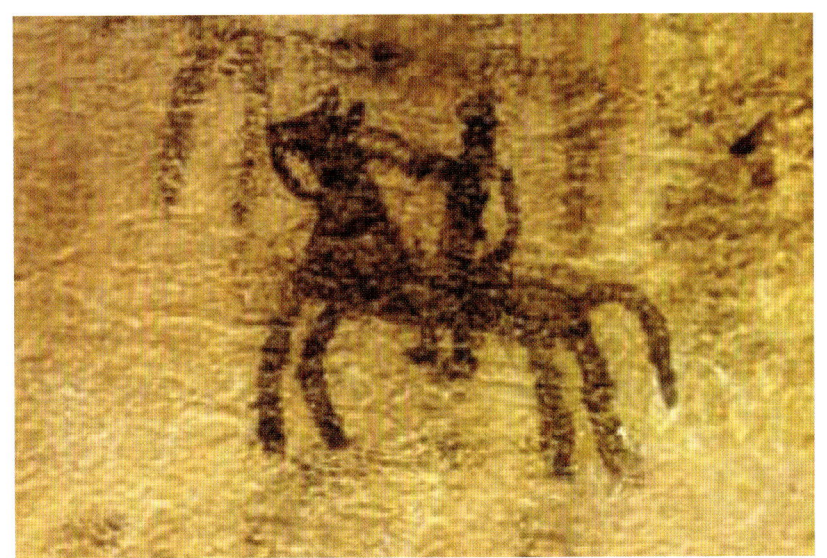

/ 1.1 / *Equestrian cave art from Persia—eighth century BC. From our earliest scribbles, the horse has been admired by humankind.* ▶

From our unkempt cave-doodling ancestors, through the various kingdoms and empires, from the high school and cavalry schools' legendary mastery, the magic in our horses keeps us riding and sweating in its pursuit (fig. 1.1). It is our Holy Grail.

Mother Nature's Perfect Design

The stance of a horse brings majesty to a space, representing the freedom, power, and grace within him. The magic of athleticism is Mother Nature's gift to *Equus*. For over 50 million years, this creature's body and mind have been honed to survive and thrive in incredibly hostile and varied environments, while evading some of the scariest predators imaginable. Horses are one of planet Earth's most determined survivors. The surprising level of athleticism that their bodies can produce is not only the prize we seek but has also been the key to their survival. Microseconds count as much as millennia in

\\\ Van Day Truex ///

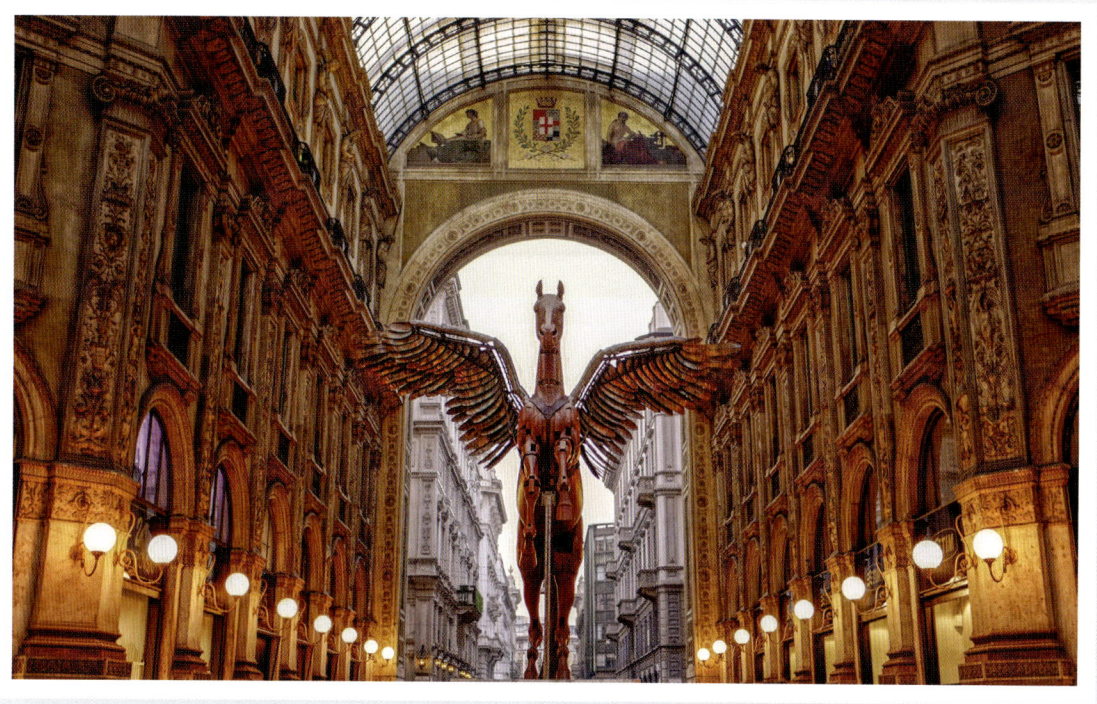

*"In design, Mother Nature
is our best teacher."*

❞

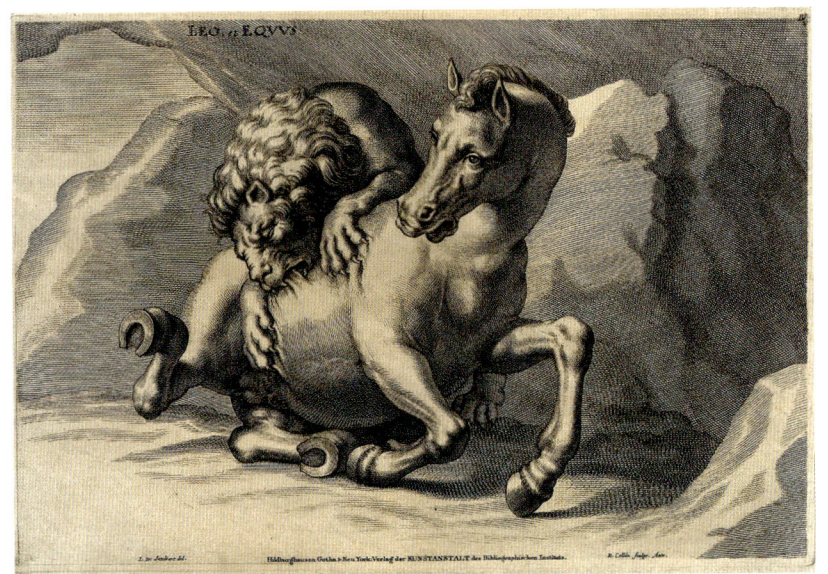

/ 1.2 / *Survival skills: Lightning-fast reactions and outstanding physical attributes have been key to Equus's long-term survival.* ▶

evolutionary terms, because if the herd is easy to catch, then soon there is no herd. To survive these frequent, and all too often final, split-second encounters with hungry, fanged beasts, the herbivore has needed to develop a finely tuned sense and sinew for incredible levels of movement (fig. 1.2).

In a situation where "close" means "curtains," a short, one-tenth of a second's head-start makes all the difference when a wolf or lion (or veterinarian!) gets too close. This is why nothing can leave the room faster than a horse.

With this legacy and these skills that allowed them to be so wonderfully adapted to their environment, our horsey friends roamed the planet in relative peace and harmony for a very long time. Then, one day, we turned up.

The Uninvited Guest

While equines were merrily minding their own business, we humans clearly saw their talents and have been dragging these cooperative creatures around the world ever since. This, of course, has taken these herbivores way, way beyond their comfort zone.

Thankfully, these days we have moved on to thundering around in machines, so at last we can give horses the respect they deserve and concentrate upon what is best for them, putting their welfare parallel to our own.

As with other people, to best help a horse and deliver assistance where he needs it most you can simply look at what is easy and what is hard for him. His strengths and weaknesses will tell you a lot about what particular aspect of his body he is not using enough and that may well be holding the rest of him back. Ironically, when we objectively assess

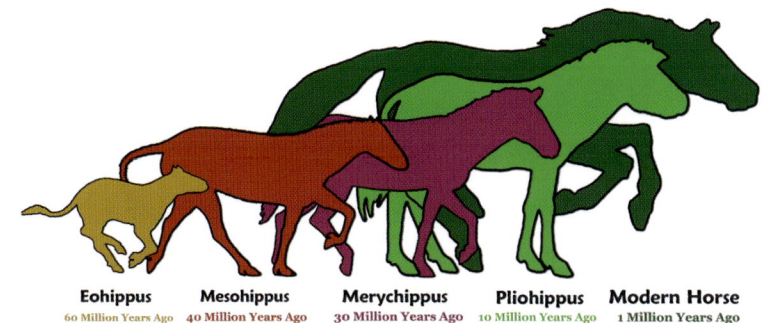

◀ / 1.3 / Many variations have come before, yet nature never did make the horse's back strong enough to carry a human.

what *really* holds a riding horse back we have to admit something quite awkward, and that is—from a design, strength, and balance point of view—the horse's body is simply not designed to carry a person. For 49.9999 million years the design worked very well indeed without people jiggling around on top.

As fate would have it, the most convenient place for us to sit on a horse is possibly the weakest of all. The horse's back looks strong from the ground but has a lot to carry as it is. Every design has its purpose and its limits, its strong and weak points, and when we sit on a horse's back we exceed the natural design capabilities…and this changes the horse's posture.

/ **1.4** / *The backing process: We desensitize the horse's mind to being ridden through gradual training, but realistically, his body has a huge challenge to face…it has to carry a person.* ▶

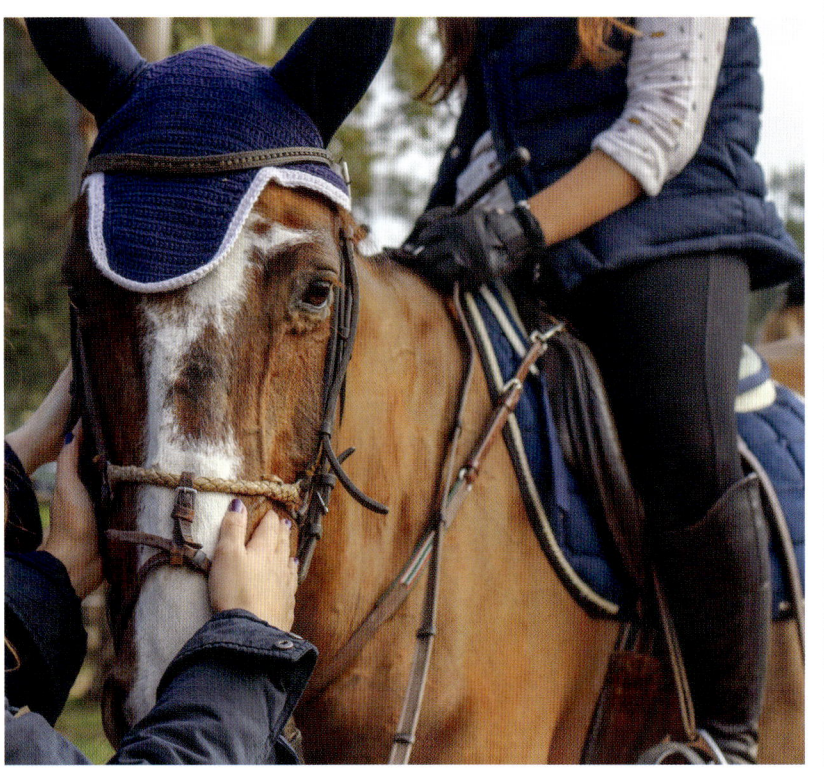

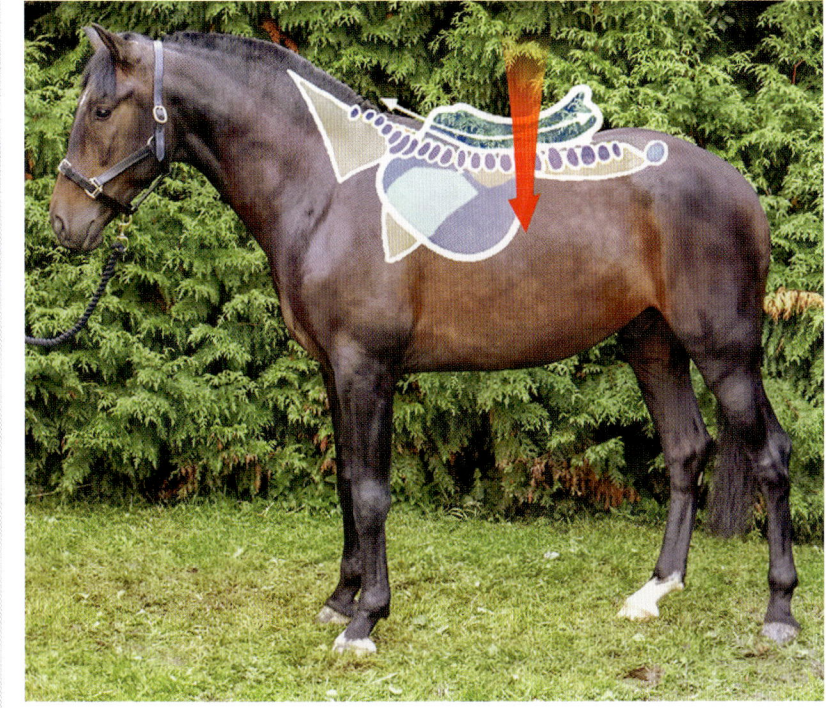

◀ / **1.5** / *The rider's weight exerts a constant downward force on the horse's back.*

Oops.

Sitting on the horse's rear end or withers would be perhaps better for the horse, as both those areas are supported by limbs. But because his back can flex like a Slinky, just sitting on it is enough to alter its delicate alignment.

When we start a youngster, we tend to focus upon the psychological aspect of the task. This makes sense because we have just crawled onto the horse's back like a panther, so trying to convince him not to run for the hills and never allow us to come near him again becomes the primary concern, usually for some weeks.

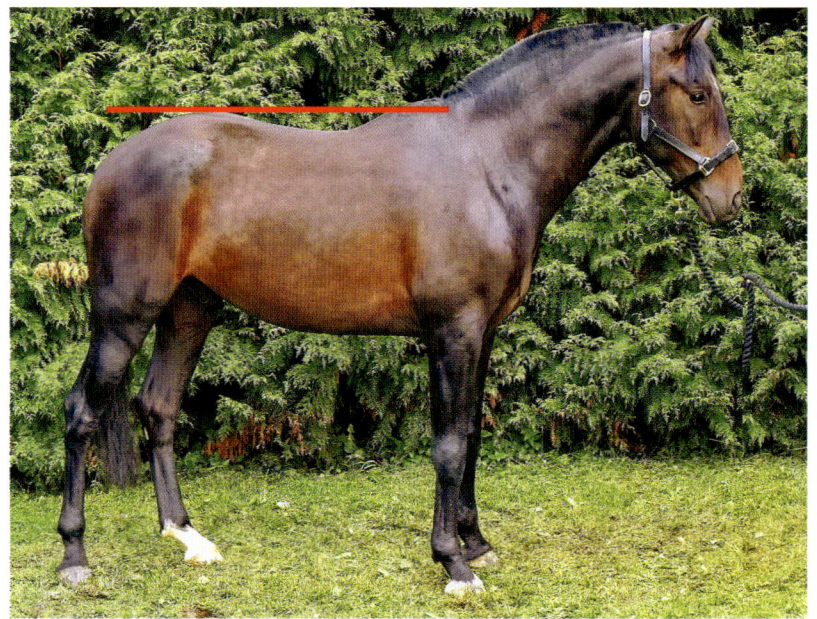

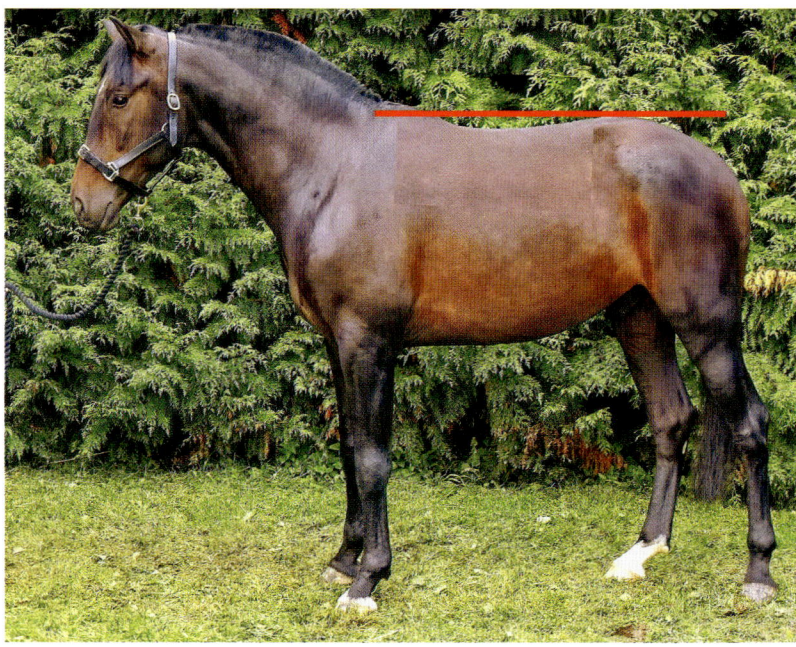

/ 1.6 / The rider's weight causes a very slight habitual dip in the horse's back (top) as compared to his natural conformation (bottom). ▶

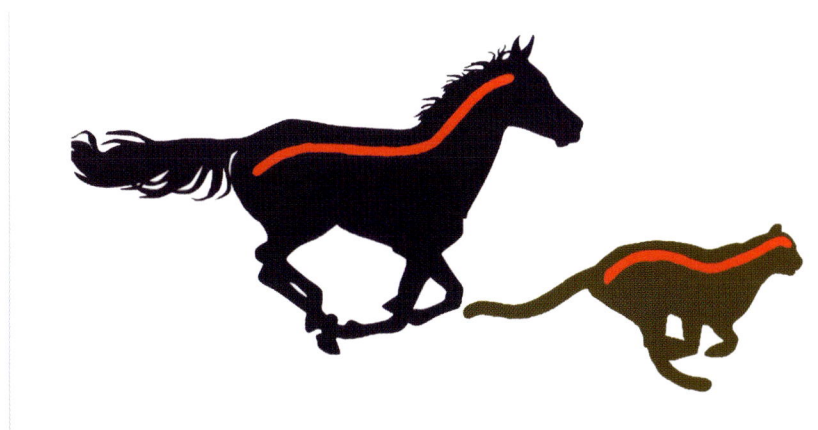

◀ / 1.7 / *The vertebrate's spine must flex freely if the animal is to be athletic, balanced, and agile. A rigid spine limits power; a flexible spine increases power.*

Once this misunderstanding has been cleared up, and we have explained that we only want to run around the countryside a bit, the horse usually becomes less hysterical about our presence on his back and his education can begin. But although his mind is calmed and you can now ride the young horse, his core muscles are far from strong enough—just by sitting there you put a critical dip in the middle of his back (figs. 1.5 and 1.6).

Without anyone really thinking about it, this back posture sets in as a habit, right from the start. Although modest and not obvious with a saddle in the way, the spine is a precision instrument and even a slight downward curve is enough to limit the mobility of this very clever and sensitive mechanism. Changes here affect the whole horse, inside and out, in both body and mind. Just like in other vertebrates, the horse's back must be able to flex, twist, and stretch to be fully athletic (fig. 1.7). When it can't, we see a shadow of what this amazing creature can really do.

\\\ Muhammad Ali ///

Muhammad Ali

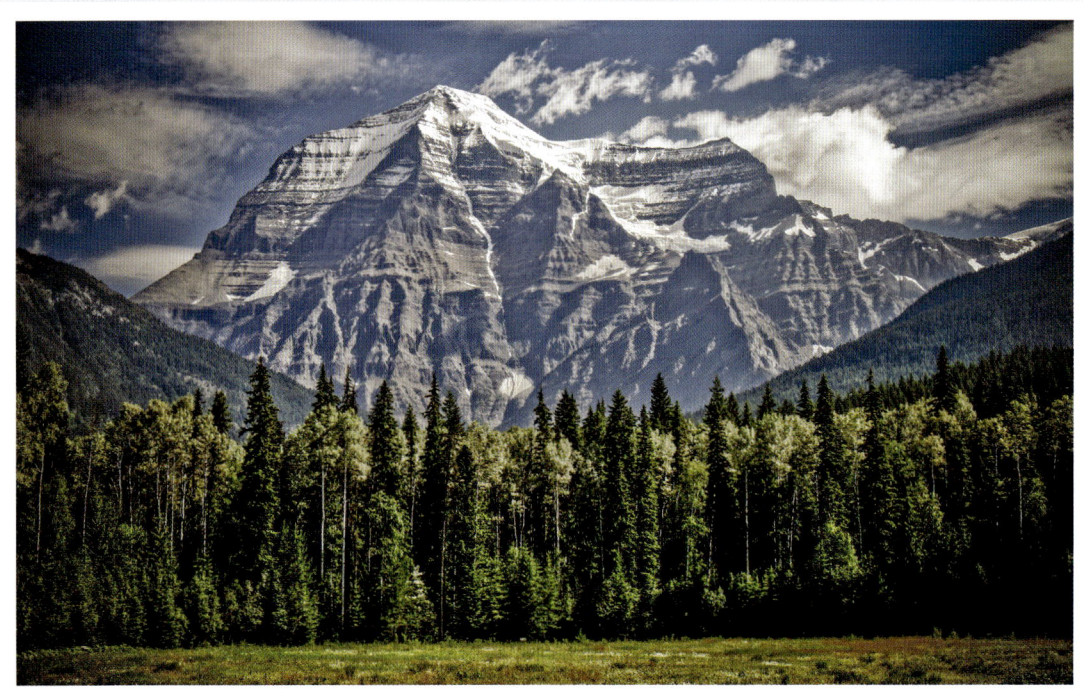

*"It isn't the mountain ahead
to climb that wears you down,
it is the pebble in your shoe."*

❝

Valegro in the Field, Dumbo in the Arena

With just a small dip in the back, a good horse will look, ride, and feel like a bad one. It is not his choice or fault. Unfortunately, it doesn't take much to lock away the magic from a mechanism that is covered in nerve endings. Even a small pinch causes the horse to avoid using part of his back—not by choice, but instinct.

When the horse lacks strength in his core muscles, his back can no longer be "round" (no matter how the horse's head is positioned), and he becomes literally "hollow" under the saddle. When this happens, you may find yourself managing a whole herd of riding problems that are, in fact, not as unrelated as they may appear.

This, in part, explains why whatever breed and name is written in the horse's passport, poor spinal posture leaves even spectacularly talented horses without lightness and grace under saddle. Without a fully functional chassis, your Rolls Royce will drive like an old Renault.

As Helle Katrine Kleven, physiotherapist and author of *Physical Therapy for Horses*, states, "The goal of training is to strengthen the horse's body so that he can carry us with his carrying muscles." From a rider's point of view, if the horse's own body cannot produce lightness and grace easily, you are left struggling with a collection of circular training issues that never go away, no matter what you do. You can also be sure that if for some reason you are not comfortable riding a horse, it is no picnic for him either. Unfortunately, this private and discreet creature is not always easy to read, even if he is having physical trouble, because he is instinctively convinced that his life depends upon "putting on a brave face."

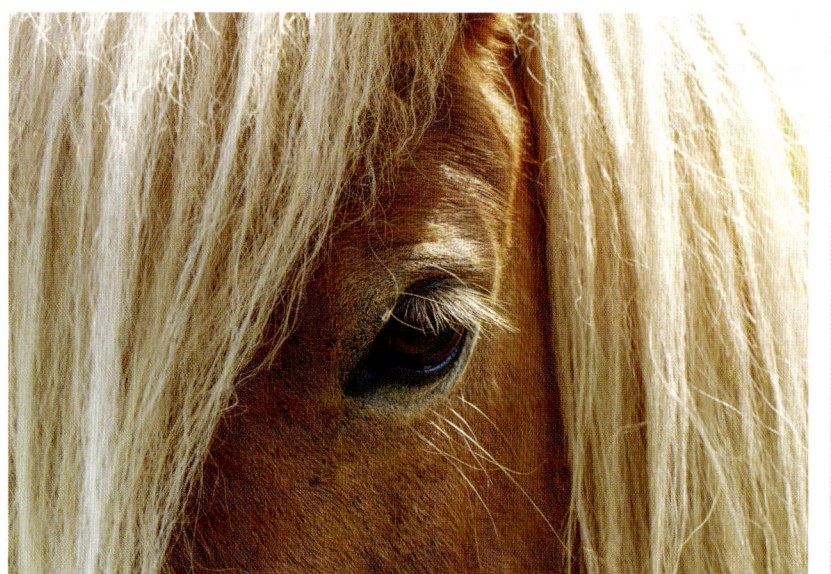

/ 1.8 / Horses "speak" with "silent words." They are sensitive, emotional, and very, very discreet. ▶

The Silent Language of the Herbivore

Our herbivore friends certainly feel emotion as fully as we do, but their communication style is very different from that of our usual mammalian companions. Most mammals we interact with, such as cats, dogs, and family members, are pack creatures—when in difficulty, we cry for help and protection. We are "programmed" to express discomfort loudly until assistance arrives. But the horse has no such instinct. In fact, it is the opposite.

Our "herbie's" predators evolved to spot the opposite of fast food. They preferred easy-to-catch prey. Their eyes were tuned to identify the old, young, or lame; the slower the better. The horse evolved to take this into account by developing excellent acting skills. Diligently disguising their difficulties, and acting as if they are ready to gallop at any moment, they take themselves off the menu for the day. Therefore horses have survived the eons by being quiet and pretending that they are fine, especially when they are not (fig. 1.8). Unfortunately, this has led to a huge and longstanding misunderstanding between human and horse, as we have taken their submission as a sign of acceptance, which is far from the case.

Freely vocal as we are, humans assume there will be a warning when the horse is in pain, a complaint of some kind. Nope. Never. *Jamais.* Sadly, suffering in silence is what horses do. They are world-class at it. But just because they don't scream the house down to express themselves does not mean they aren't communicative. Quite the opposite. With the need to be discreet, they have developed a highly complex and very expressive form of communication that is *physical.*

Showing You in Every Step

In their subtle "tiger-proof" language, horses are real talkers. Their body language is chatting away all the time. Coded in every step are subtle indicators—such as bend, stride length, body angle, ear direction, and even a confident rear—that constantly inform the herd about an individual's well-being and ability to escape if needed (fig. 1.9). This information is crucial for a herd leader to arrange everyone for the best chance of herd survival while mooching across the plains.

Since horses express their strengths and weaknesses through this language of movement, if you look very closely at how they move, they will show you exactly where they feel stiff or weak, allowing you, the "herd leader," to help them exactly where needed.

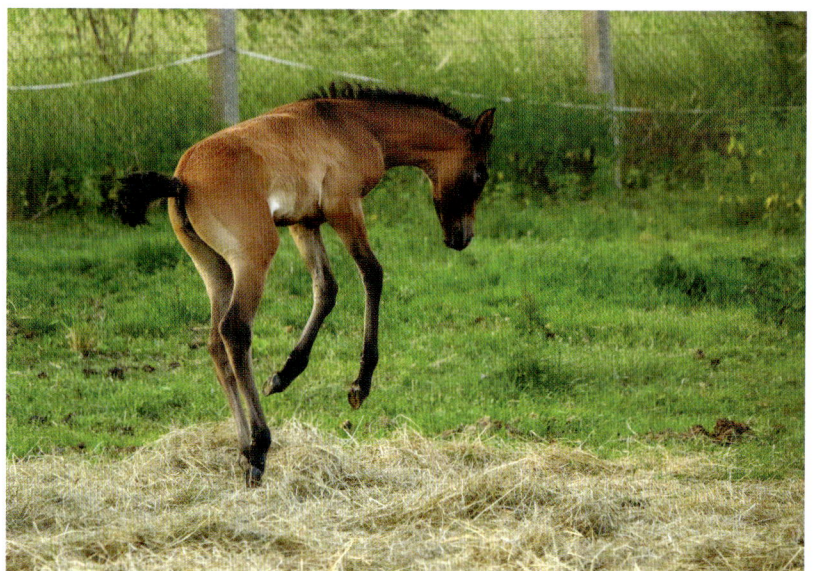

/ 1.9 / *Movement is the horse's language. Wellness is communicated to the herd by displays of agility, as demonstrated by this frolicking foal.* ▶

Riding "Feels"

Riding should be easy, intuitive, and relaxing. But when a horse's back has become habitually hollow or tense it can become a very effective ejector seat. Instead of a gently rocking, wave action that lifts and connects with you, the action of the locked back becomes harder and bigger, throwing you into the air a little—or sometimes a lot.

Despite what you may be told, this type of movement is impossible for a relaxed rider to follow, and it is very important that riders don't blame themselves when they can't sit on their horses for this reason. That makes as much sense as critiquing an automobile driver when his car has a flat tire. With little alternative, riders can find themselves gripping, leaning, and holding on in order to follow a horse's movement. This must not be mistaken for having a "good seat" by a long shot!

\\\ Winston Churchill ///

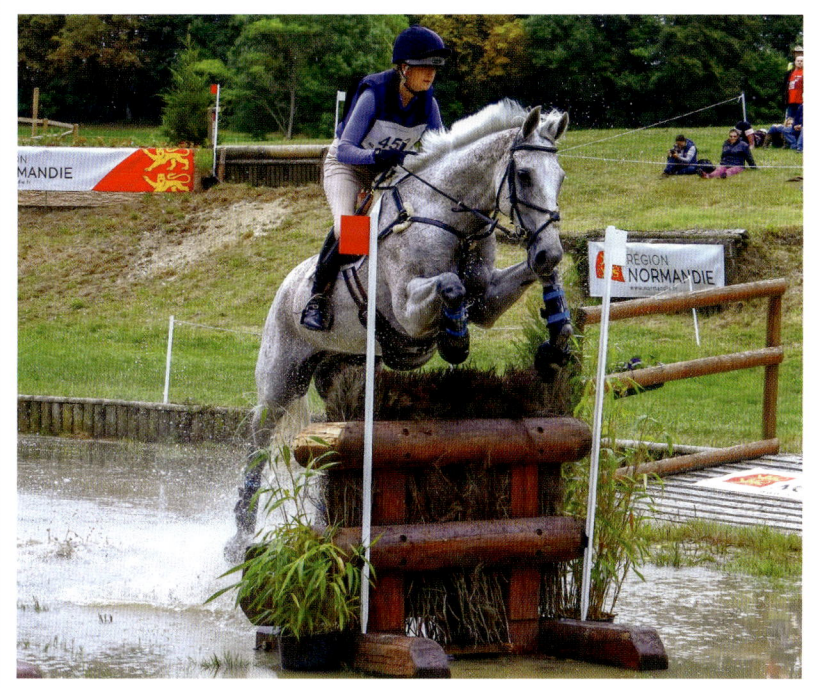

*"When you are on a great horse,
you have the best seat
you will ever have."*

When a horse has a weak core and a hollow back, he will show some typical characteristics that you can *feel* from the saddle:

- An uncomfortable, crooked gait.
- Bad steering.
- Heavy or fussy contact.
- A significant difference between the left and right directions.
- Too slow to go or too hot to stop.
- A high head.
- Lazy, crazy, or grumpy.
- A lack of progress over time.

If a horse is moving in a slightly ungainly way, he is not feeling very athletic or happy, even when he is not displaying any big signs of protest. You can easily end up living with these symptoms, working around them, even physically trying to stop the horse from expressing them by using bits or straps, which considering the cause, isn't fair at all.

Taming the "Snorting Beast"

Humans have developed many methods of training horses over the millennia, each with a different breeding program, skill requirement, and objective born of their demanding times. It is therefore very important to match the method to the breed for which it was conceived. As French dressage master François Robichon de La Guérinière was careful to note, "Others make a point of trying to attain the precision and poise they see in those who have the ability to choose from a great number of horses, those qualities found in only a very small number of horses. This leads to a circumstance in which these imitators of such studies mortify the spirit of a noble horse, and remove from it all of the goodness of temperament Nature has given it."

The two main systems behind European equitation traditions, the Classical School and the Military School, use methods that had no need for concern for the horse's core, which is why it is never mentioned in classic texts.

The Classical School plays with the highest possible quality of equitation (fig. 1.10). From Ancient Greece to the Renaissance Royal Courts, the Classical School is that of dancing, prancing, and precision. For centuries royal stud farms carefully selected only the best stallions for their beauty and agility. The Spanish Riding School,

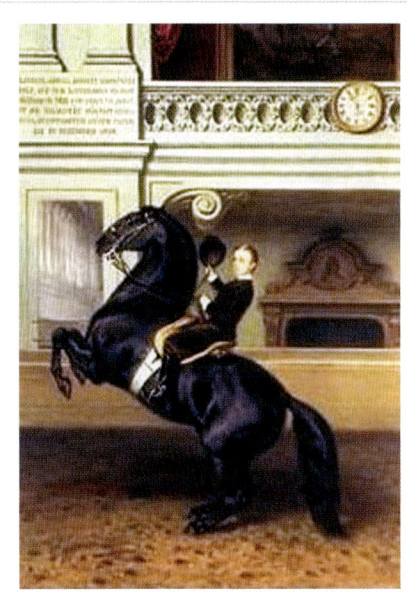
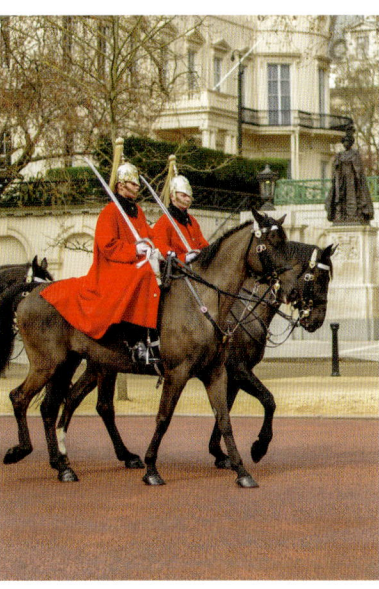

◀ / 1.10 / *Renaissance royalty practiced the purest form of equitation under the aegis of the Classical School while carefully selecting equine athletes (left).*

◀ / 1.11 / *The Military School bred a stable, solid, and useful horse (right).*

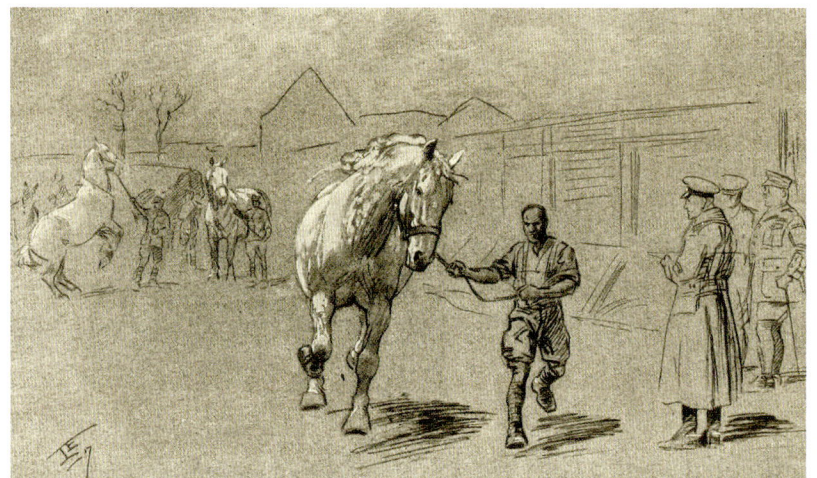

/ 1.12 / The strong and calm military-bred horse was trained quickly and purposefully, using equipment to channel his body into performing a job. ▶

for example, selects as few as three young Lipizzaner stallions, from hundreds, each year. This is one method of keeping standards high. In this case it also ensures the first and most effective training tool becomes selecting only horses that naturally find self-carriage easy; thus the horses have a strong core and healthy back from the start.

The Military School is very different. Forged in harsher times with clear requirements, the warhorse needed to be tough, easy to handle, and able to pull a carriage in the morning and a cannon in the afternoon. European cavalry horse breeders deliberately crossed the "hot" and fast Thoroughbred horse with native, heavier, and stronger "cold-blooded" breeds to create a horse with a balance of these traits. This is the "Warmblood" we see today (figs. 1.11, 1.12, and 1.13).

Military training can be a one-size-fits-all system by default. With millions of horses needed and little time to waste, training methods tended toward equipment to position the horse's posture.

Unfortunately, the military tradition of physical and mental "submission," and reliance on straps, lever bits, whips, and spurs, continues today, even though we all have plenty of time and should know better.

Although it may seem that by using equipment to put a horse's head, neck, or back in a certain place, we are "showing" him where to put it, this simply doesn't work. Many of us will admit having tried it at one time or another, and when we removed the restricting rein or bit, we had the same problem as before. Any manner of restraining the horse's head in an effort to shape and "mold" the outside of the horse will fail, because his head does what the back is doing—not the other way around (fig. 1.14). "For a horse to be in balance," stated Portuguese master Nuno Oliveira, "it has to be relaxed, which is why it must not be compressed."

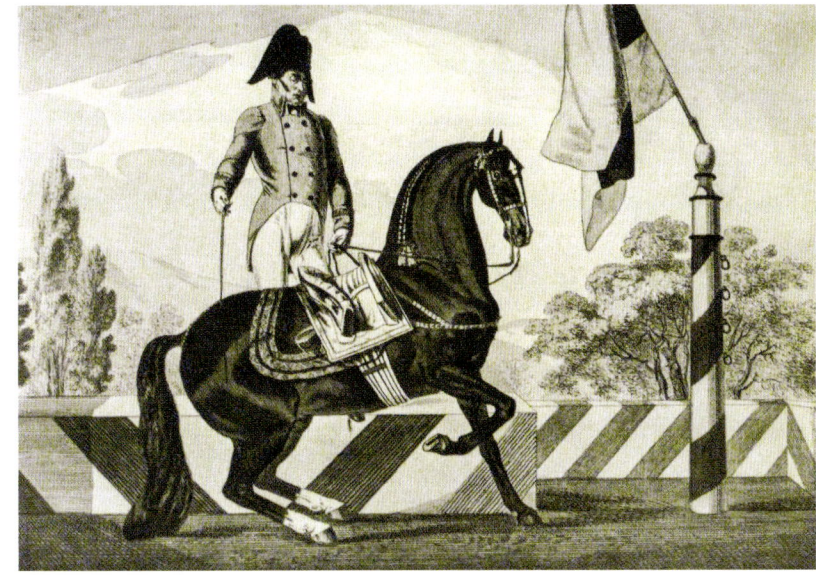

◄ / *1.13* / *The sensitive and elegant classically bred "dancing" horse responds best to subtlety, touch, and intuition.*

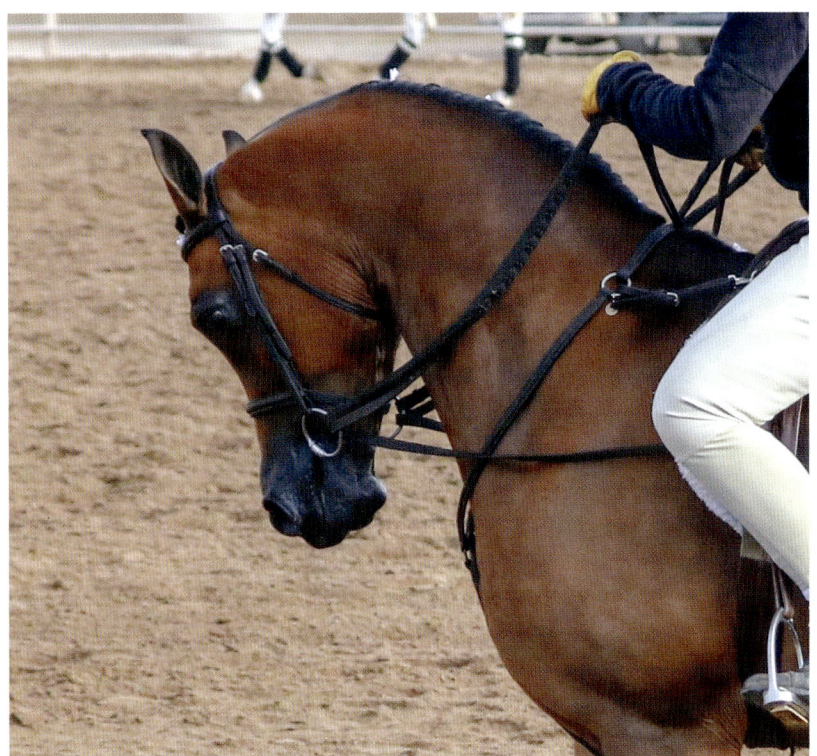

/ 1.14 / "Shaping" the outside of the horse with restrictive equipment gives temporary control but at the price of almost everything else. ▶

Restrictive equipment is not a cure; it is a cage. Granted, the horse does occasionally snort like a beast, and this may have caused our ancestors to treat him as such, but again, *these days we know better*. We now know that deep down horses are just like us: Athletes can only blossom when they have been released.

Releasing the Natural Athlete

The most beautiful of athletic performances are the ones that show a natural fluidity. Fortunately, Mother Nature's "signature" is already in the horse's core, and that magic I mentioned at the beginning of this book is there, in every horse, just waiting to be awoken. The horse's core can turn him into a dancing machine.

The vertebrate design is a masterpiece. It has speed, strength, agility, and the template scales from big to small, from mice to moose. As time has shown, the equine version is a world-beater of sure-footedness and speed. This is not a luxury or rarity for the species. All horses are equipped, as standard, with the best traction control and ABS the world has ever seen, and when faced with an oncoming puddle while at gallop, auto-braking, too. This is Nature's original 4 x 4.

So rather than artificially shaping a horse into a cookie-cutter outline, you can get a better and happier athlete simply by developing the natural gifts already within him. Following the designer's blueprint, of course, you can align, release, and train a horse from the *inside* so the magic of his core transforms him on the *outside*. "Proceed so that

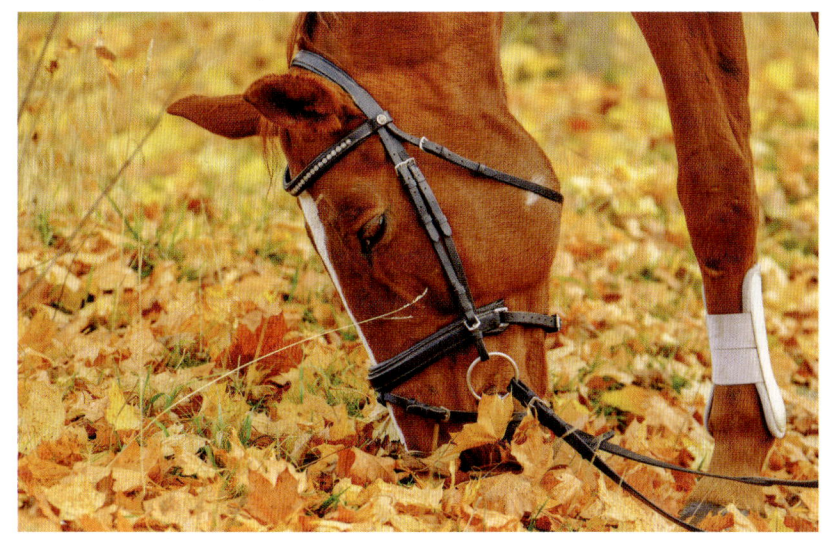

◀ / 1.15 / Dr. Peter Stadler, Professor of Equine Surgery at the Veterinary University of Hanover, Germany, says: "By preserving and promoting its natural abilities, the horse will be brought into a shape and carriage that allows full development of his strength."

the horse finds himself moving willingly into the exercise, and not by force," Oliveira reminds us.

Deliberately developing the body's abilities from within is the philosophy behind many Eastern traditions of human physical development. These often focus less upon rushing around madly, which is how we break things, but instead sensibly favor a low-impact conditioning of the body that listens to the athlete throughout the training process. Developing the horse's core resonates very well with this approach. The core's main defense is to shield itself with muscle tension, which is why it is virtually impossible to improve the core while doing any fast or concussive work. This means it is a really good idea to begin the horse's training session with low-impact exercises. And there is one specific way we can help the horse that is very unique to his physiology: We can help him by *releasing his core.*

The Core Release

The horse's spine is long and bendy—like a Slinky, as I mentioned earlier. This means that it can easily become slightly "kinked" in its groove, and when that happens it stops moving and the horse's core stops functioning.

A *Core Release* is something we have all felt as riders. It happens when the horse's spine naturally aligns deep within his body and drops into its correct "groove." The horse's back immediately rounds and the head and neck drop into a Long-and-Low Outline (see p. 130), "hanging" weightlessly in front of you. This is an important effect and something we will be using in many of the exercises that follow.

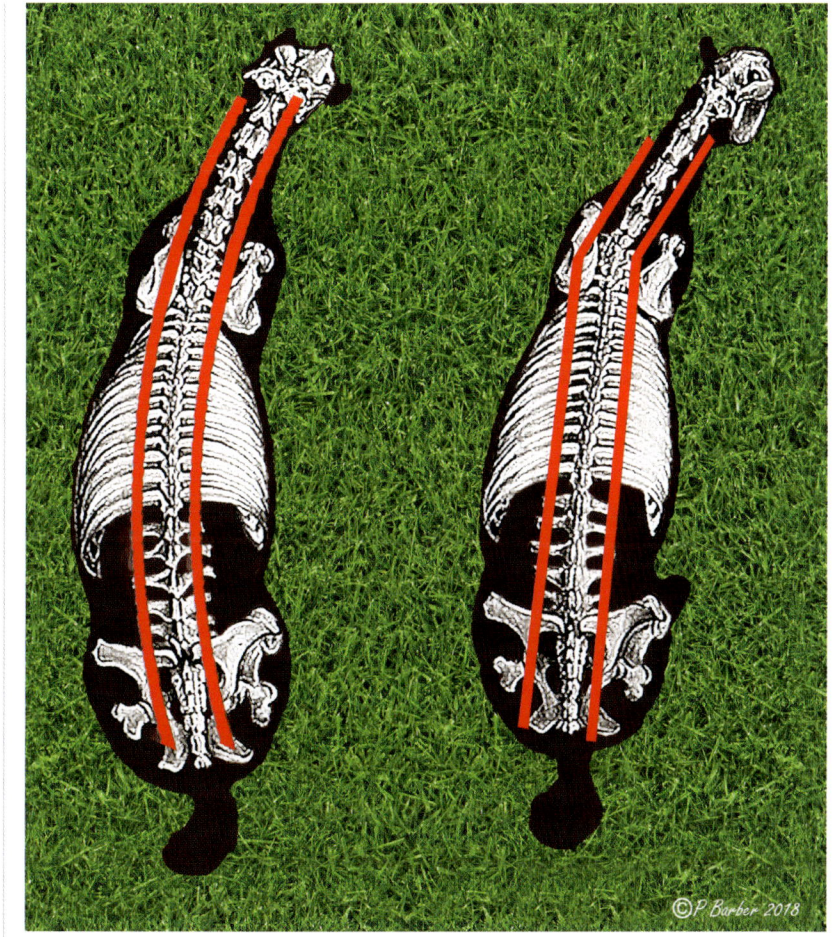

◄ / **1.16** / *The horse's spine shown on the right is stuck because it is "kinked." If we help the horse to align the spine as a uniform curve, as shown on the left, his core will immediately release and fall into place.*

If the spine is blocked in any way, the delicate "lifting parts" in the horse lock in order to become "stabilizers" instead, thus stiffening the horse's body. Once blocked in the core, a horse that really ought to sit a little more on his hocks will instead plunge onto the forehand—and traditional training techniques won't help. This can be entirely avoided, however, by performing simple exercises to deliberately release the core before anything more energetic is attempted.

This really helps the horse begin a schooling session feeling loose and agile, and it prevents tension before even making the first trot step.

The Horse's Generous Spirit Is Our Greatest Gift

Fortunately our horses' minds are as magical as their bodies. As herd members, they have wonderful instincts for cooperation and teamwork, and that is the only reason they allow us to ride them. If there remains any doubt about the generosity of this species, you need only witness what happens when a horse wants to get rid of his rider: It is fast and hard, with the rider losing any and all illusion of control in under 0.06 seconds. This is rare, thankfully, yet only because the horse is one of the world's most magnanimous and trusting spirits.

It is very important to hold this in mind during the training of a horse, particularly as his reactions may sometimes seem distinctly uncooperative! His perspective is different from ours and being "difficult" is not in his nature. There is always a reason when he shows negativity, and he deserves the benefit of the doubt, 100 percent of the time.

There are three main reasons a horse will not try to do as we ask:

/1/ **HE CAN'T.** When the horse is not strong enough to perform something, or if he feels it may hurt his body somehow, he will try to avoid it. This is natural and to be entirely forgiven, even if we end up on the ground because of it. The jump, the corner, the arena, even the saddle can be triggers of negative anticipation, tension, or pain that will be followed by some form of self-preservation.

\\\ James Herriot ///

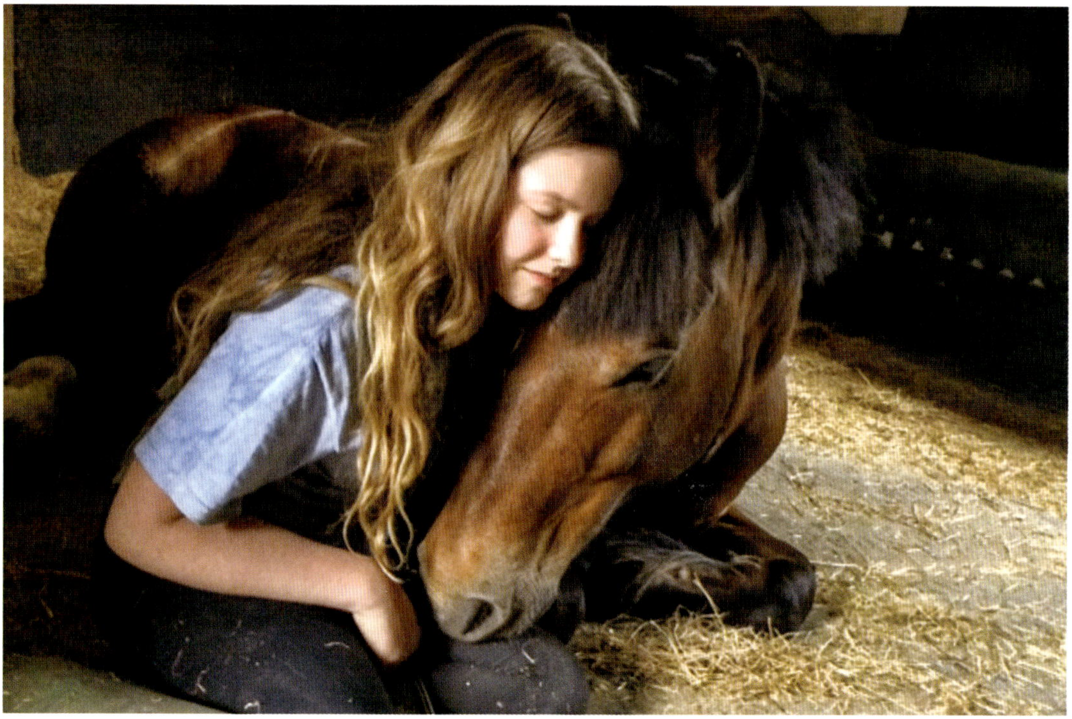

James Herriot

"I hope to make people realise
how totally helpless animals are,
how dependent on us, trusting
as a child must that we will be kind
and take care of their needs."

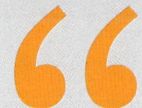

Alois Podhajsky

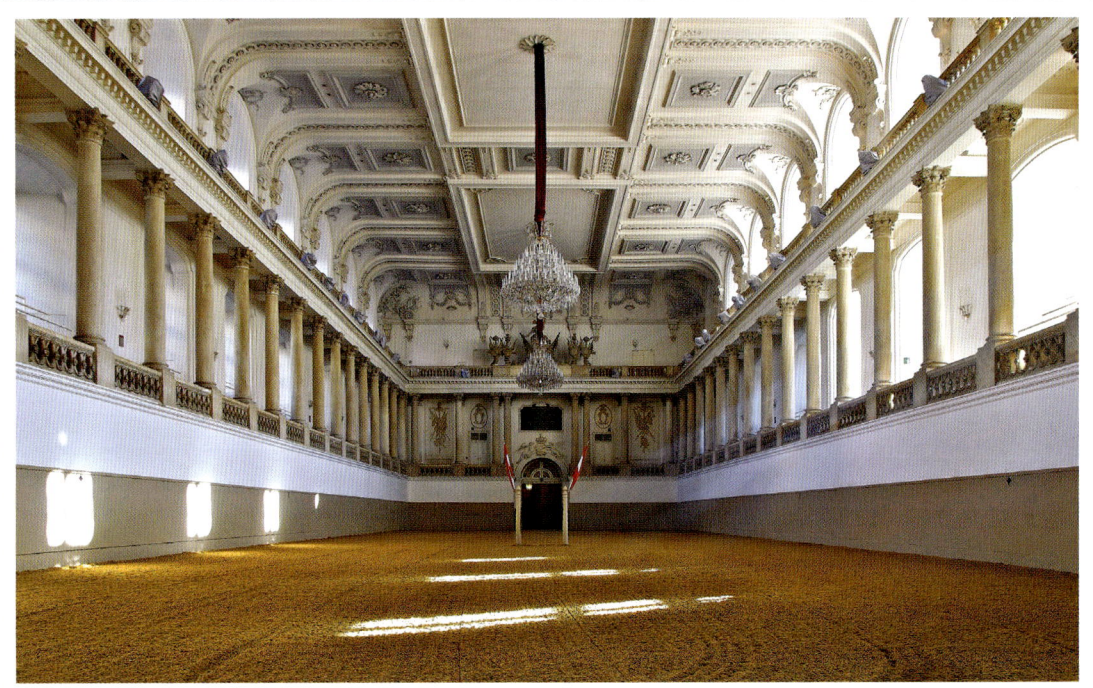

*"Whenever difficulties appear,
the rider must ask himself does the horse
not want to execute my demands
or does he not understand what I want,
or is he physically unable to carry them out?
The rider's conscience must find the answer."*

/2/ HE DOESN'T UNDERSTAND OR IS FRIGHTENED.

There is no programming or software installation with *Equus*. This herbivore is, and always will be, semi-wild and highly instinctive with a world view designed around grass, carrots, and foals. Our requests, therefore, can be very confusing to them.

/3/ BOTH ANSWER 1 AND ANSWER 2. Often, the horse can't do it or understand what you want, and/or is frightened, to boot. This makes progress virtually impossible.

Our horses are never being "difficult"—they are actually telling us something. The horse can only try to respond to the aids based upon his life experience, which can be limited, so being ridden can become a huge guessing game of pressures, noises, and memories that can easily overwhelm him. The trouble is, horses aren't very good at guessing games, and if we forget to offer them clear and straightforward choices, they will always fall back on their instinct, which can easily be mistaken for naughtiness. Frenchman Claude Bourgelat, founder of the world's first equine veterinary school in 1771, said, "In order to be able to execute what is asked, the horse has to understand what the rider wants him to do, so the rider must teach him step by step how to do it."

With such a naturally willing partner, communicating with the horse on his preferred terms will produce the most beautiful results. If you concentrate on helping him to be supple and free rather than obedient, you give him the best chance to connect with you and show you his magic. And then he will jump over the moon for you. ■

\\\ Simon Cocozza ///

Simon Cocozza

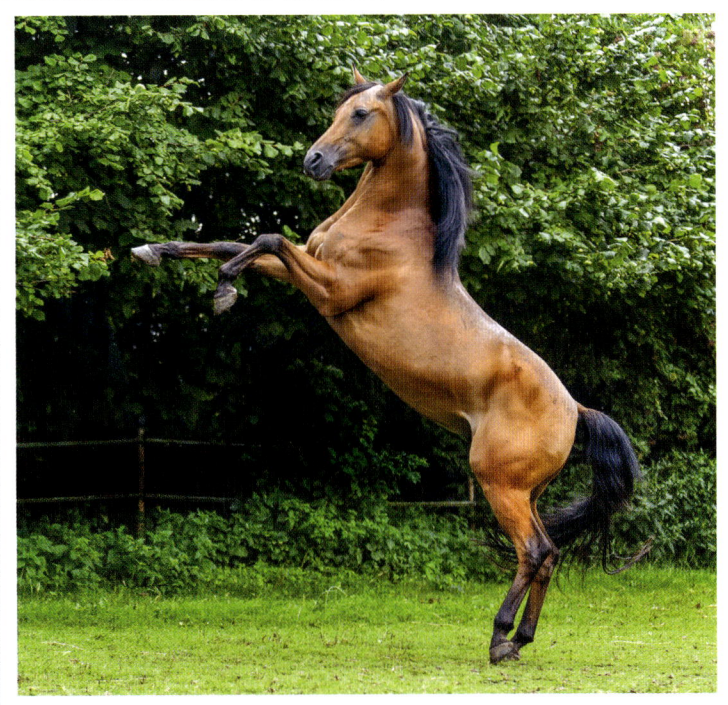

"The horse's core is a maze of muscles, bones, and 'stringy stuff' arranged in a very, very clever way. So clever that this mechanism can launch a 1,000-pound horse into the air from standstill with no warning whatsoever."

2

The Source of the Force in the Horse: The Core

Able to produce such magic, the horse's core is a masterpiece of concept and design. The big muscles on the outside of his body *thrust* the horse forward. The core muscles, on the other hand, play a *lifting* and *carrying* role, sending the body upward and maintaining posture from the inside. When working correctly, these two systems give the horse that wonderful feeling of "roundness" in the back that only comes when the whole body is moving correctly (fig. 2.1).

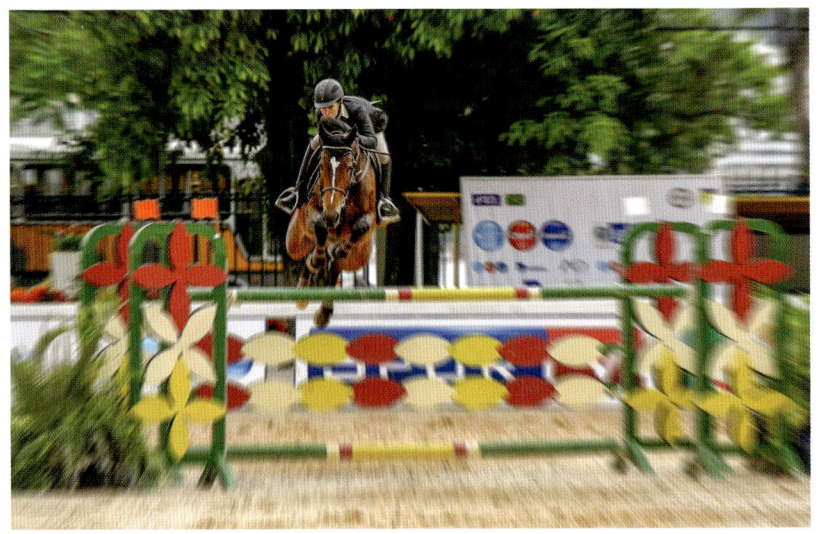

/ 2.1 / *Defying gravity: A jumper getting the balance right between his thrusting and lifting muscles.* ▶

The horse's core is a maze of muscles, bones, and "stringy stuff" arranged in a very, very clever way. So clever that this mechanism can launch a 1000-pound horse into the air from a standstill with no warning whatsoever. This is its party piece, after all, and shows how well the system works.

The horse's core has many jobs:

- Controls posture.
- Creates suspension and elevation.
- Connects all the big body parts.
- Controls balance.
- Manages the center of gravity.
- Powers the "roundness" of the back.
- Dictates jump height and bascule.
- Creates the alignment needed for straightness.

"A strong core will improve your technique, strength, and stamina, and complement everything you do," notes Susan Trainor, classical ballet dancer and choreographer.

The horse's body has three main sections that are controlled by the core (fig. 2.2):

- **Section 1: THE FRONT END**—the shoulders, chest, and neck.
- **Section 2: THE MIDDLE**—the back and belly.
- **Section 3: THE REAR END**—the "lower" back, hindquarters, and hind legs.

Each large section of the horse's body contains its own special function that centers around its section of the spine (fig. 2.3). Each of these spinal sections moves differently, does a different job,

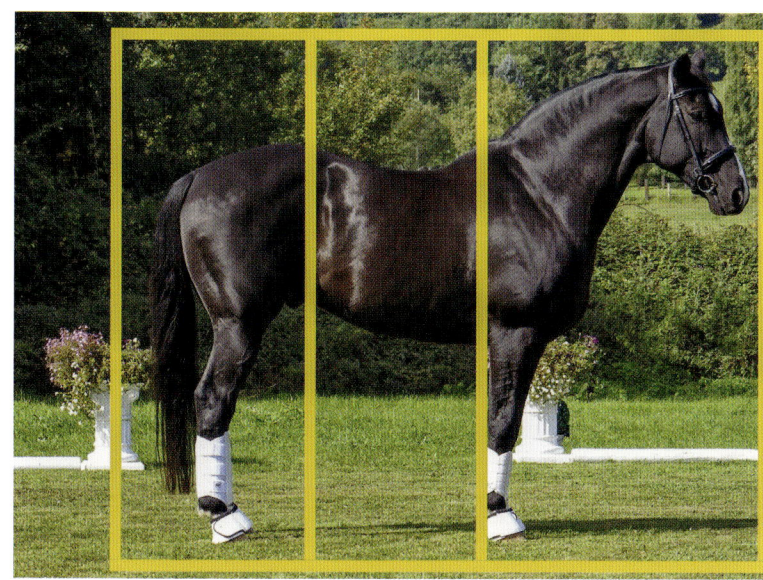

◂ / 2.2 / *The horse can be divided into three main body sections—front, middle, and rear—as each one has a different job, moves differently, and needs a different type of exercise.*

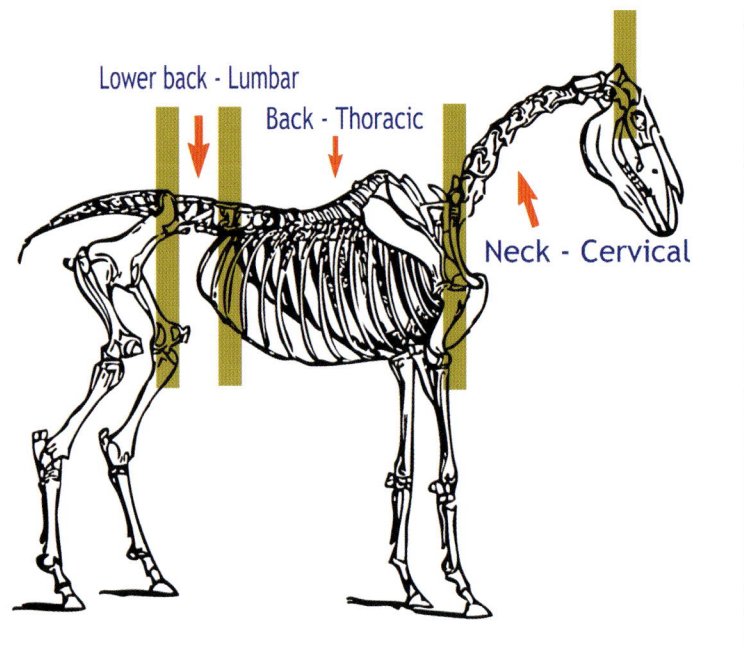

/ 2.3 / *The spine is where movement begins. Each of the spine's sections—cervical, thoracic, and lumbar—requires specific types of bend and arrangements of steps to condition them.* ▶

and needs different conditioning sequences to bring full range of motion to the full length of the horse.

/1/ **THE FRONT END** is the neck, chest and shoulders. It contains the cervical spinal vertebrae and the thoracic sling mechanism, which is made up of the muscles that attach the horse's front legs to his body, and when contracted, raise the rib cage. This section primarily gives the horse suspension and steering (fig. 2.4).

The cervical vertebrae in the horse's neck are very mobile and can move in all three directions: up and down (vertical); left and right (lateral); and twist (rotational), making this part of the horse *super* "bendy"!

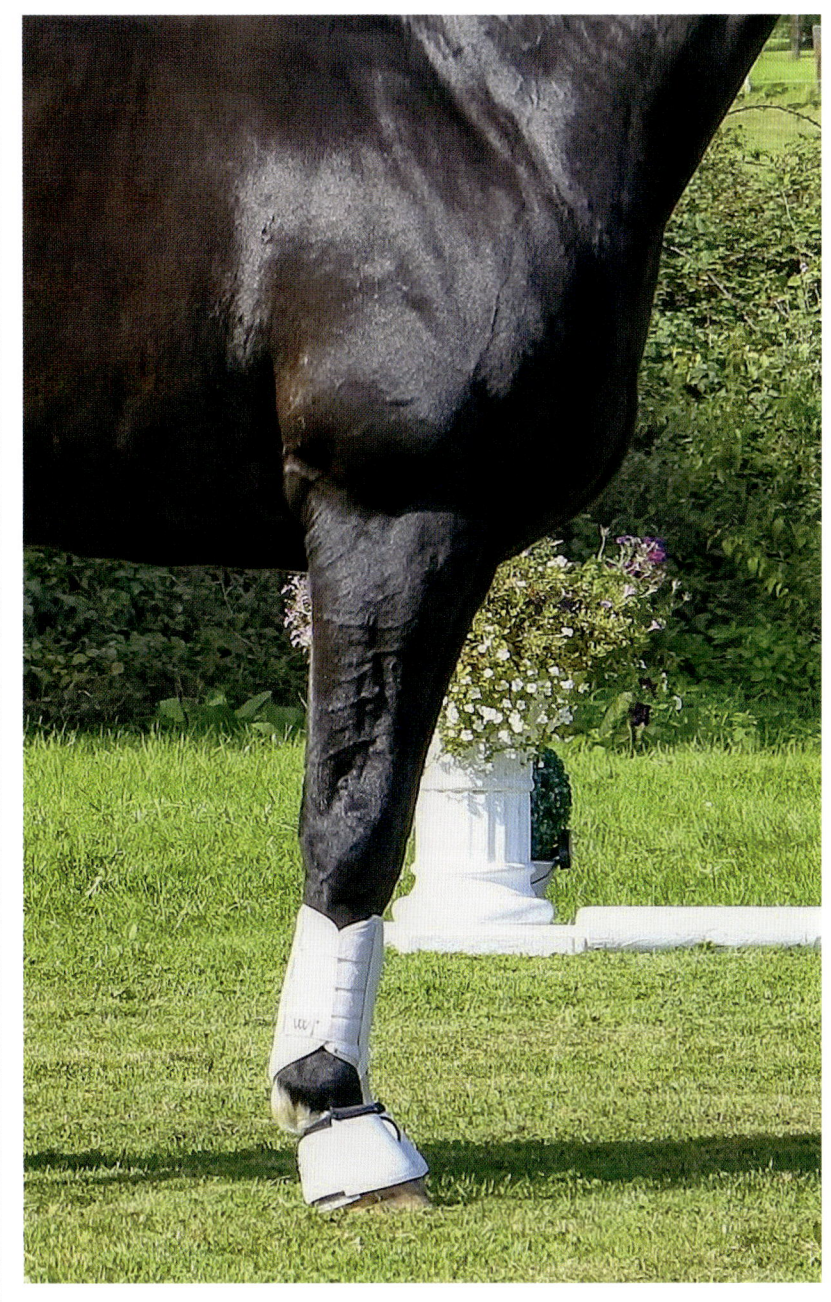

◄ / 2.4 / *The horse's shoulder contains both power and agility. When conditioned and toned correctly, the shoulder gives suspension and power steering to the horse's front end.*

/2/ **THE MIDDLE** is made up of the back and rib cage, which are attached to the thoracic spinal vertebrae. This section of the horse has the least movement in the spine, but it must perform the biggest job: It has to carry all the horse's internal organs, as well as a saddle and a rider, so it has to be very strong to work well (fig. 2.5). The thoracic vertebrae can only bend laterally, and this vital "bendy bus" effect allows a horse with a good core to wrap himself around corners from his middle, giving him the ability to stay straight and in balance under all circumstances.

/3/ **THE REAR END** is the horse's lower back, pelvis, and the huge muscles in the horse's bum. Thrust and balance lie in this very powerful body section (fig. 2.6). When functioning as designed, the vertebrae in the lumbar section of the spine can both "round"

/ 2.5 / *The saddle contact area. The horse's back has to carry the spine, the gut, and the rider, making it a stress point.* ▶

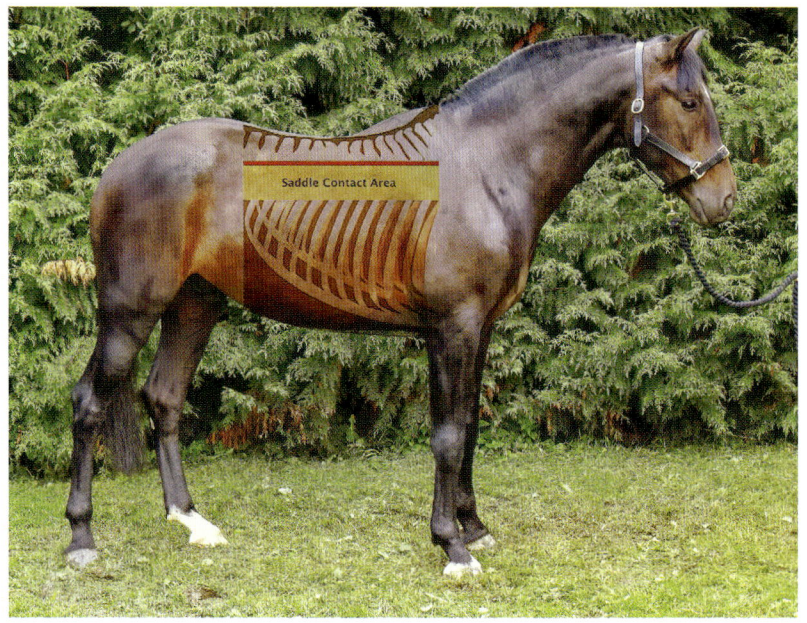

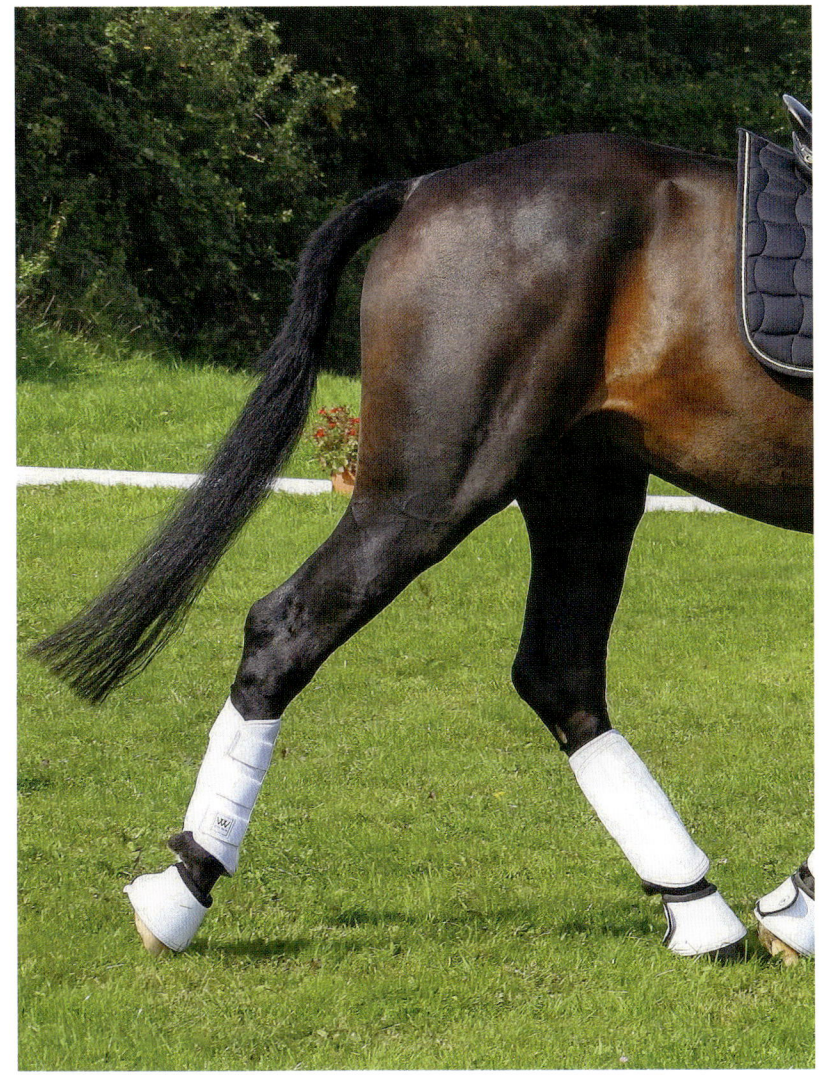

◀ / **2.6** / *Full thrust: The rear end is not only the horse's main engine but a critical component in his overall body balance.*

vertically and "twist" rotationally. This gives the horse the ability to both lower and swing his rear end at the same time. This is also called the *Pelvic Tilt*, and it is one of the horse's three *Core Powers*, which I will discuss next (see p. 44).

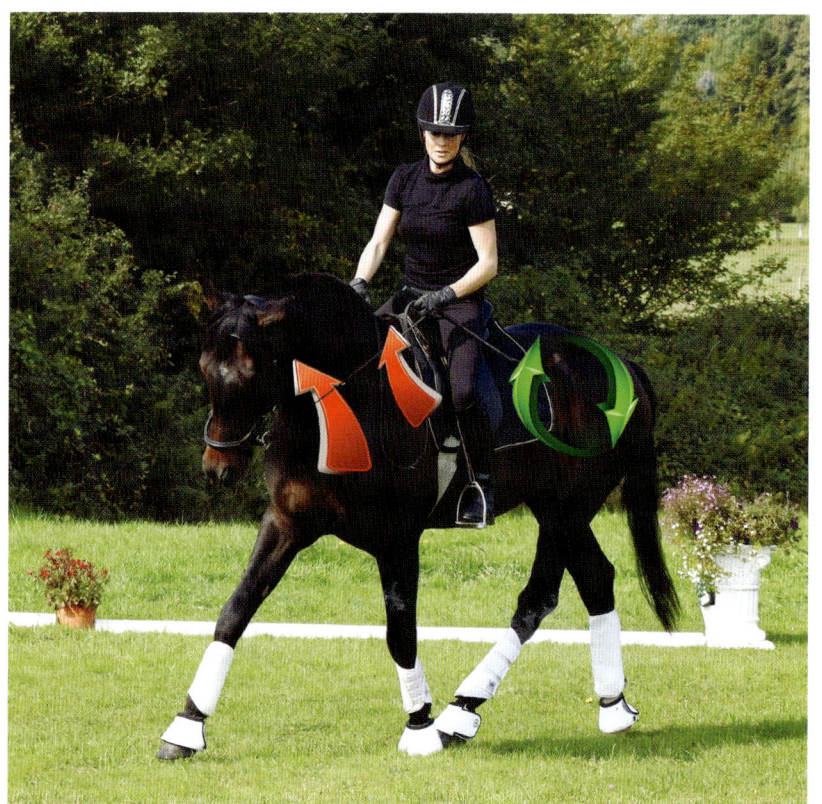

/ 2.7 / Each of the three main body sections has its own special "Core Power" that lifts and shapes the horse's posture. ▶

The Power of Three Will Set You Free

There is another important set of three as relates to the horse in motion. I call these the *Core Powers*. Nature gave the core some truly amazing skills. To be able to gallop off without lifting the head, to "sit down" and *go* without skidding, and to be able to jump in any direction—the horse has all the skills needed for evading the many predators he has faced over time. It is these Core Powers that give the horse his incredible agility, his prance…and also his ability to dance (fig. 2.7).

Core Power 1: The Thoracic Lift

"Strength without agility is a mere mass," wrote Fernando Pessoa, a Portuguese philosopher.

The front of the horse is an athletic marvel. It produces multi-directional power and reflexes so fast that it can put a hoof on your foot in the blink of an eye. The shoulder gives the horse's front end a full range of forward, sideways, and vertical directions of movement, and when working with its fellow Core Powers—Nuchal Lift and Pelvic Tilt—the whole body can defy gravity. The active part of the front end is called the *thoracic sling*, so named because the thoracic

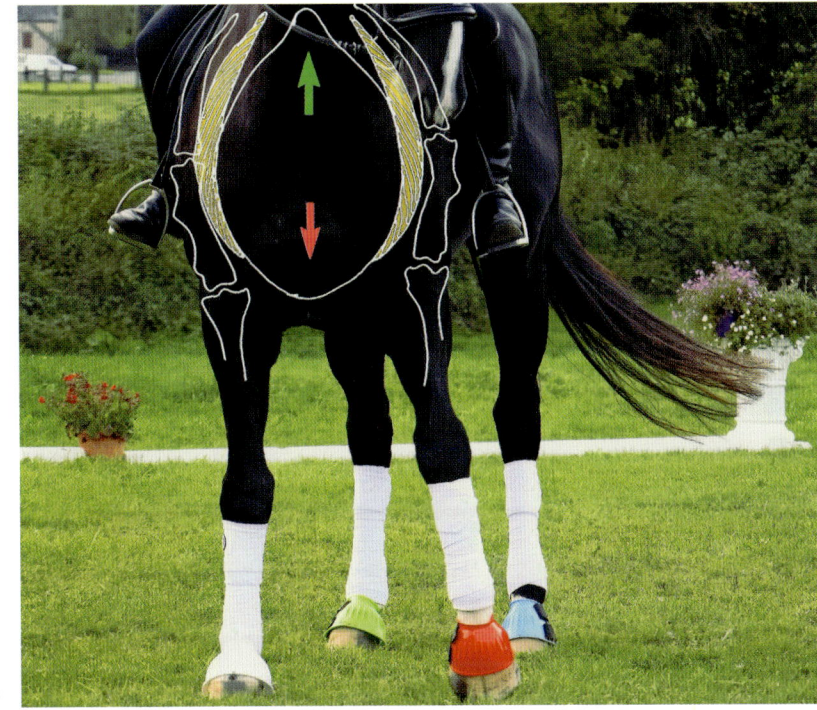

◀ / 2.8 / *The powerful thoracic sling enables the horse's chest to be raised and lowered between his shoulders, creating a powerful, natural spring.*

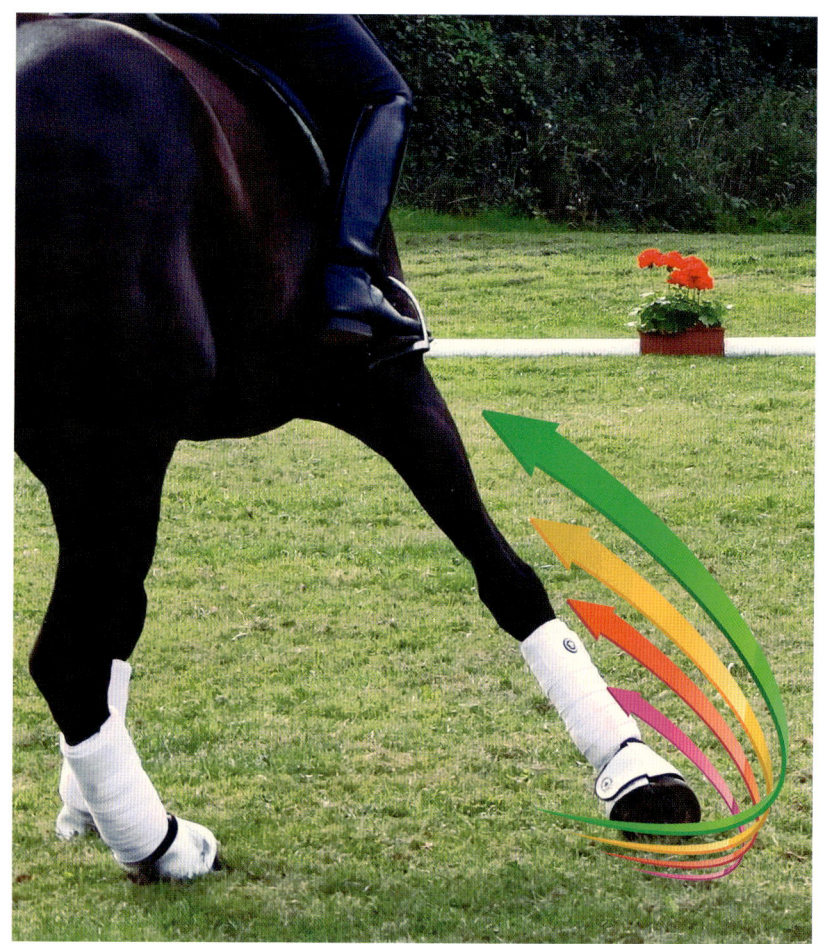

/ 2.9 / *Power, reach, and control: The horse's front legs are attached to his chest by super strong and stretchy muscles alone. The lack of a clavicle bone gives the front limbs a very large range of motion.* ▶

section of the body (rib cage) is literally "slung" between the front legs (fig. 2.8). This "floating" design gives the front legs a very large and wide range of motion only limited by the condition of the muscles that power it (fig. 2.9).

The thoracic sling creates "lift"—the Core Power called *Thoracic Lift*—giving the horse:

- The ability to raise his front end.
- A rebalancing of body weight toward the rear.
- Power and agility in the front legs.
- Easier turning and stopping ability.

As mentioned, the horse's front legs are not attached to his torso by bone, as are ours. They are held on only by muscles that make the thoracic sling function, the mightiest of which is the *serratus ventralis* (fig. 2.10). These powerful muscles get shorter and longer to lift and lower the horse's chest, acting as both shock absorbers and pistons. The Thoracic Lift is strong stuff and very effective when working well. As said at Hippika Gymnasia, the Roman Cavalry School: "The front legs push up, the hind legs propel" (fig. 2.11).

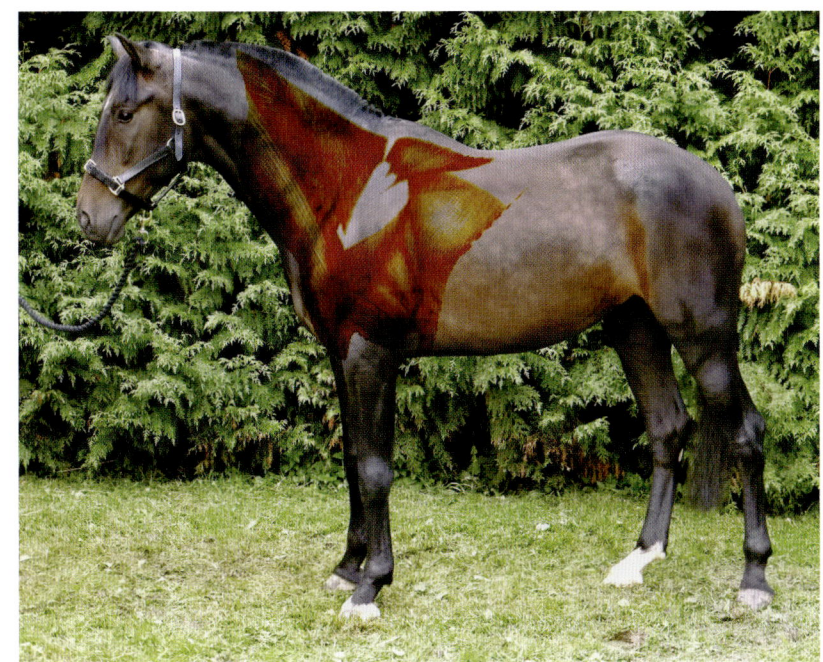

◂ / 2.10 / *The powerful thoracic sling muscles must carry, raise, and lift the horse's chest. This is the Core Power called Thoracic Lift.*

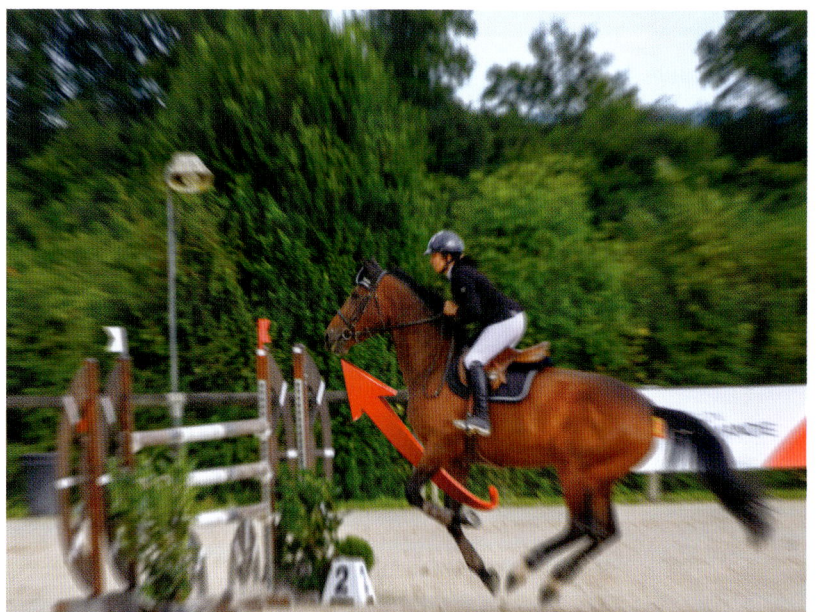

/ 2.11 / Unable to bend at the knees and push off the ground, the jumping horse's thoracic sling alone propels the horse's front end into the air. ▶

In an untrained or immature horse the muscles of the thoracic sling are relaxed and long, leaving the heavy chest sitting at the lowest point between the shoulders and making the horse feel like he is running downhill. When you ask the horse to practice front-end agility a little more intensively and regularly, it sufficiently "wakes up" the "sleepy" Thoracic Lift that is waiting inside, giving the animal a more naturally expressive and maneuverable front end.

Core Power 2: The Nuchal Lift

The horse is designed to eat grass for 18 hours a day yet to be ready to move at light speed and escape from something at any moment. For this to be possible, Nature installed a clever mechanism called the *Nuchal Lift*—the second Core Power.

When the horse finds himself in the path of an oncoming predator, having to raise the head before fleeing would cost precious microseconds. The nuchal ligament keeps the spine "round" even when the horse's head is down, thus keeping the body in balance and the back end ready to engage. It is a truly magnificent feat of engineering and an excellent natural way to help stretch your horse in a way that feels instinctive to him. "The nuchal ligament pulls and straightens the spinous processes of the withers as soon as the horse drops his head," explains physiotherapist and author of *Physical Therapy for Horses* Helle Katrine Kleven. "This arches the back up."

As the Nuchal Lift encourages a vertical flexion along the horse's spine, it is an excellent training tool to deliberately "round" a horse's back very simply and naturally, by working the head and neck longer and lower. This is a vital key in the overall process of releasing and

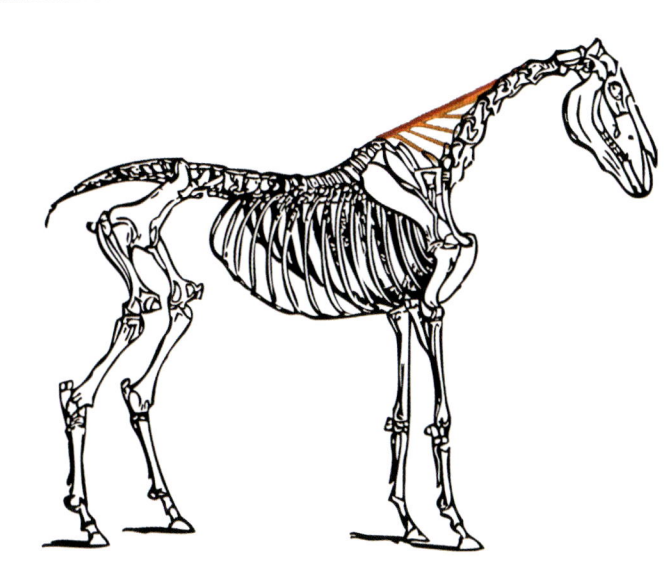

◄ */ 2.12 /* *The nuchal ligament is a clever mechanism that keeps the horse's body perfectly balanced when in the vulnerable grazing position, affording* Equus *a very quick getaway if a threat is sensed.*

conditioning the horse's core, and as such the Nuchal Lift has two core exercises dedicated to its development, which we learn in Part Two: the Core Release Volte (p. 156) and Forward, Down, and Out (p. 186).

The Nuchal Lift gives the horse:

- A rounding of the back.
- A lighter front end.
- Balanced stability.
- Alignment of the spine.

When the nuchal ligament lifts the horse's spine, the area under the saddle is raised to the correct alignment and the core can release. This also makes the saddle immediately move less, making the horse's movement much easier to follow for the rider. As this Core Power becomes more active, simply giving the horse a long rein will allow him to naturally reach a very comfortable grazing posture while in light forward motion.

Core Power 3: The Pelvic Tilt

"Core strength has the ability to produce force with respect to core stability, which is the ability to control the force we produce," explains physical therapist and professional martial artist Susan Westlake.

From the biodynamic view, you ideally want the horse to "sit" a little when you are aboard (fig. 2.13). This is old news, of course, as we all know the thrusting power of a horse comes from the big rear end

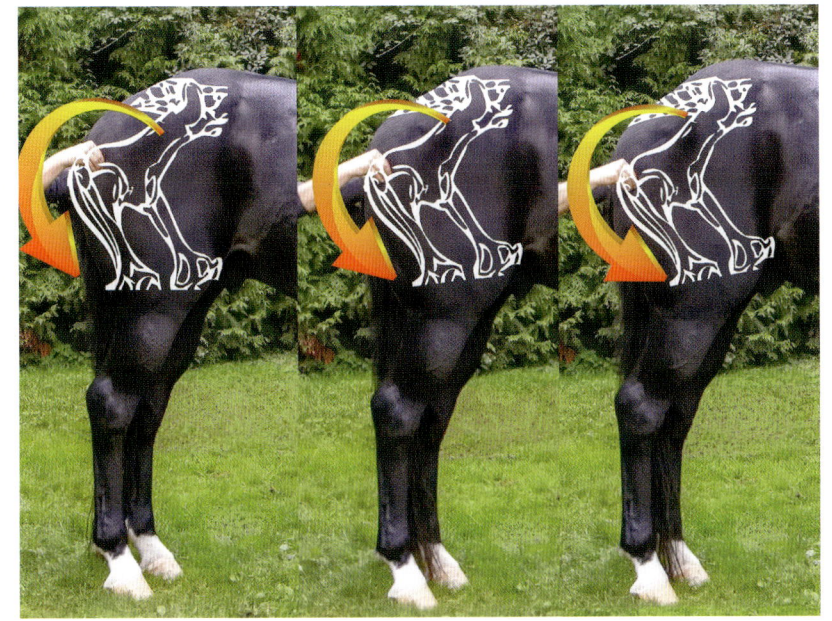

◄ / 2.13 / *The Pelvic Tilt: By artificially stimulating the hindquarters, we can see the horse tuck his pelvis under a little. This is a postural change that transforms a horse's balance while in motion.*

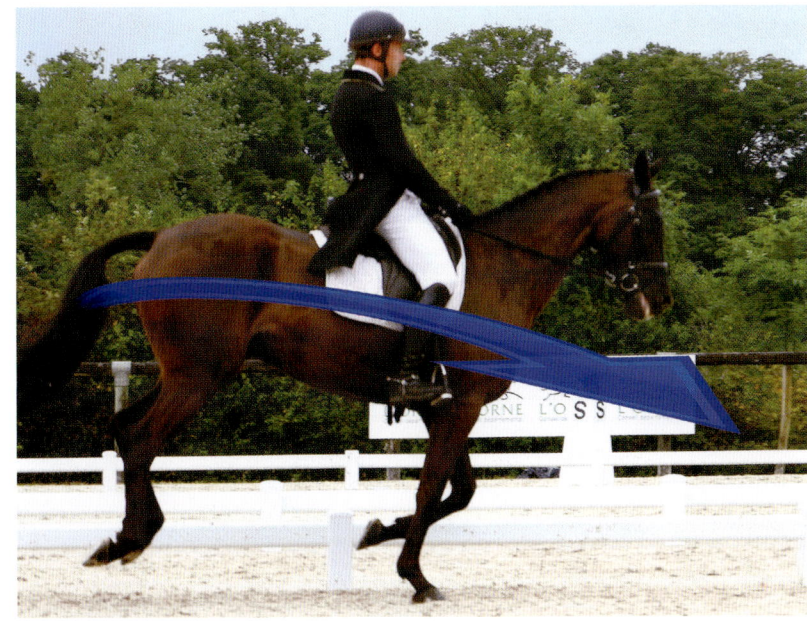

◄ / 2.14 / *When the horse is unable to "sit" into the stride, the thrust sends him forward and downward.*

behind us, but power is not always a good thing. If the angles of thrust are not correct due to poor posture, a horse can all too easily run himself unstoppably onto the forehand (fig. 2.14). To avoid this imbalance, nature installed a lower-back mechanism that can both flex vertically and rotate, acting like the "gearbox" of the horse, channeling the power just where it is needed by putting the hind limbs further under the body (fig. 2.15).

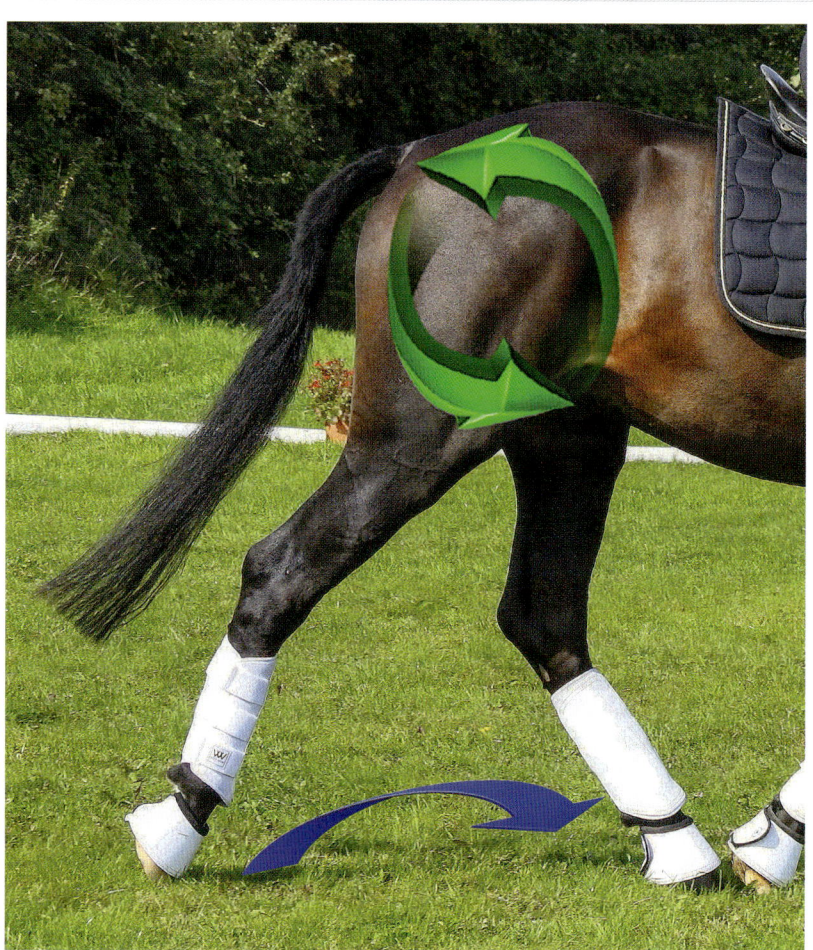

/ 2.15 / The Pelvic Tilt Core Power comes from the horse's lumbar spine and rotates the pelvis, allowing the hind legs to step farther under the body. ▶

■■ Core Conditioning for Horses

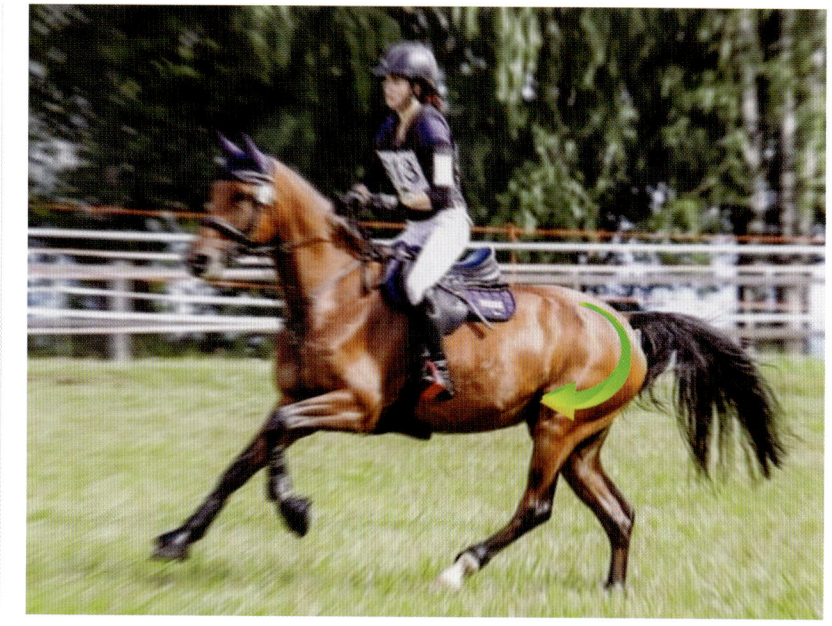

◄ / 2.16 / *A horse that has good hind limb engagement will be more balanced and easier to ride.*

When working in conjunction with the other Core Powers of Thoracic and Nuchal Lifts, the Pelvic Tilt can correctly send all the thrust from behind in an upward, as well as forward, direction. The result is a balanced, uphill stride (fig. 2.16). As dressage master Dr. Gustav Steinbrecht wrote in his classic *The Gymnasium of the Horse,* "By temporarily bringing the weight of the forehand backward, toward the horse's center of gravity, he is not only able to exert a downward pressure on the thoracic and lumbar spine, as with a lever, but he can also transmit this effect to the hind legs, if he brings them sufficiently underneath the body."

When you can specifically and deliberately train the horse's core to be proficient in all three Core Powers, you give the horse a good chance at becoming as self-balanced and athletic as he can possibly be. However, we must also accept that this kind of power can have a dangerous potential, and that the force in the horse can indeed have a "dark" side.

The Dark Side of the Core

As wonderful as the horse's body is when fully athletic, when a horse's posture is incorrect and he is expected to work under a rider, all that power can push and press things that were not designed to be pushed or pressed (fig. 2.17).

If there are misalignments in the spine during physical demands, they will gradually produce niggles, stiffnesses, and eventually pain in the back. Silently (and entirely forgivably), this will make a horse reluctant to bend or move in any way that utilizes these sensitive areas, and the Core Powers will be used to lock the areas in self-defense. As this generous

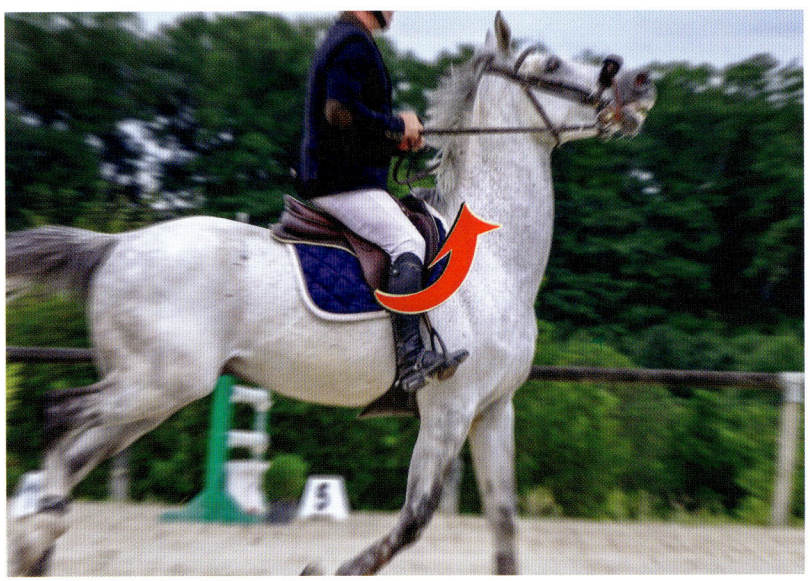

/ 2.17 / *Flexibility gone wrong: All too easily, the horse is asked to perform with poor posture, and his body bends in all the wrong directions.* ▶

\\\ Yoda ///

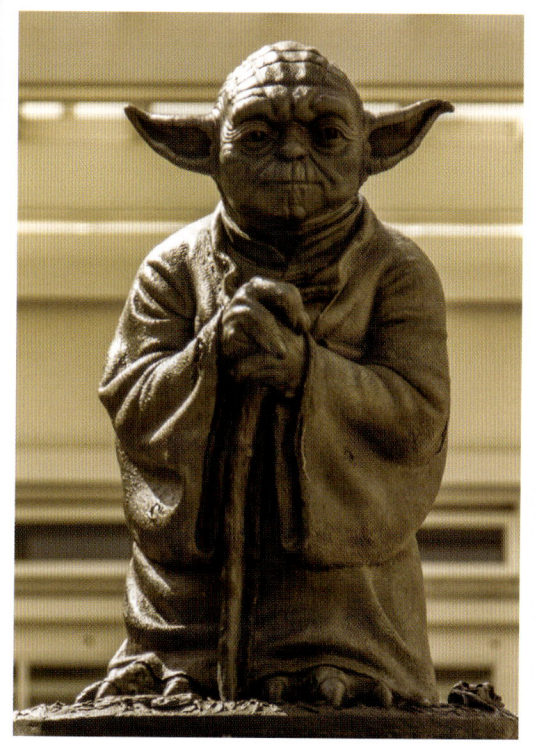

*"The dark side
clouds everything."*

❝

and discreet creature begins down the road of negatively internalizing his power in this way, you don't necessarily know. The horse is still being ridden, still performing, yet silently harboring a growing restriction. To stand a chance of reversing this all-too-common twist of fate, you must be brave enough to look the dark side in the eye.

Why the Horse Can Lose the Force

"What we know is that pain inhibits normal muscular activation [in the horse] and can actually lead to inactivation of normal muscular pathways," says Dr. Sarah Le Jeune, a professor of equine sports medicine in Belgium. "Pain can result from actual injury, excess tension or from imbalanced muscular development."

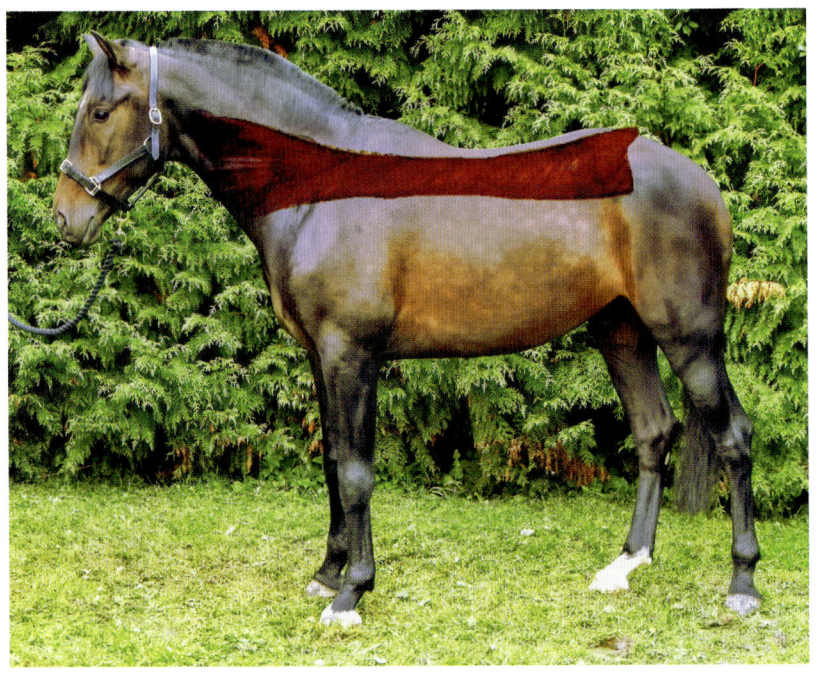

/ 2.18 / The longissimus dorsi is the biggest and most influential back muscle. It connects the horse's front end to his rear end. ▶

In a way it is helpful to see the horse's skeleton as a machine. All machines have very precise mechanisms that work well, if they are set up "just so." It is as true for a horse's body as it is for everything else in your life—if just a little part is stuck, the whole thing becomes a hot mess.

When the horse begins to feel discomfort in his back, his instinctive reaction is to stabilize the area by tensing the two big *longissimus dorsi* muscles. The *longissimus* muscles run the whole length of the horse, from deep in the neck to the pelvis (figs. 2.18 & 2.19). They are immensely strong and after they have been triggered into tension, the horse's back tightens by reflex. We must remember this is not a choice on behalf of the horse—it is part of his instinct, and he simply can't help it.

The dipped—and now tense—back can't bend in any direction, making the horse stiff and hard to

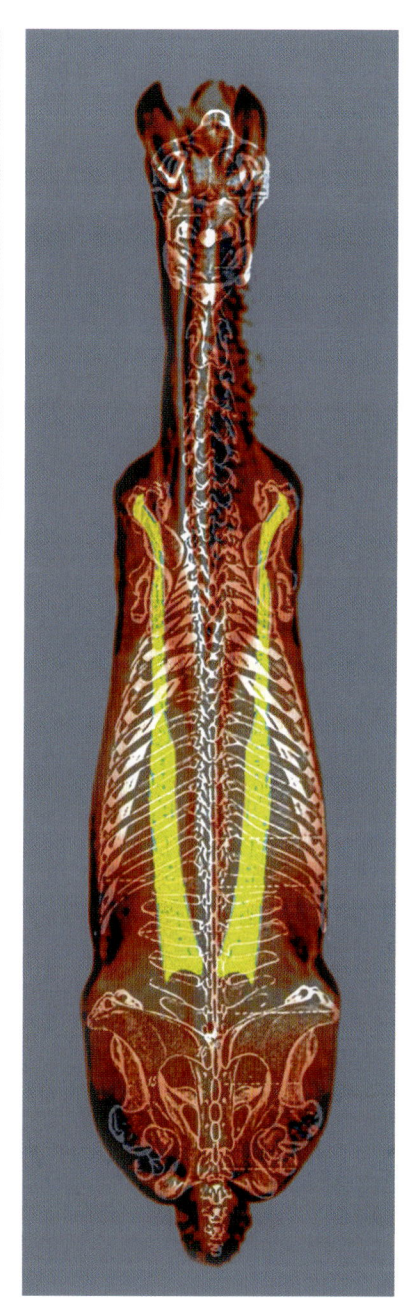

◄ / 2.19 / *The muscles beneath our saddles: There are two* longissimus dorsi, *one either side of the horse's spine. They not only have to do their job moving the horse, they also must directly take our weight.*

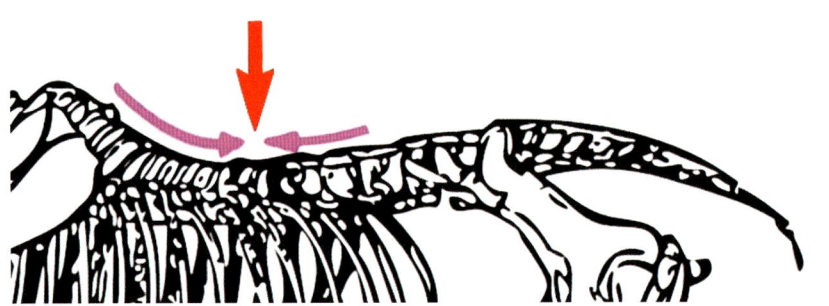

/ 2.20 / A "hollow" back: The most common site of back pain in the horse is the weakest, least supported part of the back. ▶

ride, creating a whole little family of complications that cannot be solved as individual issues, despite appearing to be so. The components of the three Core Powers need complete freedom to work, and when the back becomes tense, they simply lock themselves. The angles they require to do their jobs become unachievable. And, without a supple back, the horse's gaits consequently lose their elegance, amplitude, and ease.

The more energetic the demands are, the more the tension builds. The horse stoically compensates for the loss of his back's movement by using his amazing legs more and more. This unfortunately puts more stress on them than they are designed to accommodate, which only increases as the horse finds ways to keep going over time. This wonderful animal is so resilient that he will even compete, with success, despite having deep muscular and geometrical imbalances. One can only guess what the individual could achieve if unrestricted.

"When doing postmortems on horses," writes Grace Fairburn, a British equine locomotion therapist, "it was found they consistently had asymmetry of the *multifidus* core muscle. Most alarmingly, the study highlighted the under-diagnosis of back pain in athletic horses; when seven were examined, six had severe pathology" (fig. 2.20).

\\\ Stephen R. Covey ///

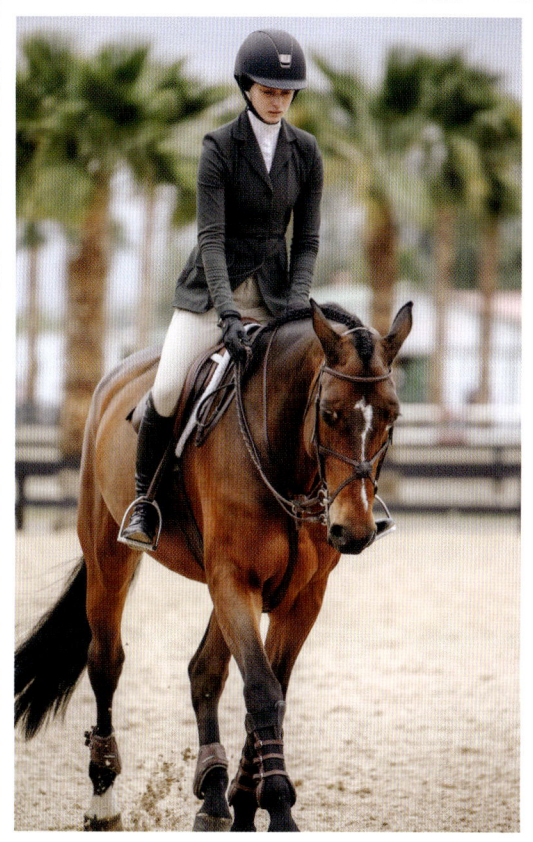

"If the ladder is not leaning against the right wall, every step we take just gets us to the wrong place faster."

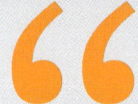

This "syndrome" spirals downward if not corrected. As the horse does not really understand where the pain is coming from and the rider is often viewing the symptoms as training issues, time goes by, and while the horse's core becomes weaker, the wrong muscles get stronger. Gradually, this takes away a horse's sparkle.

The horse's body is such an adaptable design that this "trade" between tension and ability can be tolerated and stabilized in most horses while still allowing a high quality of life. However, for those asked to perform strenuously with poor posture, the tension will continue to build.

Advanced Negative Back Tension

When back issues are only muscular, the horse has room for relaxation and respite between rides. Unfortunately, the design of the horse's spine is not on our side.

/ 2.21 / "Inside" where we sit: Each vertebra has a vertical bone called a spinous process sticking upward. Some are naturally very close together, even without the rider sitting on them. ▶

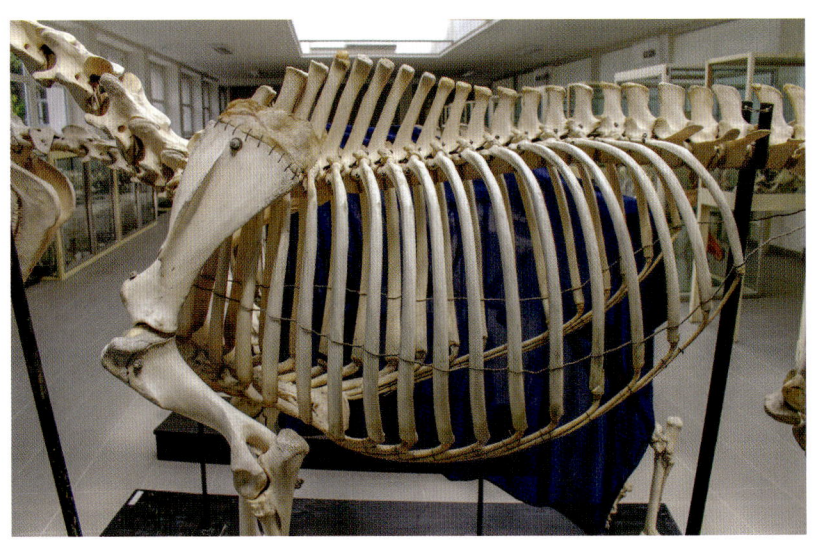

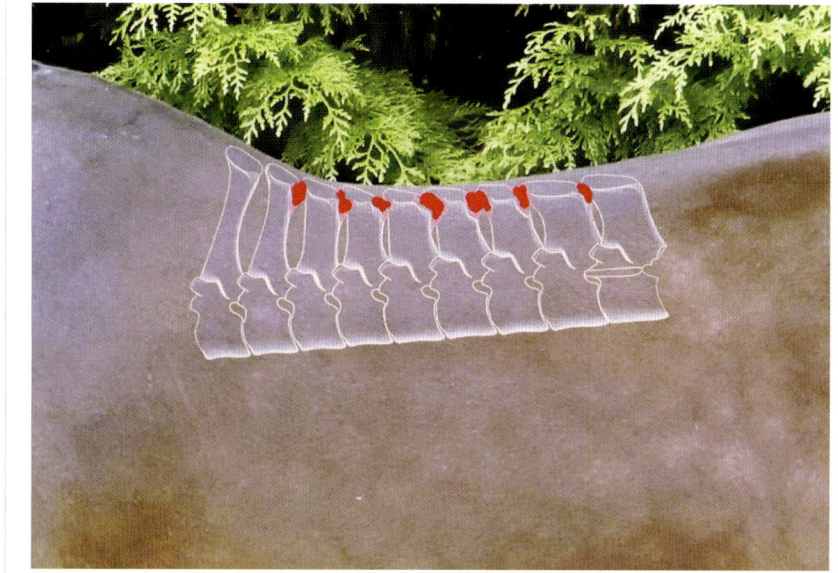

◀ / 2.22 / *If the spinous process "heads" touch—a state called "kissing spine"—the horse's back becomes understandably very painful and tense.*

Each of the back vertebrae has a bone sticking upward called a *spinous process* that can cause a riding horse a lot of problems (fig. 2.21). In some locations the process "heads" are only millimeters apart, so if the horse's back dips farther under the power of a very tense *longissimus* muscle, these heads begin to compress together (fig. 2.22). This is called "kissing spine." (A misnomer if there ever was.) If there is testimony to the patience of the horse, it is that even with this happening in the back, many still allow a rider on board. If this were rare, it would be less distressing.

In German veterinarian Dr. Matilda Holmer's 2005 inaugural dissertation to Munich Veterinary University, she set out to find the prevalence of compressed spinous processes in normal riding horses. She took the pre-sale X-rays of 295 healthy horses to see how the average horse's back copes with our demands.

"For this purpose X-rays of the spines from 295 younger and older horses were evaluated, from which the clinical examination showed no sign of an existing back disorder; however, the X-rays were made in connection with pre-purchase examination," she wrote. "Of the 295 examined horses, there were only 25 horses (8.5 percent) that had no pathological findings on their spine… 270 horses (91.5 percent) all had pathological findings on at least one vertebra, 51 percent on several."

When the *longissimus* muscle begins to spasm, the force of compression is so high it can even "kink" the spine (fig. 2.23).

The better our technology gets, the clearer these problems become. Thanks to advanced scanning, we can now track the progress of previously overlooked deep inflammation in standing horses to see the effect of training as an ongoing process (fig. 2.24). This new data proves that horses' back issues are somewhat of an epidemic, tragically being expertly hidden by the "victims."

The military-type principles behind back problems such as I've described have much to answer for. The concept of using restrictive

/ 2.23 / When advanced back tension persists, the vertebrae themselves can be forced out of alignment. This is called spondylosis. ▶

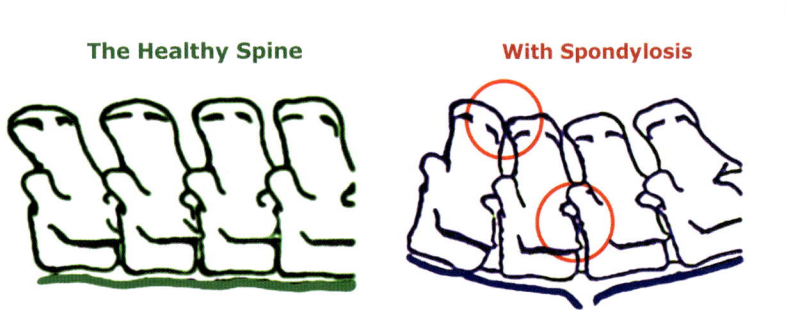

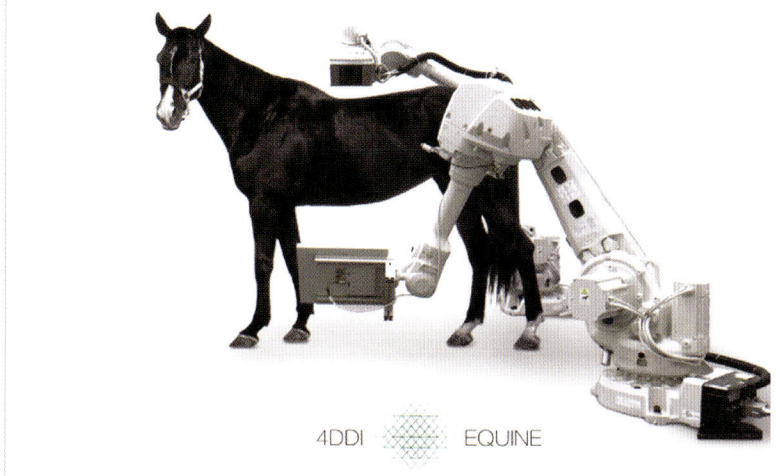

◀ / 2.24 / *Technology like that of the Equimagine™ Helios Four Dimensional Digital Imaging CT Scanner (4DDI) allows us to now see deep within the horse as part of his healthcare, allowing inflammation or pain sites to be detected early and injury prevented.*

equipment while driving ever more forward is hurting horses' backs too often. Our horses are our friends, and we want to help them live pain-free, as well as perform well with us as their partners. In this spirit we can and should always look for ways to not only make their job easier but also to help them through any difficulty they may meet in training in a proactive manner only. Prevention is a crucial part of the change we see ahead.

When considering options for preventive and corrective work to help our horse's backs become stronger, we can draw inspiration and experience from the human practices we have grown up trusting. This is possible because horses and humans are made of the same stuff, feel in the same way, and most intriguingly, need exactly the same kind of help. ∎

\\\ Barry H Gillespie ///

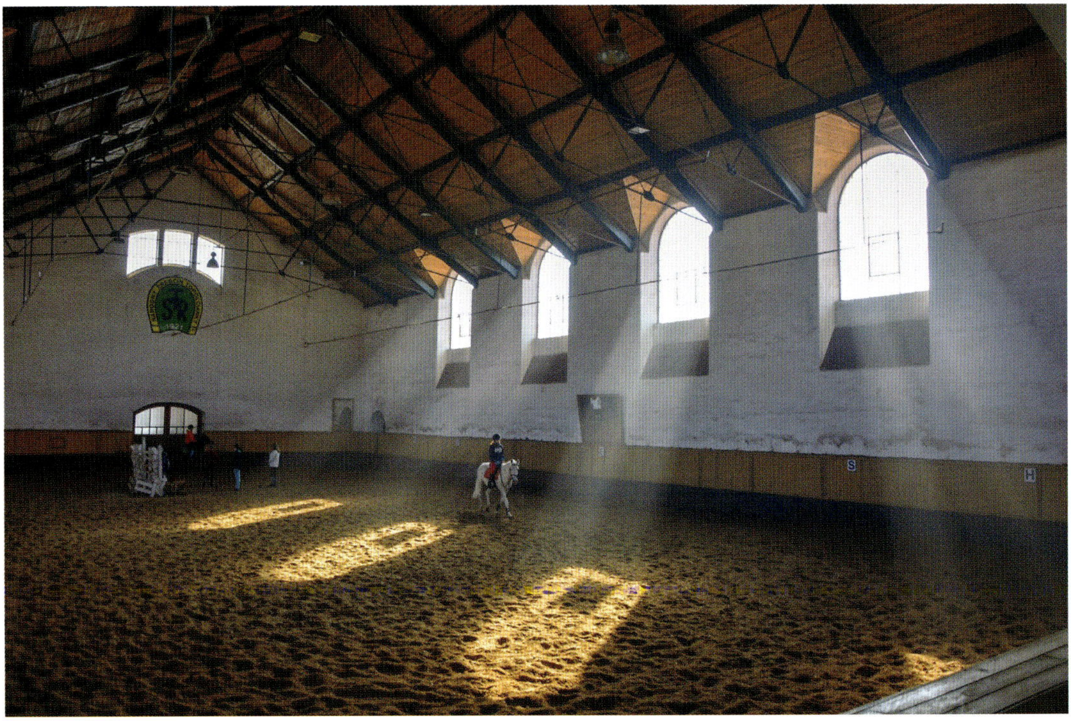

Barry H Gillespie

"The path isn't a straight line, it's a spiral. You continually come back to things you thought you understood and see deeper truths."

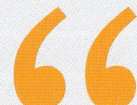

3

Horses Are People, Too

Humans and horses are currently trained very, very differently. Perhaps our propensity to scream has, over the millennia, inspired those with sensitive hearing to develop ethical ways to improve the human physical condition as pleasantly as possible. The squeakiest wheel gets the oil.

In spite of the horse's flying hooves and bluster, he is as much flesh and blood as we are, so rather than train horses as if they are different from us, far more interesting things happen when we train them as if they are of the same template. Despite *Equus'* occasional Godzilla impressions, deep down they need just as much preparation, explanation, and encouragement as we do.

The Human Touch

A few thousand years of "on-and-off" civilization has taught humanity a thing or two about our own bodies and what they can and can't do. Countless centuries of being quite horrible to each other have shown us exactly what our limits and capacities are. We have discovered that it is a lot quicker to break an athlete than make one, and that one foolish moment can take away years of dedication and potential; so it is better to take time and care to prepare the body for sport, rather than pushing the limits only to find the breaking point (fig. 3.1).

Nowadays, we have sympathetic and intelligent methods to train floppy humans into healthy, happy athletes without making them scream and run away. Here are some training principles that have been fully tested on humans:

3.1 "No pain, no gain?" Quite the opposite: Good training is rooted in science, good judgement, and respect for the athlete. ▶

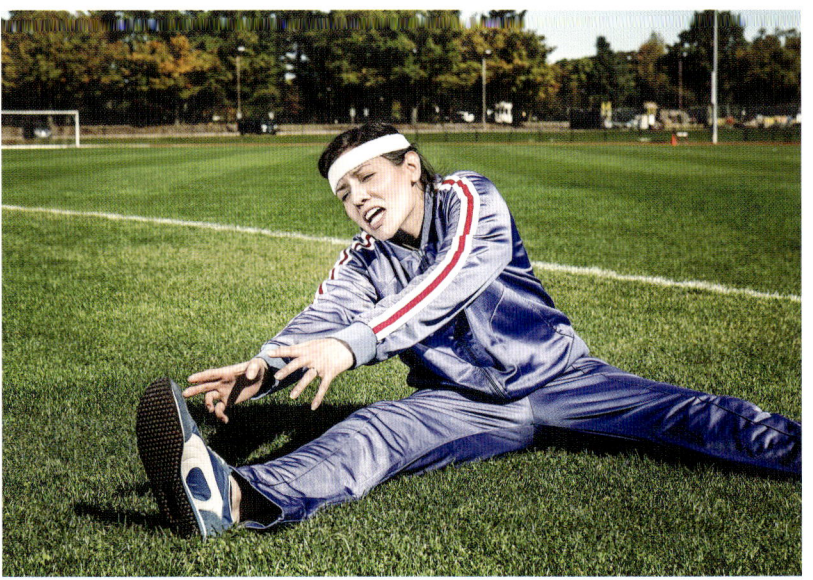

\\\ Morihei Ueshiba ///

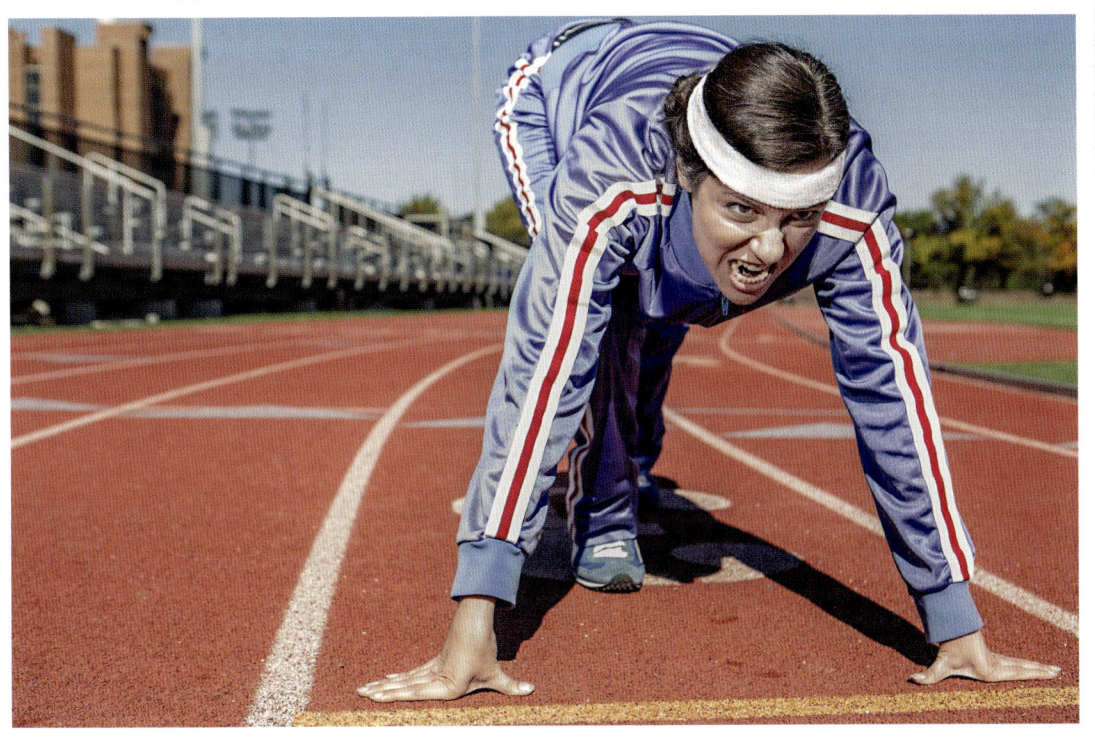

"The purpose of training is to tighten up the slack, toughen the body, and polish the spirit."

- Preparation is very important for performance and injury prevention.
- Never push the body or mind too hard.
- Isolate weak areas and focus on strengthening them.
- Discomfort in training is acceptable but pain is not.
- Rest, heal, and eat well.
- Performance comes from trusting the coach, environment, and equipment.
- Remember, we are all individuals.
- When "blockages" are met, take time to clear them rather than try to train through them.
- Ambition should never outweigh compassion.

Preparation before exercise is at the top of the list for a good reason. Start badly and progress becomes an uphill game. If body or mind is pushed into attempting something before feeling ready, we risk a physical or motivational injury that will create an even bigger obstacle later on. Knowing where the limits are without crossing them is the critical human safeguard. This is the first and perhaps the most important step for all athletic endeavors: the Warm-Up.

Using the Warm-Up to Condition the Core

"Whilst some injuries are true accidents in the sense of being unavoidable, many are the result of your body being unprepared for tasks that you have set it," says Hazel Fish, dance teacher and physiotherapist. "There is an unwritten law among both elite athletes and casual exercisers that a warm-up prior to exercising is essential for any program to be successful, and is an important part of prevention of injuries."

Dancers don't just dance and hurdlers don't just hurdle. If all it took to warm up a human for the performance of a lifetime, the Bolshoi would take a quick jog around the theater and then leap into the first act. This is far from the reality. The dancer athlete's warm-up is precise, methodical, and deeply traditional for one simple reason: Skip it and the "Dark Side" we discussed in the last chapter awaits (fig. 3.2).

The benefits of the Warm-Up include:

- Increased circulation to all muscle groups.
- Increased body temperature to optimal.
- Triggered muscle memory.
- Boosted "body confidence" in one's ability.
- Gymnasticized three Core Powers—fully and in three directions.

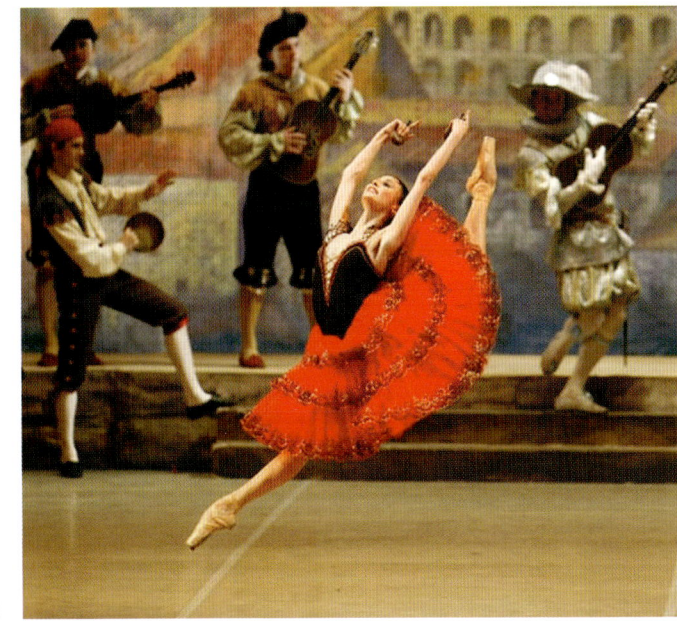

◀ / 3.2 / Russian ballerina Svetlana Zakharova of the Bolshoi Ballet performing. It is the dancer's warm-up that is the foundation of her performance.

With both horses and humans, using core conditioning exercises as the Warm-Up performs three functions in one. With a mixture of static (on the spot) and dynamic (while moving) exercises, the body is not only stretching, it is also slowly warming from the inside while connecting the large body parts together through the core. As the body's physical center, everything else depends upon the core acting first and freely. Anyone who has swung an axe or hit a ball with a bat will know instinctively that any movement not instigated by the core will be powerless. So, for the same reason, if a horse is to be ridden well he must be sufficiently warmed up through the whole body, most particularly the core, or we will not see his best.

As five-time Olympian British dressage Rider Carl Hester notes, "Working-in is one of the most important aspects of dressage. You want your horse to be long, round, and stretching before you start more taxing work, to get the muscles in front of and behind the saddle soft and working—gymnasts don't hop straight onto the top bar!"

/ 3.3 / *Warming up is a vital part of training. Humans take great care to supple the body's core before doing anything strenuous or elegant.* ▶

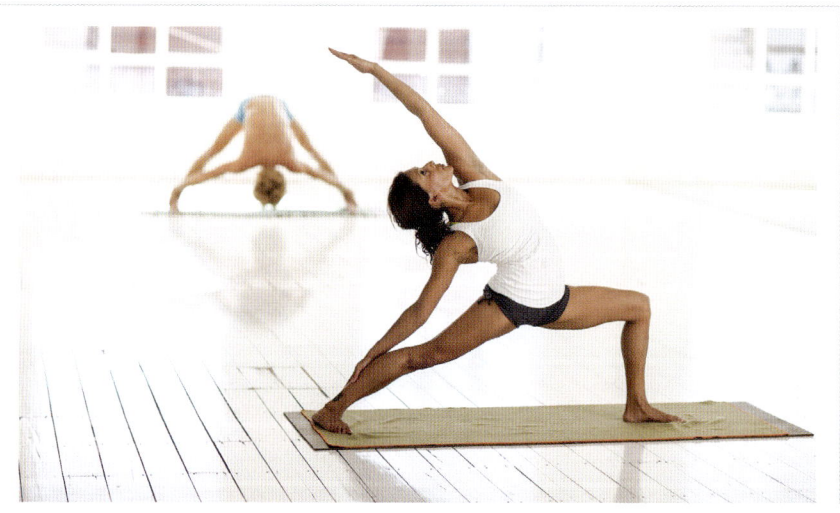

\\\ Dashama ///

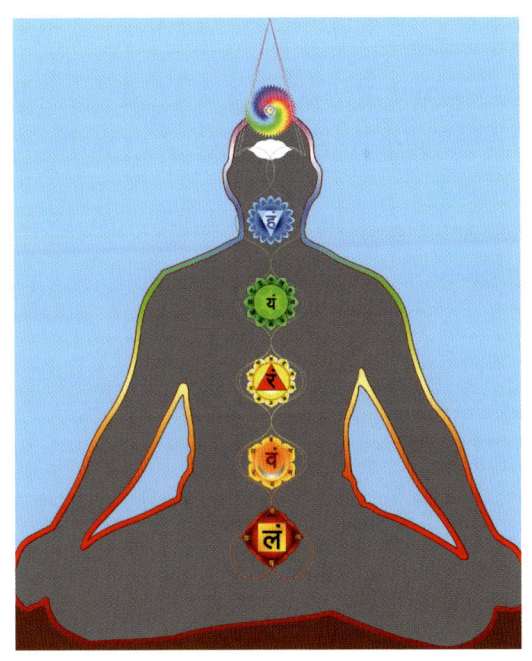

"Core yoga poses are one of the most important aspects of yoga practice. Without a strong core, everything else is weak."

One of humanity's most popular methods of warming up the body through its core is the ancient tradition of yoga.

Yoga: Kind to the Core

The amazing art of yoga is said to be between 5,000 and 10,000 years old, so it has probably been fairly well tested by now.

Yoga's very special quality is to gently take the "imperfect" human body, slowly reach inside, and improve every single little piece of the vertebrate bio-puzzle until the whole thing is restriction-free.

What yoga does for the human core:

- Improves posture and core strength.
- Increases flexibility in the spine.
- Encourages ideal skeletal alignment.
- Increases range of motion throughout the whole locomotory system.
- Encourages good body connection and coordination.
- Heals old tissue damage with replacement muscle, circulatory, and neural support.

As a result of its slow but deep approach, yoga's static stretches can gradually convince old and even painfully stiff areas to let go and start moving again. The key is giving the body as much time and repetition as it needs to gain enough confidence to let go of its defenses. Yoga's dynamic exercises can then develop the ability to maintain balance while in motion—slowly at first until flexibility develops all on its own. Both static and dynamic yoga exercises are commonly seen in

\\\ Amit Ray ///

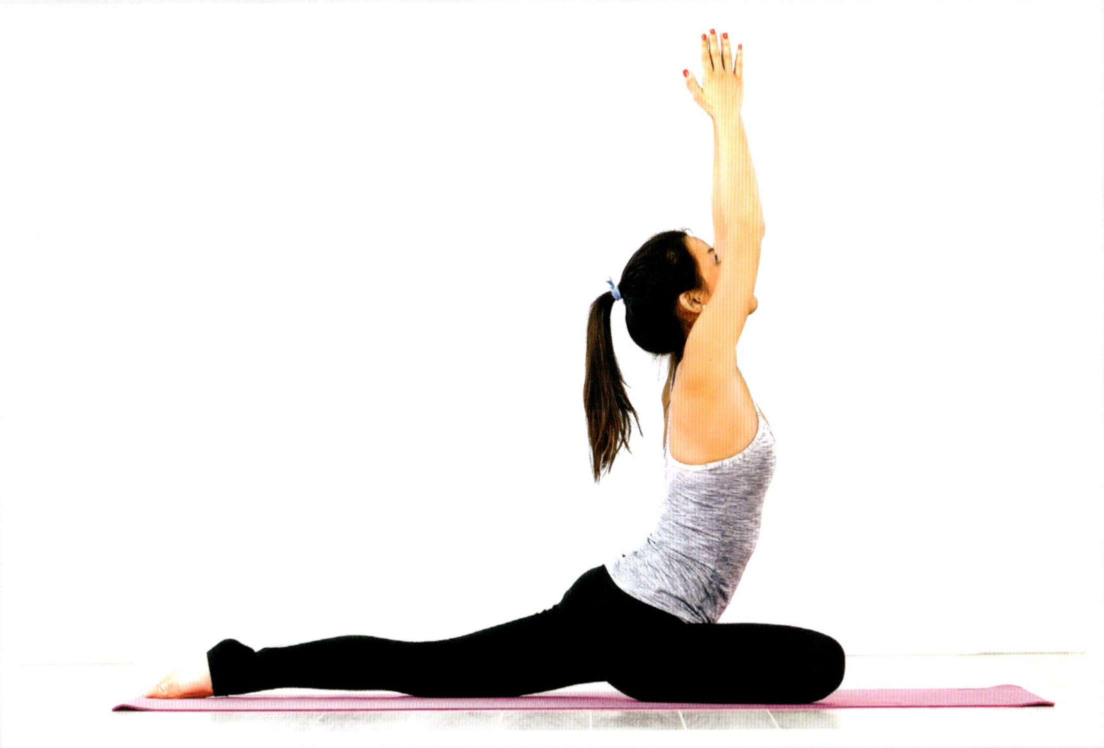

"Yoga means addition—addition of energy,
strength, and beauty to body,
mind, and soul."

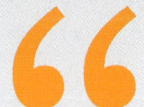

the warm-up of almost all human performances for these reasons. And as luck would have it, yoga's core warming principles can be applied equally to our forelocked friends.

Yoga: Created for the Horse

There is no doubt how good the practice of yoga is for people. The results and benefits can be identical for our horses—for all the same reasons and more.

Yoga pays particular care to avoid triggering tension, and this is an extremely useful property when applied to the horse's needs. The particular physical and psychological qualities of horses make the low-impact, measured, and repetitive theme of the yoga movements ideal for helping our horses start a training session in the best possible way (figs. 3.4 & 3.5).

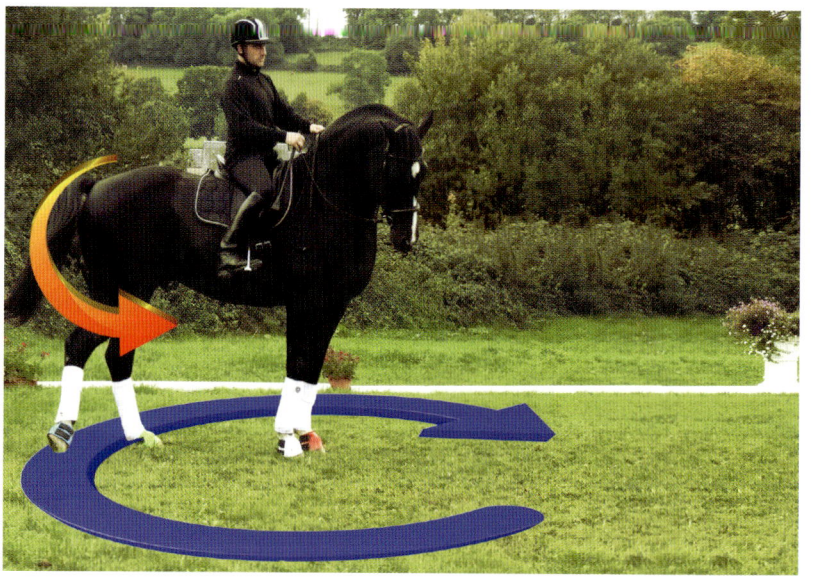

/ 3.4 / *It's about range of motion: yoga's low impact movements can awaken the horse's core without him breaking a sweat.* ▶

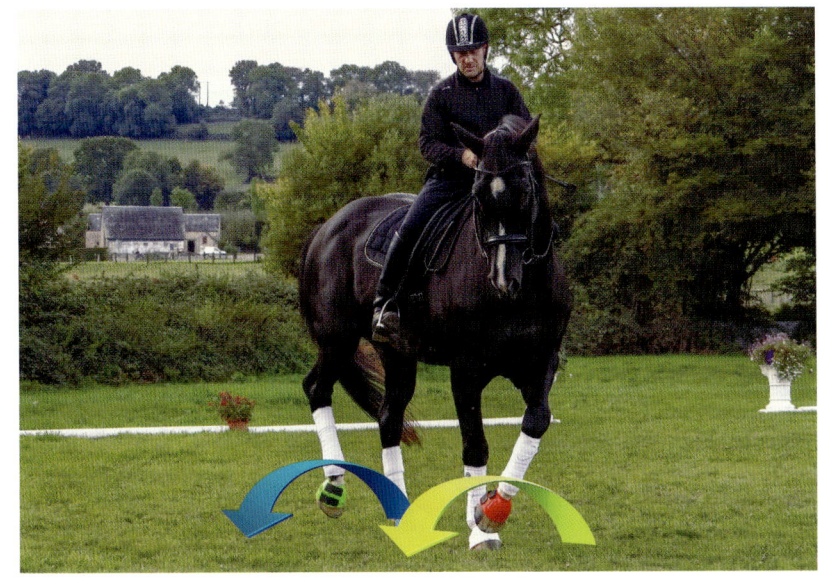

◂ / 3.5 / *Like us, when the horse practices coordination exercises at a comfortable speed, body confidence and technique improve without triggering tension.*

The equine's spine is particularly responsive to yoga's principles, because it uses a full range of lateral, vertical, and rotational movements to deliberately reach every little joint and muscle along its length, activating all the components of this complicated three-dimensional bio-puzzle.

A yoga warm-up offers the horse these physical benefits:

- Releases the core.
- Stretches the spine laterally, vertically, and rotationally.
- Clarifies communication.
- Increases all-round range of motion.
- Repairs old stiffnesses and blockages.
- Improves circulation.
- Improves coordination.
- Increases body confidence.

As American dressage Olympian Christine Traurig reminds us, "Relaxation means that the horse is physically and mentally tension-free."

This approach is thankfully as kind to the mind as it is to the body.

Yoga for the Horse's Mind—The Happy Place

Holding the horse's attention is not always easy. Designed to spot predators before they strike, keeping their attention on our aids can be a challenge, considering one of you thinks he can see a velociraptor behind the chrysanthemums at C!

Horses tend to only give one subject their focus, and you really need that to be you. When he does, you have a wonderful opportunity to connect and move as one. When he focuses on something scary, you become nothing more than a passenger on a half-ton of panic.

So, having a method of helping the horse into a "happy place" is not only less dangerous, it will also keep him in the "Learning Zone." Let me explain.

The horse's state of mind can be:

- Asleep ("Sorry, did you say something?")
- Alert (The Learning Zone.)
- Nervous ("Something in the hedge is watching me!")
- Survival ("Whoosh!")

\\\ Bertil Voss ///

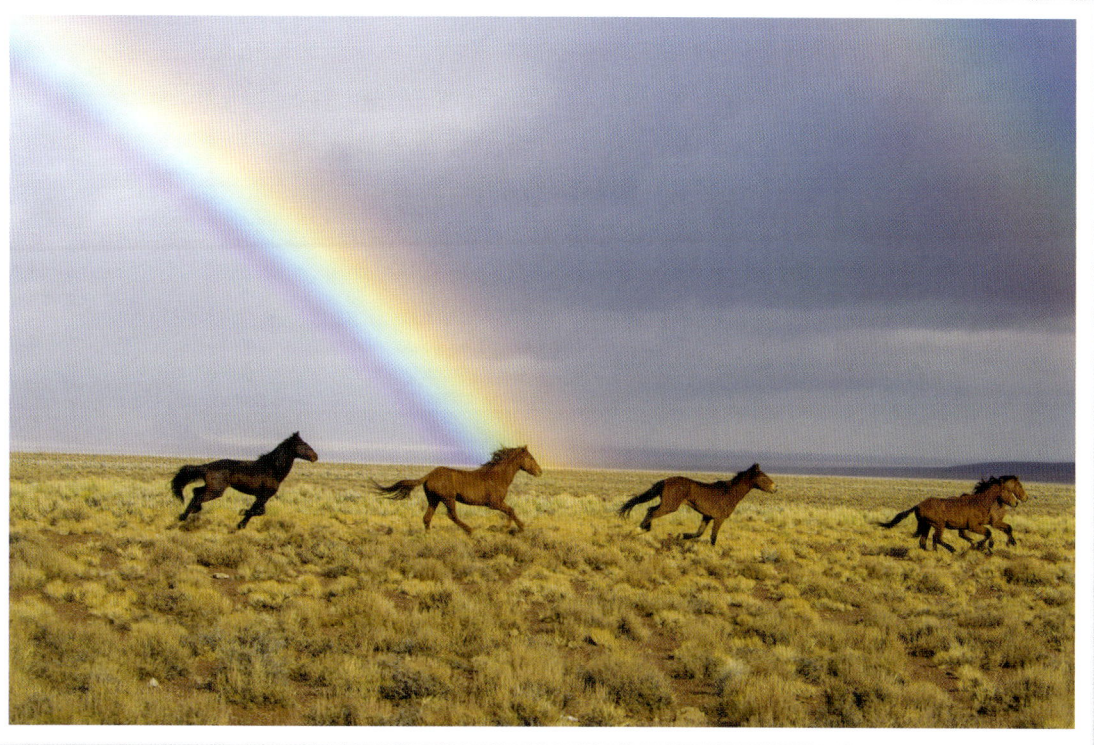

"You must let the horse be a horse."

„

Riding a horse in any other state than "Alert" brings complications to the day. The "Asleep" horse will do a zombie impression; the "Nervous" horse will frazzle your nerves; and the horse in "Survival" mode will put an *Equus*-shaped hole in anything in his way.

The Alert horse's reasonable frame of mind is open and interested, making it the only Learning Zone. The Asleep, Nervous, and Survival horses are not "learning"—they are reacting and need our help to bring them back into the Learning Zone. For this, yoga-inspired exercises are the perfect answer (fig. 3.6).

"The practice of yoga makes the body strong and flexible," explains American yoga teacher Megan Ridge Morris. "It also improves the functioning of the respiratory, circulatory, digestive, and hormonal systems. Yoga brings about emotional stability and clarity of mind." Yoga-inspired exercises help the horse's mind find the Alert Learning Zone in a multitude of ways:

- They are slow, methodical, and therefore calming.
- They are motivating and proactive.
- They are simple to understand.

/ 3.6 / "Yoga" means "union" in Sanskrit. Yoga principles can heal, soothe, and connect—just what every horse needs. ▶

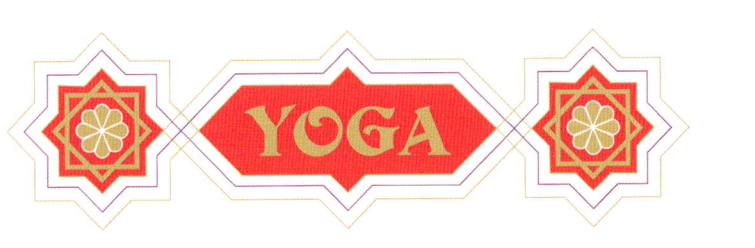

Core Conditioning for Horses

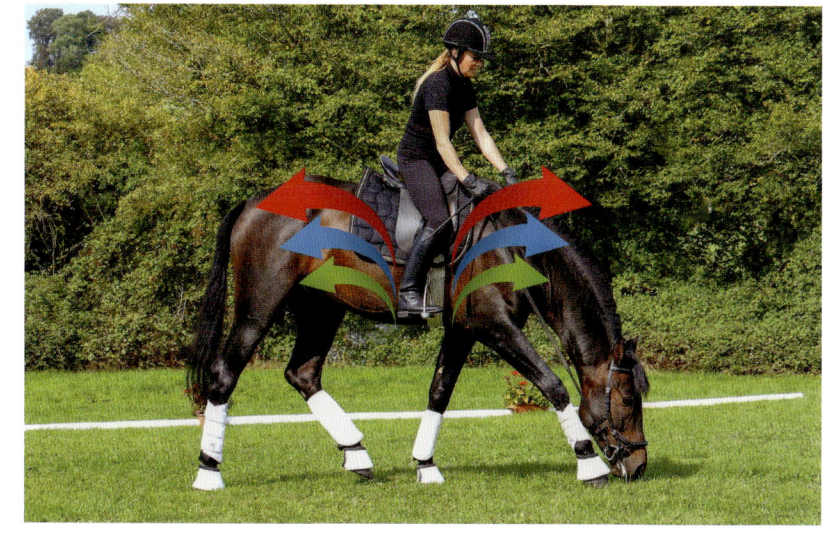

◄ / 3.7 / *Yoga-inspired warm-up exercises condition the core, focus your horse on you, and feel good!*

- They improve aid "clarity."
- They improve rider trust.
- They focus the mind on something good.
- They feel good!

Performing yoga-inspired movements to warm up a horse can bring a collection of wonderful effects (fig. 3.7). Special exercises practiced from both the standstill and a free walk give the horse and rider a perfect opportunity to find a calm, centered place to work the basics out together while suppling at the same time. As many of the movements I will teach you require the horse to concentrate carefully, this approach also helps to focus your horse on you and your shared "game."

In the next chapter I will show you how to assess the condition of your horse's core before choosing a core conditioning and warm-up plan comprised of yoga-inspired exercises that will bring out his best self. ■

\\\ George Morris ///

George Morris

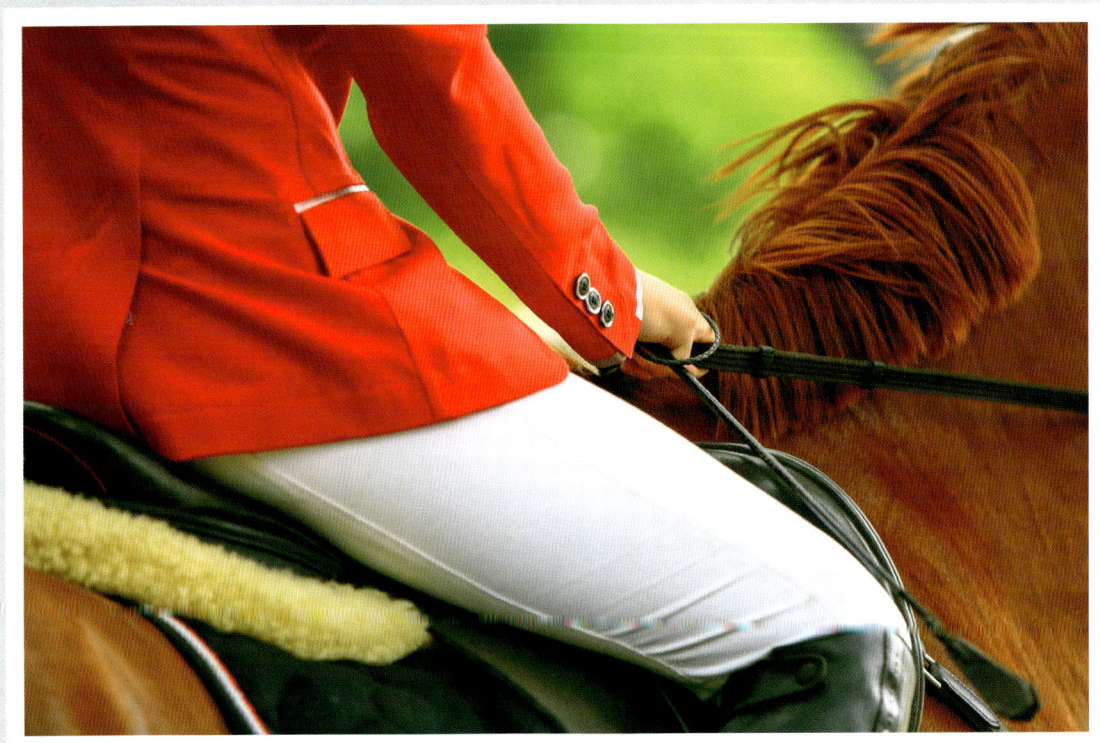

"Think of riding as a science, but love it as an art."

❝

4

Assessing the Horse's Core and Choosing a Warm-Up Plan

The born athlete is very rare. Most are made by will, effort, and experienced guidance, so there is no reason why every healthy riding horse should not be the best version of himself and on jolly good form. To do this we need to find out precisely what his core strengths and weaknesses are by giving the horse a "Core Score." This is a system I have developed to more accurately interpret the patterns of the core-related movement you experience from the saddle. These are called "Core Indicators" and will help you decide your horse's overall Core Score.

The Core Score

From harmony to horror show, horses vary infinitely in their rideability. Some float and "read your mind," while others feel as if you are riding a bicycle down the Spanish Steps with loose handlebars. Whichever end of the spectrum a horse may be, he will tend to have a general "way of going." This habitual posture is, of course, an entire checklist of his core condition for all to see.

I have put together an easy-to-follow Core Score chart listing typical Core Indicators to help decide your horse's core condition by giving him a Core Score of 0 to 5.

Core Score 0 is our goal and indicates a horse that has achieved near perfection in gait technique and that will be an excellent

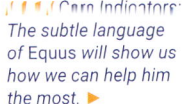 Core Indicators: *The subtle language of* Equus *will show us how we can help him the most.* ▶

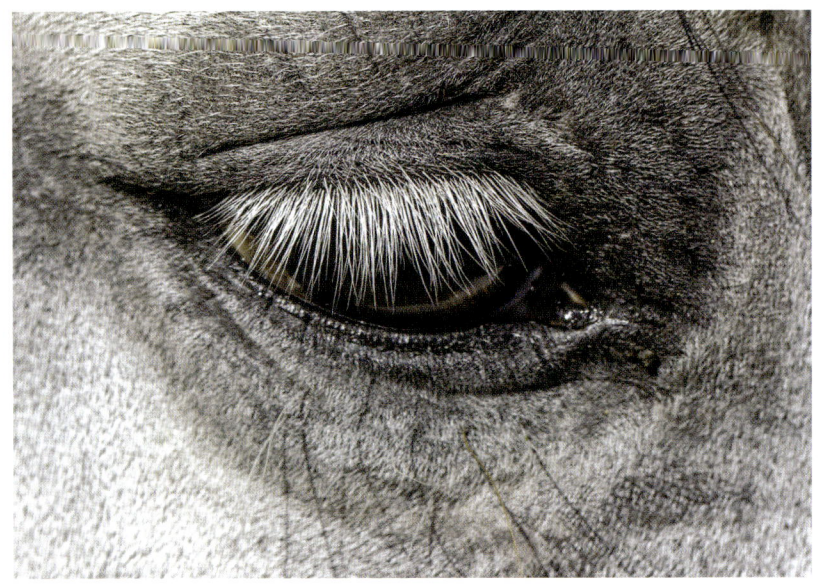

riding partner. A Core Score of 4 or 5 is a horse in need of our help and kindness.

Core Condition Indicators

What follows are my five Core Indicators to evaluate the riding experience you get from your horse (fig. 4.1). Each one should have a Core Score, which you can determine using the chart found on pp. 96 and 99.

/1/ **RIDEABILITY**—How easy is this horse to ride?
/2/ **SUPPLENESS**—How flexible is he?
/3/ **SOUNDNESS**—How stable, agile, and regular is he?
/4/ **HEAD, NECK, AND MOUTH**—How supple, soft, and light is he?
/5/ **THE RIDDEN MINDSET**—Is he alert, lazy, or crazy?

Core Indicator 1: Rideability

This is the most important and easiest Core Indicator to assess. A horse with a Core Score of 0 has a very strong core and as a result he will go extremely well under saddle (fig. 4.2). This horse will feel as if he is an extension of your own body. He will stay round on his own, stop, turn, and go like dancer Mikhail Baryshnikov after a good night's sleep.

At the other end of the spectrum, the horse with a Core Score of 4 or 5 has a weak core and poor posture, putting all the wrong angles into the horse's locomotive system. This makes the gaits look and feel very disconnected.

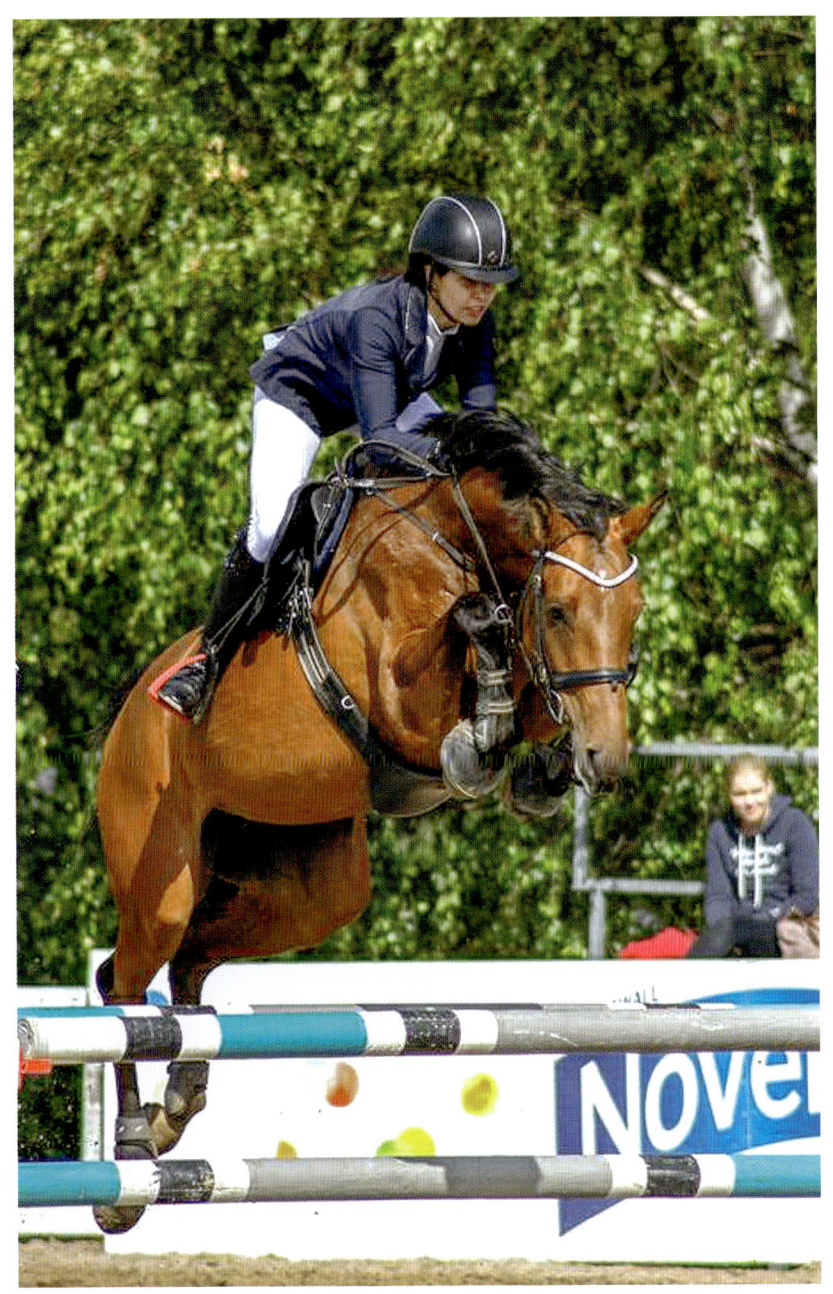

/ 4.2 / *Rideability is one of the many factors that must be in place to have a truly great connection between horse and rider.* ▶

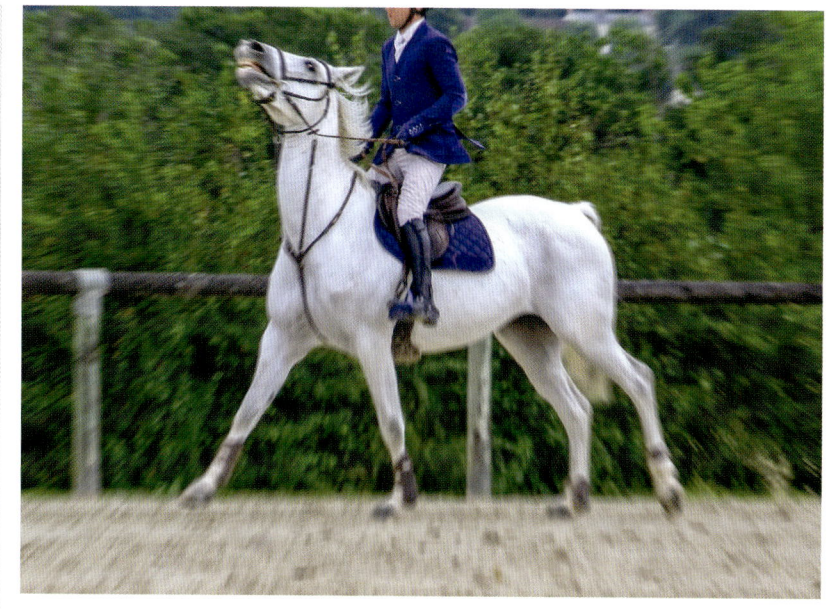

◄ / 4.2 / When the horse has a weak core and a Core Score of 4 or 5 for the Rideability Core Indicator, any equestrian sport will be hard for both horse and rider.

RIDEABILITY CORE SCORE

- **0–1** Easy mover, elegant, and intuitive.
- **2** Good, useful, and mobile.
- **3** A limited yet reliable ride.
- **4** Uncomfortable and uninterested (seek veterinary advice).
- **5** Unpredictable, lazy, or crazy—possibly for good reason (seek veterinary advice).

Core Indicator 2: Suppleness

Suppleness can be described as every little joint and muscle in the body working optimally, like the inside of a Swiss watch.

A Suppleness Core Score of 0–1 indicates that a horse is very flexible throughout his body (fig. 4.3). He can bend through corners, "sit"

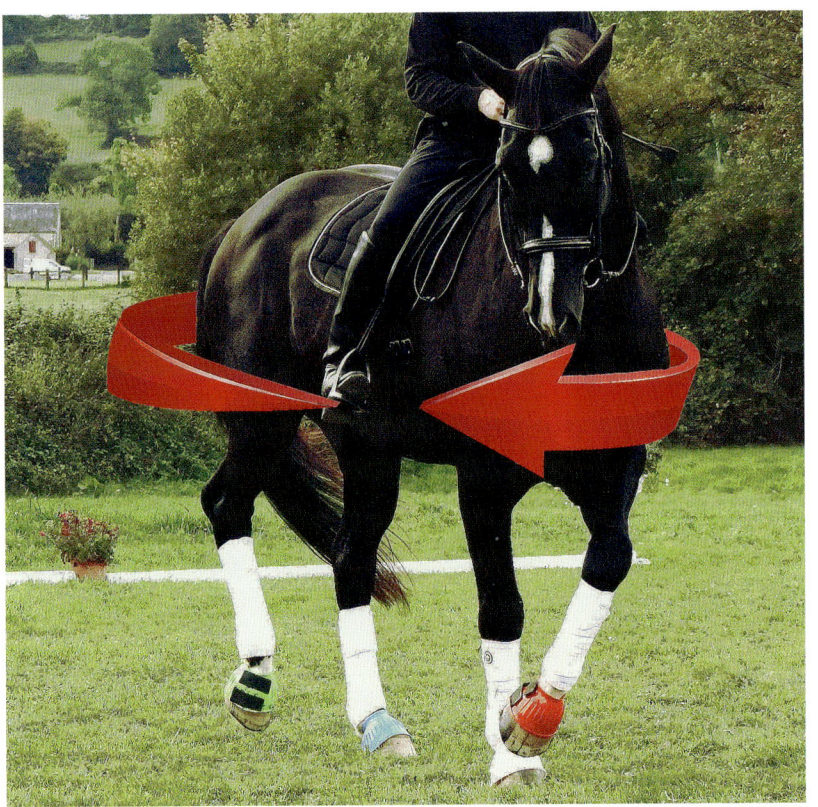

/ 4.3 / Bending through the body is the door to everything harmonious, subtle, and graceful. ▶

in transitions, and manage his center of gravity perfectly, giving the rider a very smooth riding experience.

For the purpose of assessing the horse's Core Indicators, we can consider suppleness and straightness as being from the same source (fig. 4.4). If the horse's core is scoring a 4 or 5 for Suppleness, the horse is not able to use his whole back. So, to get the job done, he will bring his bottom to the inside with a swing action (figs. 4.5 & 4.6). This plays a significant role in determining what his limbs can or cannot do, and limits how much the rider can help or even follow.

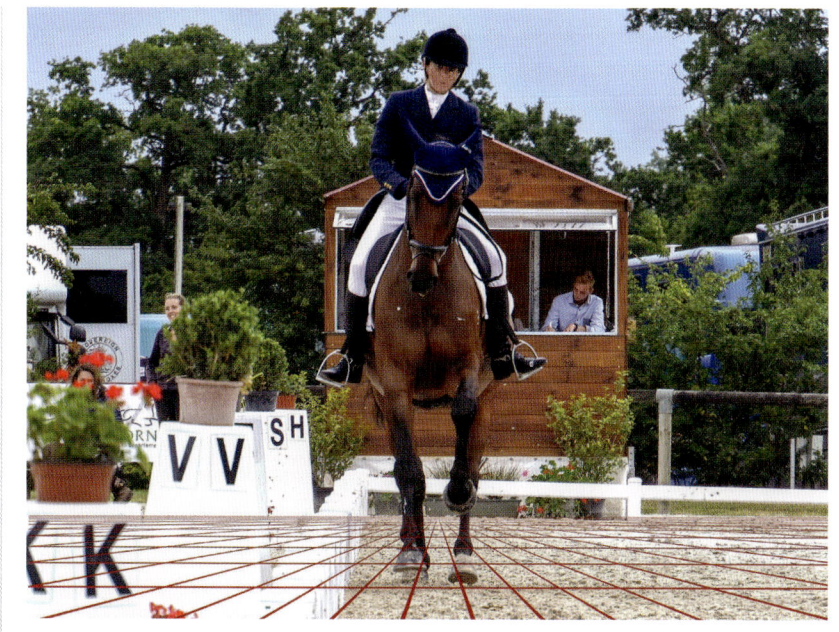

◄ / 4.4 / *Straightness: When the horse's back is completely supple and released, straightness comes automatically.*

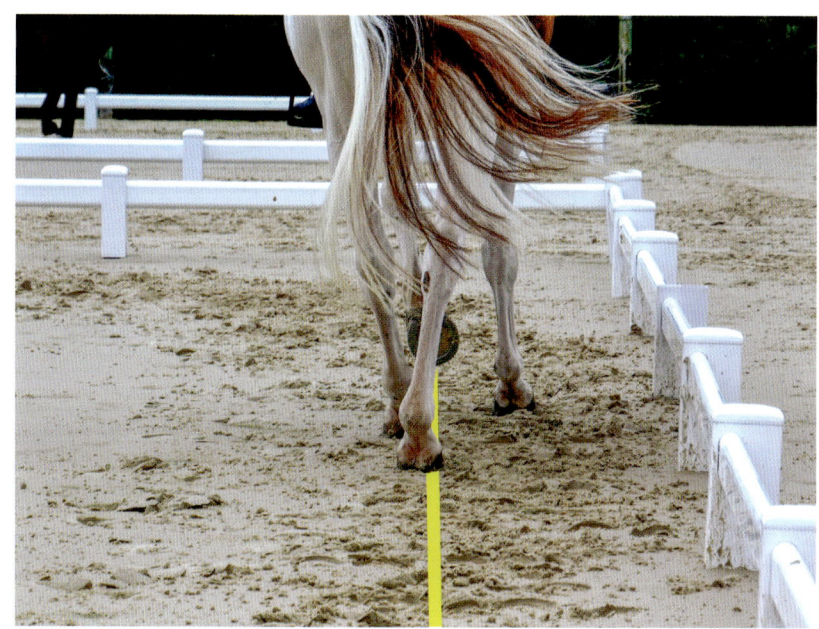

◄ / 4.5 / *Crookedness: A horse with a Core Score of 4–5 for Suppleness with a hollow back has to bring his rear end to the inside of the front end, making him crooked.*

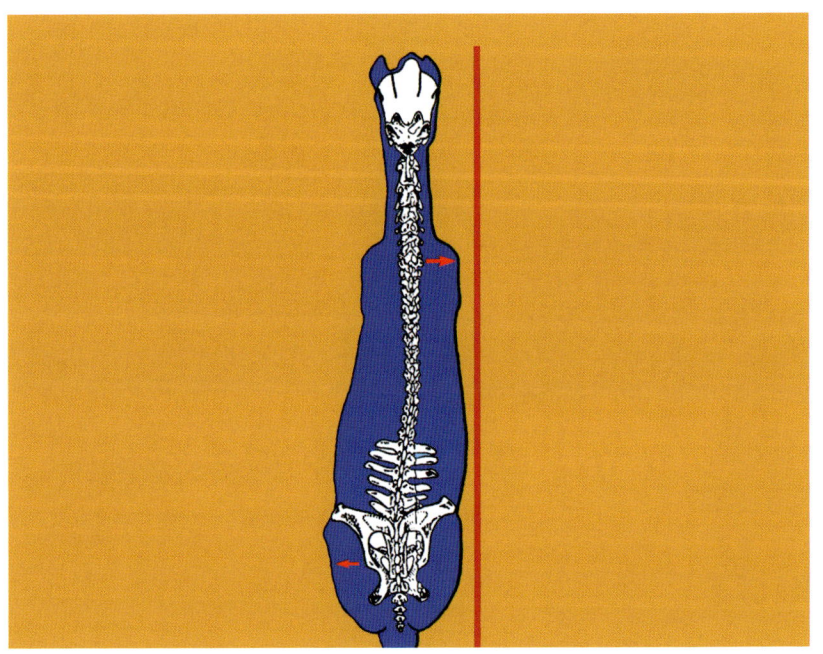

/ 4.6 / *The horse's spine can easily find itself crooked in several places.* ▶

From a biomechanical perspective, the more crooked the gait, the less balanced and rideable the horse is, and as time goes on, the body muscles up unevenly, compensating as best it can for the lack of alignment and function. The horse's body can't take this indefinitely.

SUPPLENESS CORE SCORE

- **0–1** Straight and balanced, easy to sit on, and intuitive to ride.
- **2** Bends well, crooked slightly on straight lines and particularly in medium gaits or extensions.
- **3** Has one better direction, flat paces, and some sticky transitions.
- **4** All gaits, paces, and transitions feel stiff, crooked, and on the forehand (veterinary exam recommended).
- **5** The horse fights to remain crooked and hollow (veterinary exam recommended).

Core Indicator 3: Soundness

In an assessment of the horse's core condition, Soundness is best thought of as regularity, athleticism, and coordination in all that a horse does.

When a horse displays a Core Score of 0–1 for Soundness, he is extremely regular and surefooted. This horse will rarely trip or injure himself, and he will feel secure and stable from the saddle.

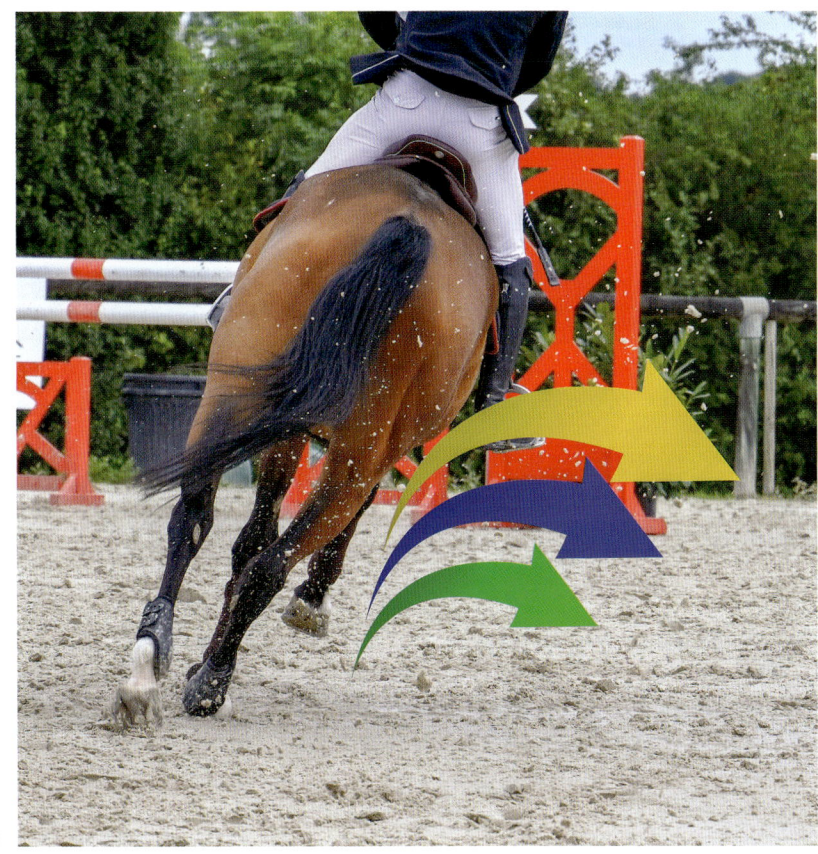

◄ / 4.7 / *Leaning inward: The horse's limbs have to take too many unusual forces when misaligned. This makes the horse unlevel and irregular in his stride.*

The horse's limbs are heavily dependent upon the structures they are attached to. If the horse is crooked, the legs have to work slightly askew. This produces a horse that leans into turns like a bicycle, putting one-sided forces along the skeleton (fig. 4.7). An imbalanced gait will, over time, show wear in the overloaded areas of the horse's body.

> **SOUNDNESS** CORE SCORE
>
> **0–1** *A full four-square double metronome. Straight, surefooted, and never unlevel.*
> **2** *Sound, regular, straight, and balanced, with only an occasional stumble.*
> **3** *Sound yet slightly irregular in lateral movements and corners.*
> **4** *Unlevel, particularly in lateral movements and corners; can have leg injuries (veterinary exam recommended).*
> **5** *Appearing almost lame and very unbalanced in motion, usually with some limb issues (veterinary exam recommended).*

Core Indicator 4: Head, Neck, and Mouth

The horse's head, neck, and mouth may appear to be separate from his core, but their behavior is, in fact, a reflection of his core health (fig. 4.8). Whatever is happening with the core, the "bits that stick out the front" will tell us everything we need to know.

A strong core enables the horse to be fully balanced and mobile throughout the body, leaving the head and neck weightless and free. The horse with a Core Score of 0–1 for the Head, Neck, and Mouth seeks a sensitive and stable relationship with your contact. His head, neck, and mouth are soft and flexible, both laterally and vertically, allowing the head and neck to be raised or lowered without resistance or any alteration in his body balance.

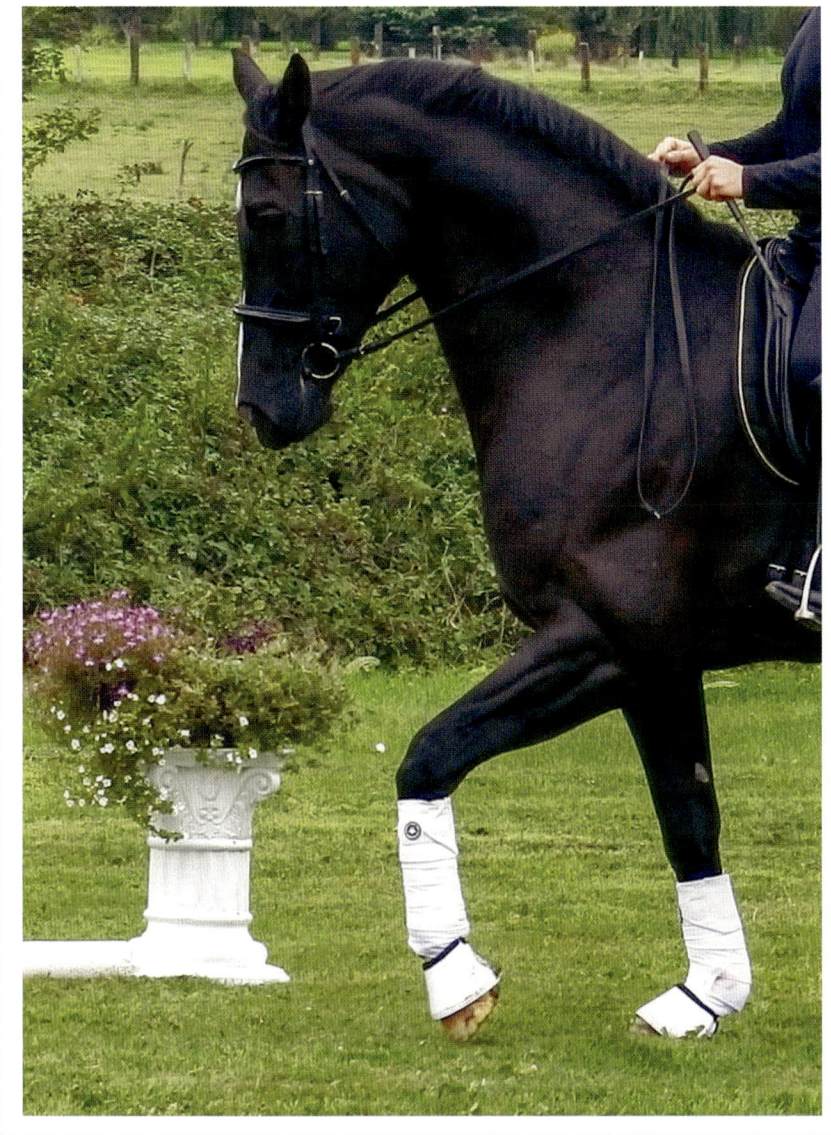

◄ / **4.8** / *A horse with good core condition will offer a soft, steady, and still contact.*

Alternatively, the horse with a weak core will have a very hard-to-ride front end. The mouth becomes hard, the neck stiff, and the head carriage either too low or too high (figs. 4.9 & 4.10). When a horse is

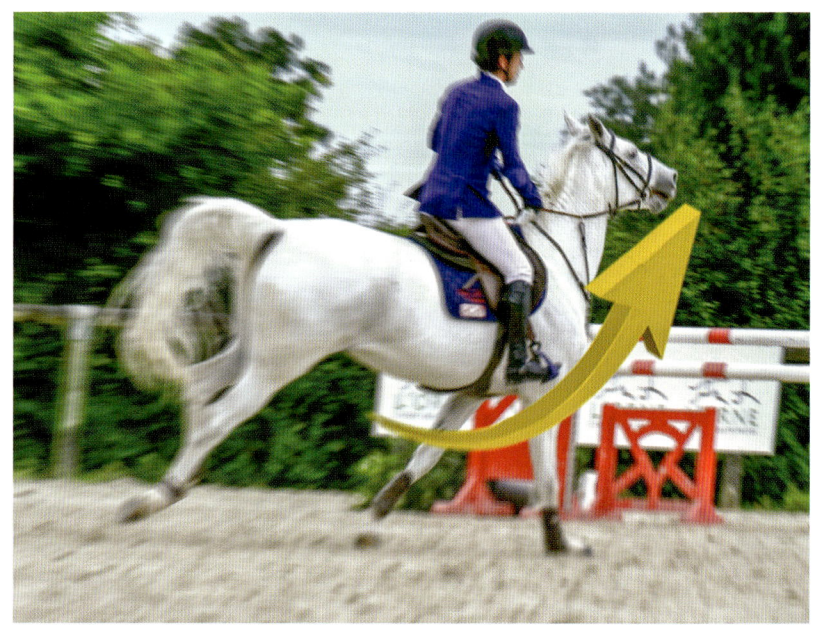

/ **4.9** / *When his core is not functioning well, the horse may come above a healthy head-and-neck position...* ▶

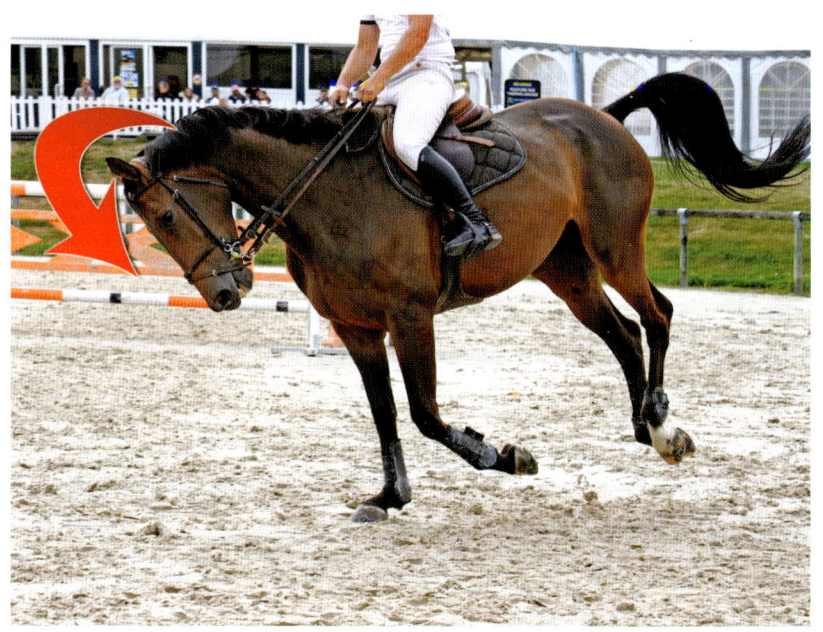

/ **4.10** / *...or below or behind it.* ▶

Core Conditioning for Horses

this hard to ride, we need to remember that our own experience in the saddle is a picnic compared to that of the horse, and as such, lower our requirements accordingly.

HEAD, NECK, AND MOUTH CORE SCORE

0–1 Light and soft with a full range of flexion and bend available to rider.
2 Good, steady mouth; can be a little strong in the contact.
3 One rein tends to have a stiffer, stronger contact.
4–5 Bend in the neck impossible on one or both side(s) and the head raises or lowers too easily.

Core Indicator 5: The Ridden Mindset

As the horse's body and mind are deeply interconnected, the quality of his posture and core condition have an equally profound effect upon his mind. Personality in horses varies as much as with us: some are brave souls and others are buttercups—it takes all sorts to make a world, and the state of his emotions, pain level, and other temperamental factors will change how a horse deals with everyday tasks. In general terms, a horse's overall attitude toward being ridden speaks volumes about his physical well-being under saddle. So, if a horse is physically unhappy, gradually he will lose his willingness—and quite right, too.

As a general rule, horses with a strong core are happy to be ridden because they feel good under saddle (fig. 4.11). The horse with a Core Score of 0–1 for Mindset will tend to be willing to participate, attentive, proactive (rather than *reactive*), calm, and able to learn on the go.

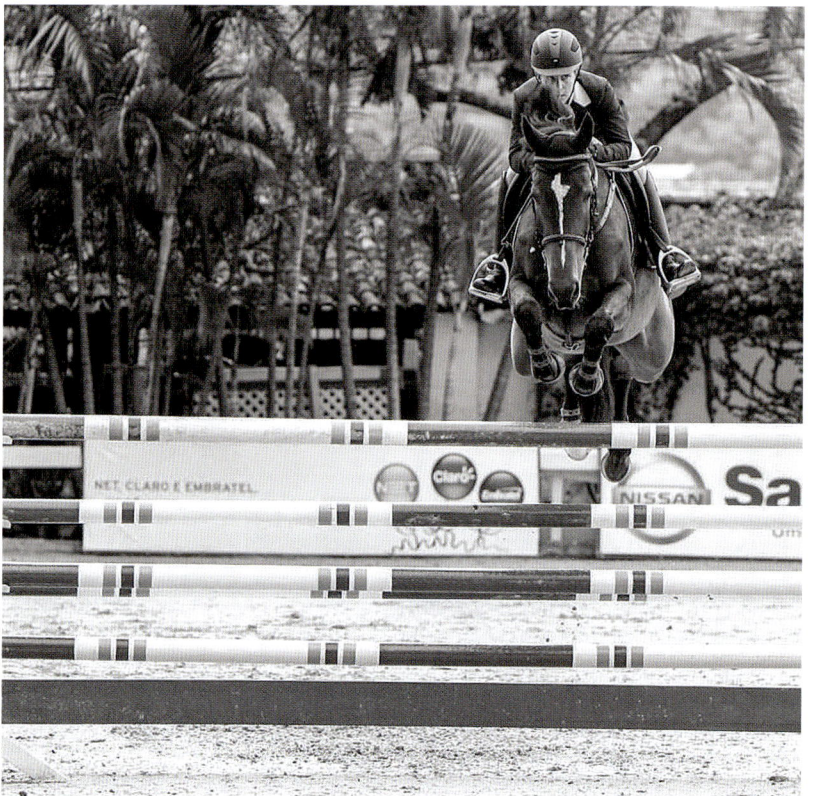

/ **4.11** / *Willingness is an indicator of core condition. When a horse feels strong and supple through his body, he can enjoy the challenge of learning, training, and performing.* ▶

On the other hand, when there is discomfort as a result of being ridden, it will gradually and proportionally make the horse disinvest, and eventually he may become quite resentful of being ridden, mounted, and eventually even girthed.

Together, the five Core Indicators I have just outlined make up the Core Score Chart on pp. 96 to 99. You are now prepared to use it to calculate your horse's Core Score. Note that there are a few other, non-ridden Core Indicators that can help you decide how your horse's is feeling inside. I describe those beginning on p. 100.

■■ Core Conditioning for Horses

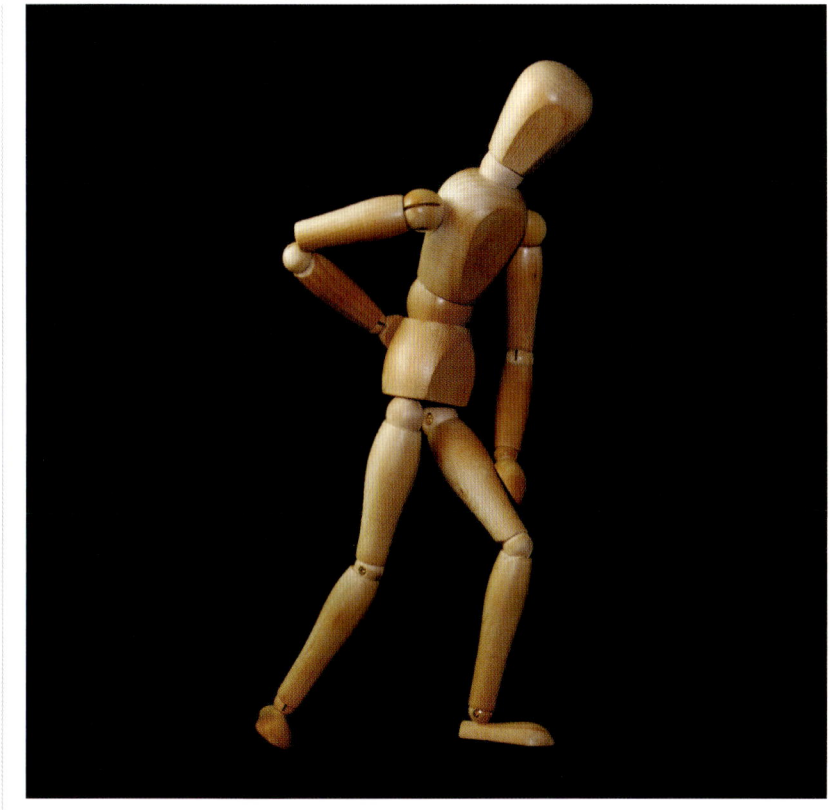

◄ / 4.12 / *When in pain, exercise for human or horse becomes an unhappy activity of self-protection.*

THE RIDDEN MINDSET CORE SCORE

0–1 *Horse:* "Let's go!" *Rider:* "Get on fresh, get off fresher."
2 *Horse:* "It's all good." *Rider:* "Good ride!"
3 *Horse:* "Okay, I will do what I can." *Rider:* "Wow, good workout!"
4 *Horse:* "That was hard." *Rider:* "I need to sit down."
5 *Horse:* "No, I can't." *Rider:* "I need to lie down."

Your Horse's Core Score

The five Core Indicators of **RIDEABILITY; SUPPLENESS; SOUNDNESS; HEAD, NECK, AND MOUTH;** and **THE RIDDEN MINDSET** each have a column in the chart on these pages. Consider these aspects of core conditioning and choose a Core Score that best describes your horse's ridden characteristics.

Using the Core Indicators

If your horse matches most of the indicators on one row, then the corresponding number is his Core Score. If he scores higher or lower for one or two Core Indicators,

THE CO

CORE SCORE	
0	• Excellent core condition • Optimal core strength, full flexibility
1	• Very good core condition • Strong core • Flexible
2	• Good core condition • Strong core

RE SCORE CHART

RIDEABILITY	SUPPLENESS	SOUNDNESS	HEAD, NECK, AND MOUTH	THE RIDDEN MINDSET
• Intuitive ride • Top performer • Comfortable in all gaits • Effortless roundness in collection and extension	• A fully conditioned back • Exceptionally supple and effortlessly round • Bends easily in both directions • Agile and flexible • Optimal movement	• Excellent health • Unsoundness is rare • High stamina and coordination • Rhythmical and regular movement • Moves easily • Multitalented	• Superb contact • Light and flexible • Easy to stop, go, and steer • Soft contact • On the bit all the time • Steady head and neck • Intuitive	• Alert • Focused, reliable, and a team player • Learns quickly • Alert, even under pressure • Very happy horse
• Excellent ride • High performer • Comfortable in all gaits • Effortlessly round • Slight preference for one direction	• Supple back • Flexible and soft • Bends easily in both directions • Agile and balanced • Excellent movement	• Excellent health • Unsoundness is rare • High stamina and coordination • Rhythmical and regular movement • Moves easily	• Superb contact • Light and flexible • Easy to stop, go, and steer • Soft contact • On the bit all the time • Steady head and neck	• Alert • Very happy horse • Focused and reliable • Intuitive • Learns quickly • Playful
• Good ride • Established gaits and skills • Gaits become bumpy and complicated under impulsion • Favors a direction	• Strong back • Bends well • One direction bends more easily • Slightly crooked in corners, extension, and collection	• Very good health • Good self-balance • Coordinated and surefooted • Some movements create tension • Dependable	• Good contact • Flexion range is good, but not light • Good head and neck position under most circumstances • Can get heavy or fussy with impulsion	• Mostly alert • Happy horse • Reliable and interested in life • Gradually improving, but slowly

THE CO

go with the average. The Core Score determines what level of core exercise your horse should begin with in the Warm-Up Plan you will choose in Part Two (p. 114). Note that when your horse is scoring 4s or 5s it is likely he is experiencing some discomfort—perhaps a lot. It is best to consult with a veterinarian before exercising your horse in this scenario. Of course, with correct medication and pain management, it may be possible to condition his core following a thorough consultation.

CORE SCORE	
3	• Basic • Functioning core • Limited back strength
4	• Poor core condition • Hollow back
5	• No core condition • Kissing spine • Back in spasm

RE SCORE CHART

RIDEABILITY	SUPPLENESS	SOUNDNESS	HEAD, NECK, AND MOUTH	THE RIDDEN MINDSET
• A rustic ride • The job gets done • Trot bouncy and uncomfortable • Modest movement • One rein takes a while to let go	• Intermittent stiff back • The back bends one way only • Resistant to some movements or transitions • Limited spine movement	• Well horse • A little stiff • Loses balance in turns and transitions • Poor topline • Leg problems • Stiff gaits • Tack seems to be tricky to get right	• Firm contact • Stronger contact • One rein heavier • Mouth can be hard • Head either fixed in place, too high, or too low • Never soft on the bit	• Intermittently alert • Content Horse • Unfocused • Disinterested or distracted often • Not improving
• Complicated ride • Hard to start, stop, and steer • Poor transitions • Uncomfortable • Basic control only • Poor aid response • Unhappy being mounted	• Blocked back • Inflexible • Hollow under saddle • Horse folds on one side and won't bend on the other • Unbalanced • Falls in/out around corners	• Limited ability • Stiff gaits • Poor posture • Haphazard transitions • Unbalanced • Not surefooted • Limb and stiffness issues	• Hard contact • Heavy, one-sided contact • Head is either too heavy or too light • Easily goes too low or too high	• Lazy or crazy • Disinterested or distracted • Temperamental • Tail swishing • Difficult to deal with • Either slow to react or over-reacting
• Unpredictable • May be dangerous • Either flat, shuffling paces or out of control • Ears back, tail swishing	• Locked back • Blocked through the body • Noticeably hollow back • Impossible to steer and stop • Rigid under saddle	• Unlevel • Either sideways and irregular gaits or very, very slow ones • Not surefooted • Unbalanced and unlevel • Horse in pain	• Contact impossible • Unpredictable and erratic head and neck position • Often very high head • Reins have little effect • Injury and stress/strain injuries	• Lazy and crazy • Withdrawn, reluctant, distant • Highly distracted, grumpy, sad, or even angry • May be dangerous • Depressed horse

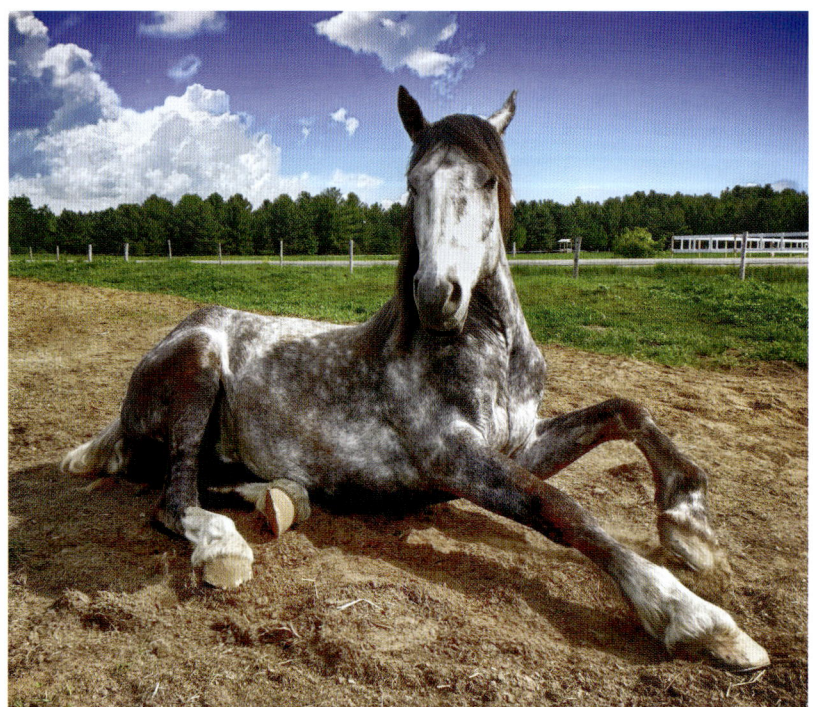

/ **4.13** / Is your horse happy and interested? A happy horse behaves "normally." This is a simple indicator of whether he is pain-free and enjoying life. ▶

Non-Ridden Core Indicators

As mentioned, there are non-ridden Core Indicators to consider in addition to your horse's Core Score. Consider these supplemental information as you make decisions related to your horse's core conditioning program and Warm-Up Plan.

Mood

As a rule, horses are an affable sort and not inclined to grumpiness. So, how the horse reacts to daily activity, such as being handled, groomed, and tacked up, gives us insight into his deeper Zen.

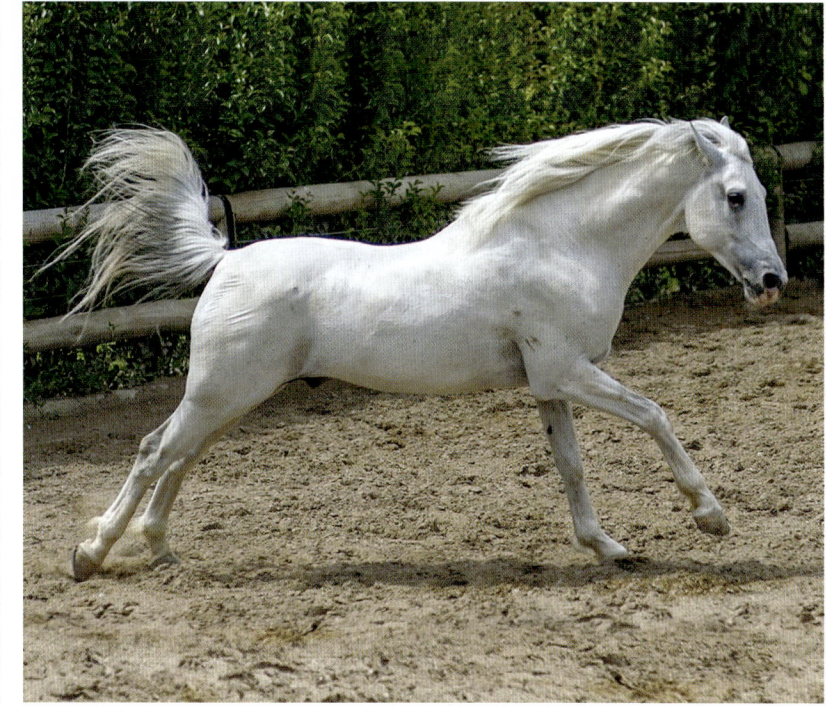

◀ / 4.14 / *A bad-tempered horse is usually in some form of discomfort or even pain.*

When a horse has good core condition and consequently feels good inside, he will usually be in a good mood (fig. 4.13). It is that simple. He will be predictable, calm, focused, and interested with an "ears forward" view of life. Being highly mobile gives him body confidence in the knowledge that he is tiger-proof today—nothing makes a horse happier.

On the other hand, the weak-cored horse knows that when the tigers come, he may be at the back of the herd. This knowledge makes him feel vulnerable, sad, irritable, or sometimes just uninterested in life. When we see "bad" behavior like this, the horse is telling us something, and we need to listen (fig. 4.14).

Joseph Pilates

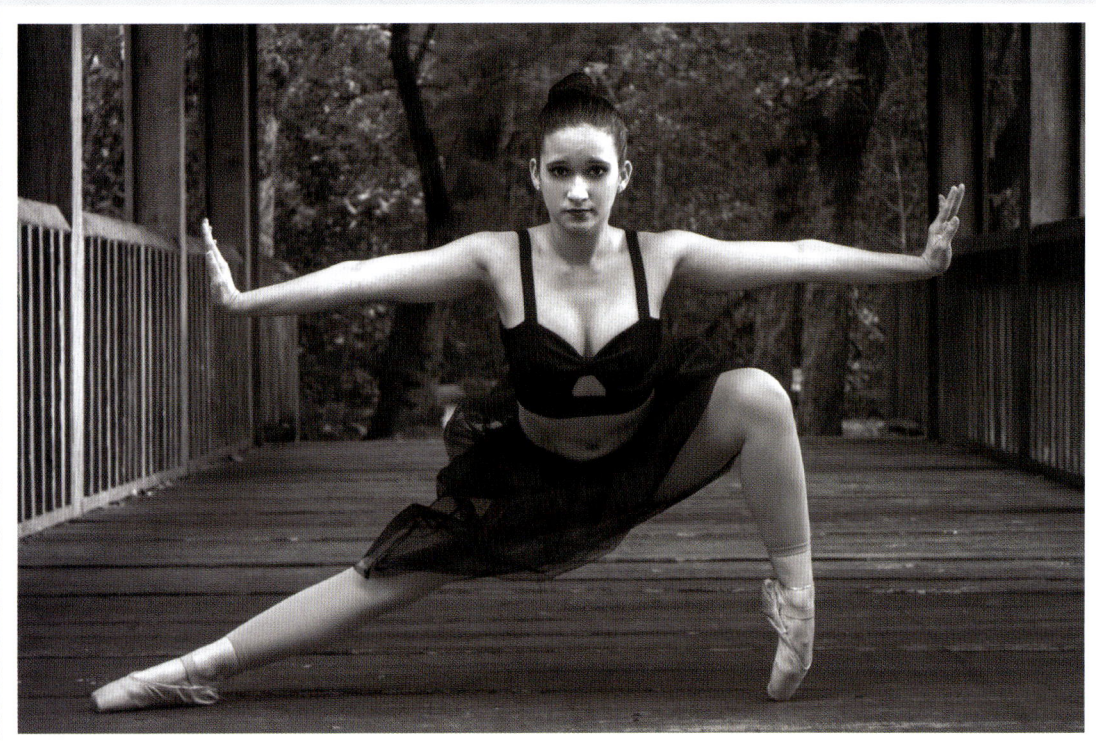

"Good posture can be successfully acquired only when the entire mechanism of the body is under perfect control."

Posture and Physical Appearance

Build and posture are very closely linked. The way in which a horse moves will build the muscles that are being used by the horse's unique gait. To have a Core Score of 0–1 a horse is using the three Core Powers correctly, and this requires the whole body to be used well (see p. 44). He will have excellent muscle distribution as a result (fig. 4.15).

Poor posture or crookedness leaves some muscles completely unused. These areas appear on the body as hollower areas, even in some cases all along the horse's topline (fig. 4.16). When you look at the horse's body-muscle distribution, it is easy to see if his gait is "skipping leg day."

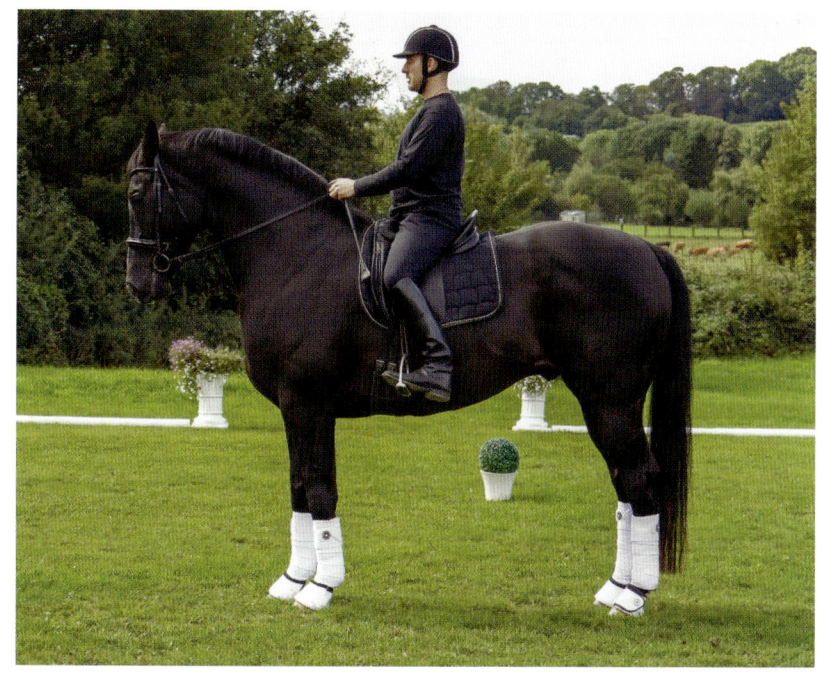

◀ / *4.15* / *A horse's muscle distribution tells a story about what he is and is not doing with his gaits.*

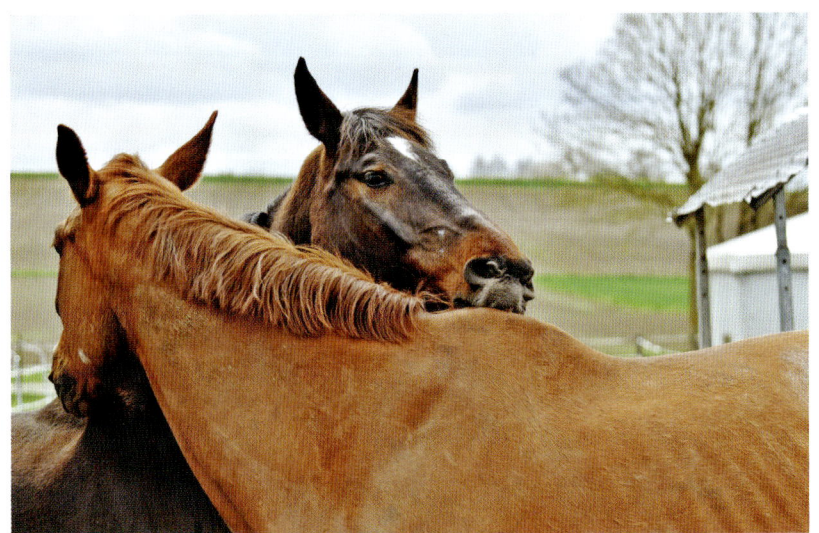

/ 4.16 / *When the horse's body doesn't move correctly, areas will show poor muscular development.* ▶

When the horse is working incorrectly because his core is weak, he will pull himself along with his front legs while paddling a little behind because the Core Powers are not able to work. This style of gait eventually appears in the horse as a strong, muscular shoulder but a weak topline.

"Xenophon was the first one to claim that horses can become only more beautiful with correct training, never uglier," noted Alois Podhajsky, one-time Director of the Spanish Riding School. "I would like to add to this that if the horse becomes uglier in the course of his work, it is the unmistakable proof of incorrect dressage training."

"Hoof Lift"

As simple as it is, when we pick up the horse's hind hoof to clean it, the horse's reactions tell us a lot about the condition of his back.

A sound horse with a strong core should do everything evenly, and he should be able to lift each hind foot equally high and hold it up for you—although not many horses can. The indication of a weak core is when one hind foot is easy to pick up yet its partner is much more reluctant to be lifted (fig. 4.17).

When the horse has back pain, being asked to stand on one hind leg requires that he bend a little throughout the body and use the muscles along only one side. If there is a problem on that side, the opposite foot will not want to leave the ground. It is important to remember that if it hurts the horse to stand on one leg at a standstill,

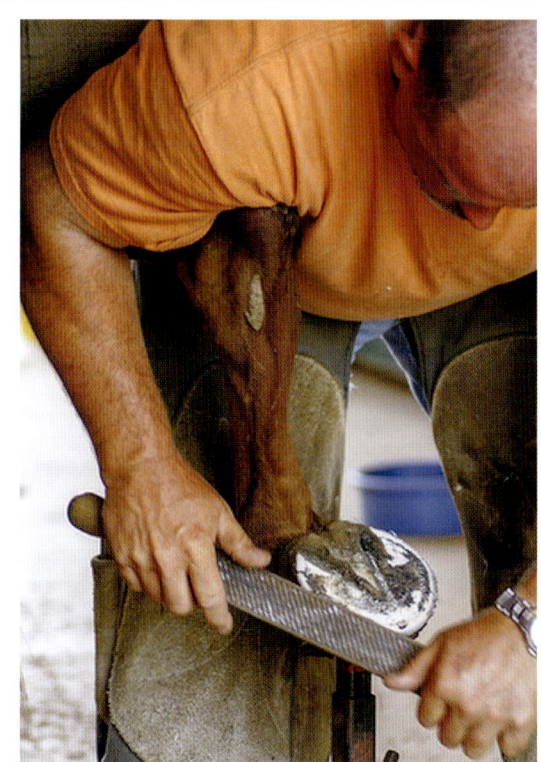

◀ / 4.17 / When the horse has a weak core and back pain, he will lift one hind foot higher and more easily than the other.

we should spare a thought for what the canter must feel like for him while under saddle.

Rolling

After having a good roll, a horse with a strong core will get up easily. He will stretch out the forelimbs to raise the shoulders, then push off with his hocks to get the rear end up (fig. 4.18). It should look reasonably effortless. When it looks like it is a big undertaking to get the hindquarters off the ground, this is often a sign that the horse's core and back may be under the weather.

/ 4.18 / *Watch how your horse gets up after a nap or a roll. Is it with a heave and a groan or like a spring lamb?* ▶

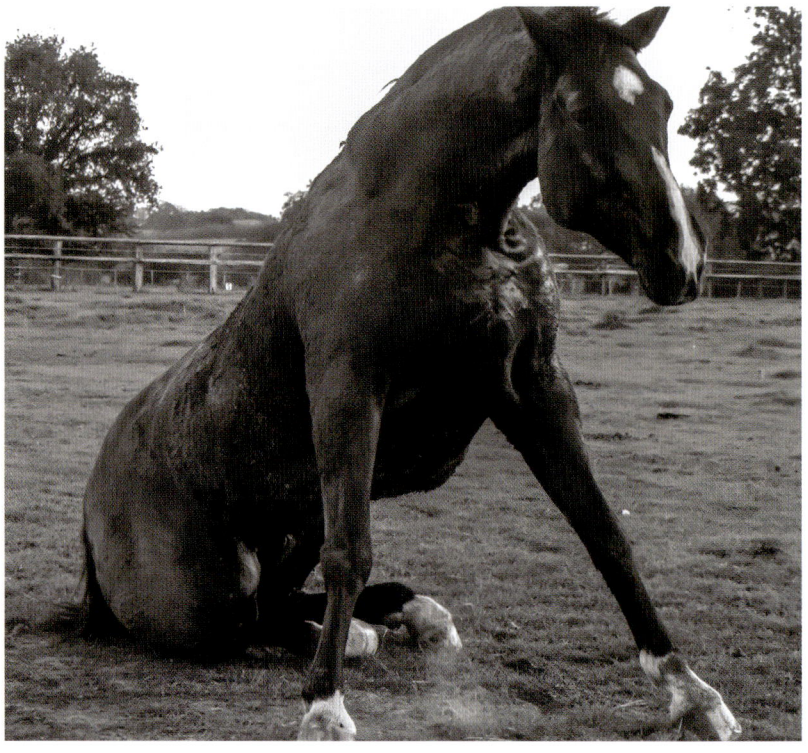

■■ Core Conditioning for Horses

Choosing Your Core Warm-Up Plan

Nobody knows your horse as well as you do, and you now have more information to use in evaluating his core condition and state of well-being. From the four different exercise plans that follow, choose the one you feel will do your horse the most good with his Core Score and Unridden Indicators in mind:

/1/ **CONNECTION**—Promotes mobility, cooperation, communication, and education.
/2/ **WELLNESS**—Promotes maintenance, good health, support, and calm.
/3/ **FLEXIBILITY**—Promotes suppleness, range of motion, and better head and neck position.
/4/ **AGILITY**—Sport mode!

The Core CONNECTION Plan

This Warm-Up Plan is all about bringing you and your horse together.

The exercises included develop a mutual harmony and improved balance. Gentle stretching along with improved aid response will make your horse more rideable as he perfects the routines. This plan is super for horses that will benefit from precision training and rounding poses with a bit of energizing fun to keep them entertained.

> ### The Core Connection Plan Exercises
>
> - **Core Release Volte** (Yoga Half-Moon Pose), p. 156
> - **Turn on the Forehand** (Yoga Half Split Pose), p. 169
> - **Forward and Back** (Yoga Balancing Table to Tiptoe Chair Pose), p. 198
> - **The Rounding Rein-Back** (Yoga Garland Pose), p. 223
> - **The Perfect Pirouette** (Yoga Thread the Needle Pose), p. 250

The Core FLEXIBILITY Plan

This Warm-Up Plan will release your steed's mobility and grace. The exercises included promote suppleness and range of motion throughout the body, using movements inspired by yoga's deepest core stretches. This plan is ideal for the horse that finds turning, transitions, and lateral work a bit tricky. It will help him become more "bendy" and balanced by releasing and coordinating the back and core.

> ### The Core Flexibility Plan Exercises
>
> - **Core Release Volte** (Yoga Half-Moon Pose), p. 156
> - **Turn on the Forehand** (Yoga Half Split Pose), p. 169
> - **Forward, Down, and Out** (Yoga Cat Pose), p. 186
> - **Limbering Leg Yield** (Yoga Revolved Triangle Pose), p. 238
> - **La Giravolta Longe** (Yoga Revolved Half-Moon Pose), p. 274

The Core WELLNESS Plan

This Warm-Up Plan will provide excellent head-to-tail maintenance, repair, or stress relief.

The low-impact and low-pressure exercises included in this plan promote a soft, stretchy, and relaxed horse. They are ideal for horses that need to learn to relax, be allowed to recover, or simply need to maintain a healthy level of balance and coordination for life.

The Core Wellness Plan Exercises

- **Core Release Volte** (Yoga Half-Moon Pose), p. 156
- **Forward, Down, and Out** (Yoga Cat Pose), p. 186
- **The Rounding Rein-Back** (Yoga Garland Pose), p. 223
- **Limbering Leg Yield** (Yoga Revolved Triangle Pose), p. 238
- **La Giravolta Longe** (Yoga Revolved Half-Moon Pose), p. 274

The Core AGILITY Plan

This Warm-Up Plan is all about action.

The exercises included focus on enthusiasm, range of motion, and athleticism. This plan is right for the horse that needs to be ready to perform, as it will help him become alert, prepared, and ready to express himself as your enthusiastic partner.

> ### Core Agility Plan Exercises
>
> - **Turn on the Forehand** (Yoga Half Split Pose), p. 169
> - **Forward and Back** (Yoga Balancing Table to Tiptoe Chair Pose), p. 198
> - **The Driving Seat** (Yoga Chair Pose), p. 211
> - **The Rounding Rein-Back** (Yoga Garland Pose), p. 223
> - **Forward, Down, and Out to Competition Outline** (Yoga Cat to Cow Pose), p. 264

Putting It All Together

You should have a Core Score for your horse, and should also now have some idea of which Warm-Up Plan might best suit his needs. To show you how it should all come together, here is an example:

Blossom is a 16-hand show jumping mare. Her overall Core Score is a 3 because she becomes crooked easily, which makes her lean around corners, and her head comes up on the approach to fences.

The Core Flexibility Plan is a good choice to help her improve bend and roundness. By looking at each of the exercises in this plan (described in detail in Part Two), Blossom's owner will know how to perform the Warm-Up at the level right for the mare's Core Score of 3.

Specal Considerations

Existing Back Problems

For horses that have a Core Score of 4 or 5, it is best to work alongside your veterinarian and other practitioners to discuss a plan of action before beginning the core exercises, as all cases have their own idiosyncrasies. Existing back problems can evoke a dangerous situation for horse and rider. Without intention, pained horses can react quickly and unpredictably, so please always use your best judgment in a preventive manner. If the professionals supporting the horse feel that yoga-inspired exercises will help, work together as a team to help bring him back on track.

> Note: When it is not advisable to mount, **Exercise 10: La Giravolta Longe** (see p. 274) is an excellent way to begin a horse's retraining without needing to get onboard.

Youngsters

"If you have to fight a dragon, you shouldn't wait until it comes to the village," says Jordan Peterson, clinical psychologist and author of *Maps of Meanings*.

Considering the data, back complications in horses are much more common than they should be. When core conditioning, such as I have laid out in this book, is done in the very early stages of training, it is much easier to strengthen the horse's core than it is after it has become "defensively stable." Incorporating these exercises early is an

\\\ Bikram Choudhury ///

Bikram Choudhury

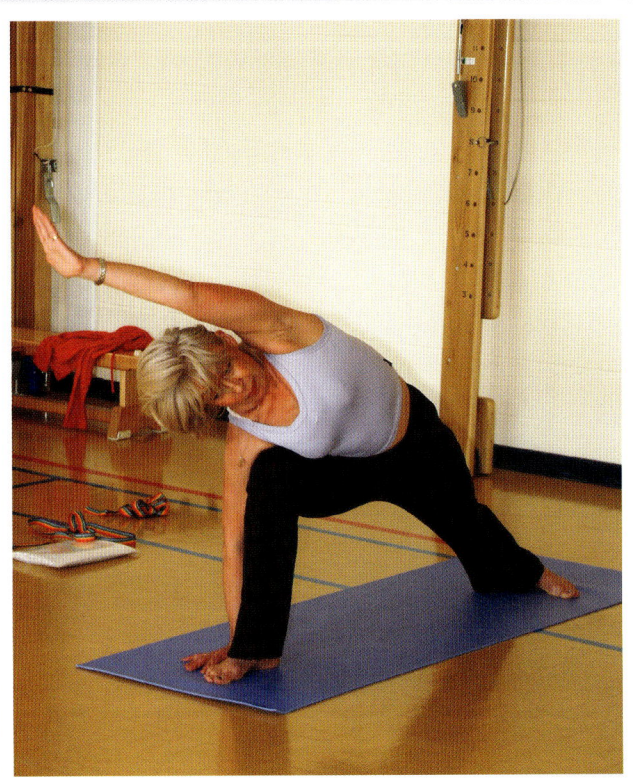

"Yoga is the only exercise in the world that you can do at any age. There is always some posture that will improve your health, mind, and soul."

excellent way to prevent much of the resistance that horses commonly display as training advances. Prevention of core weakness deserves its own book, although much can be done by using the Core Wellness Plan (see p. 109) to build the core in the youngster as early as possible.

Older Horses

With the exercises in this book, the horse never has to give more than he can comfortably offer. Yoga-inspired exercises are, in fact, ideal for maintaining mobility, quality of life, and usefulness in older horses. As with young horses, the Core Wellness Plan is ideal for older horses to keep them mobile and maintained throughout light work and retirement.

But before we get to know the exercises, I will first show you how to get the most from your Core Conditioning Warm-Up by riding it with true *Namaste*.

Namaste is Sanskrit for "my soul honors your soul." ∎

/5/ **How to Ride from the Horse's Core**

/6/ **10 Core Exercises for the Horse**

   / 🧘 / The Half-Moon Pose / 🐴 / The Core Release Volte
   / 🧘 / The Yoga Half-Split / 🐴 / The Turn on the Forehand
   / 🧘 / The Cat Pose / 🐴 / Forward, Down, and Out (FDO)
   / 🧘 / The Balancing Table to Tiptoe Chair Poses / 🐴 / Forward and Back
   / 🧘 / The Chair Pose / 🐴 / The Driving Seat
   / 🧘 / The Garland Pose / 🐴 / The Rounding Rein-Back
   / 🧘 / The Revolved Triangle Pose / 🐴 / The Limbering Leg-Yield
   / 🧘 / Thread the Needle Pose / 🐴 / The Perfect Pirouette
   / 🧘 / The Cat to Cow Pose / 🐴 / Forward, Down, and Out to Competition Outline
   / 🧘 / The Revolved Half-Moon Pose / 🐴 / La Giravolta Longe

/7/ **Happy Bendy Horsey!**

THE CORE CONDITIONING
EXERCISE

PART TWO: THE CORE CONDITIONING EXERCISES

\\\ Arthur Ashe ///

Arthur Ashe

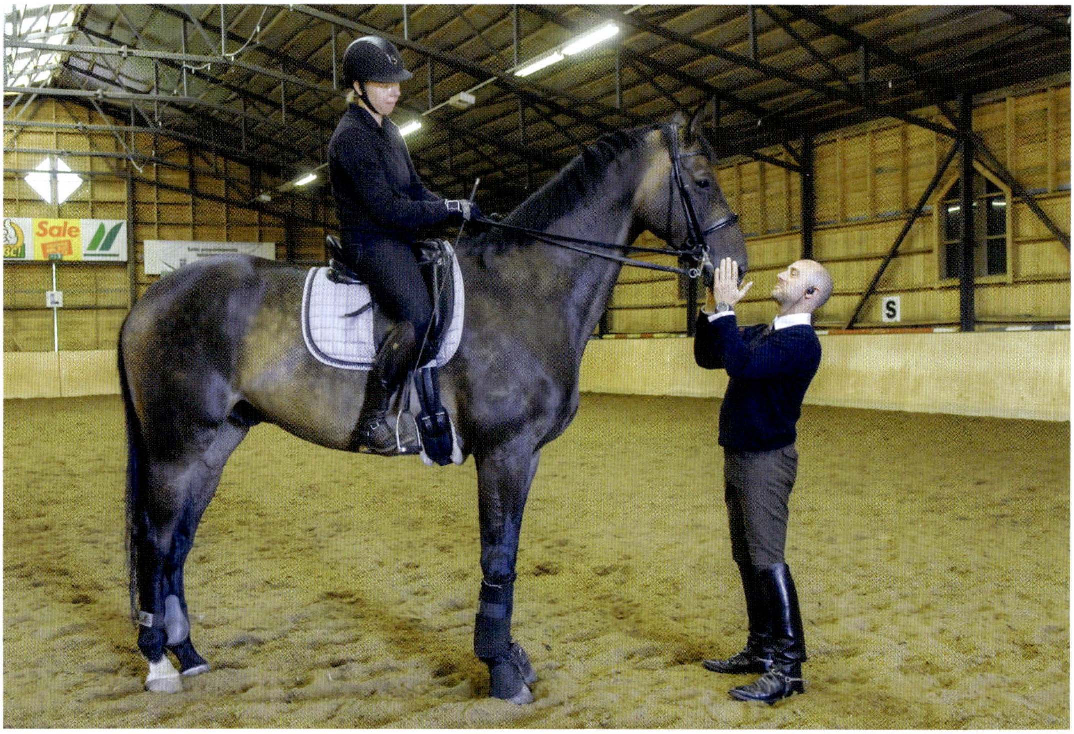

*"Start where you are,
do what you can,
use what you have."*

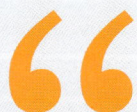

5

How to Ride from the Horse's Core

The Core Conditioning and Warm-Up exercises will improve your horse's core just by performing them. Your role as the rider is to guide your horse into doing them well. Warming up the core requires different outlines to be used, as well as several Head and Neck Positions (what I'll call HNPs going forward), so the riding style is more therapeutic than dynamic. Our goal here is to stretch, release, and encourage so we must be giving, allowing, and following. This chapter will explain how to bring out the best in your horse's Core Warm-Up. It teaches riding, yoga-style.

Unknown

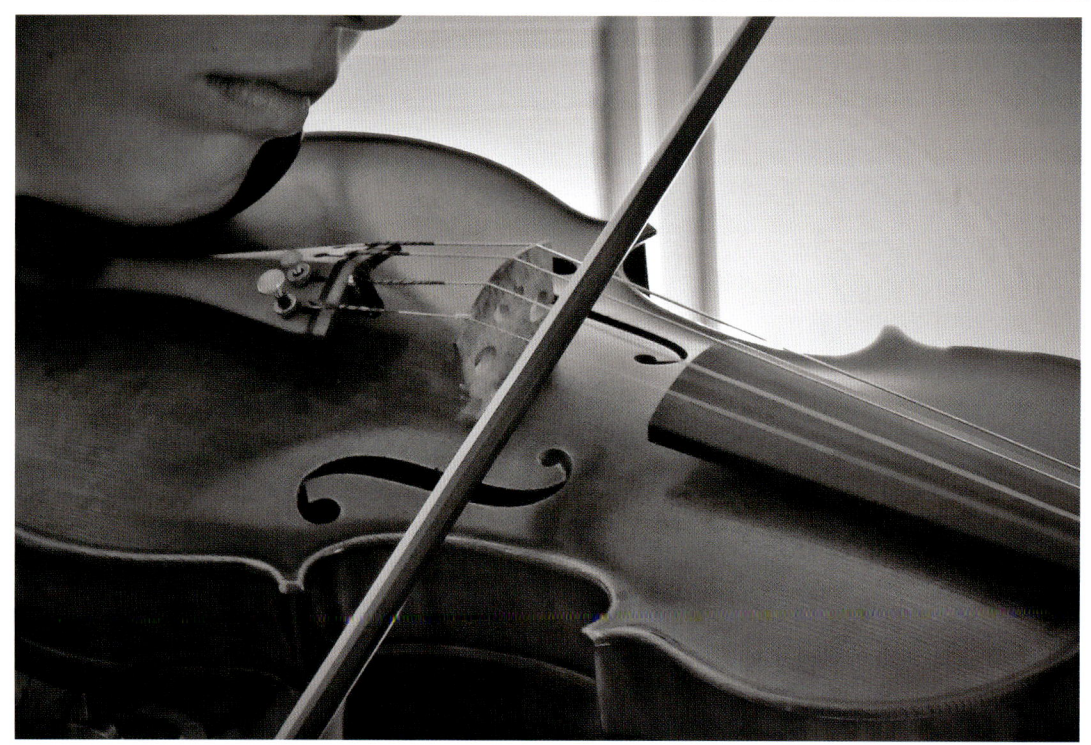

*"A horse is like a violin.
First it must be tuned,
then it must be accurately played."*

Building Blocks:
What You Need to Know for the Core Exercises

20 Minutes of Feedback

As well as an opportunity to improve our horses, a comprehensive Warm-Up is a very important feedback period. This is the first section of your daily ride where you can get to know what is easy and hard for the horse on that day, giving you a focus and a realistic level of expectation for the next part of the ride. Using the core exercises ahead, we can create suppleness, freedom, and calm from the start, improving everything that comes after. This initial phase is probably the most important part of the whole session, as a stiff horse cannot perform happily.

The ideal Warm-Up Plan is 20 minutes—an appropriate length of time to read the horse and help his weak areas come into play, slowly and confidently. A shorter time seems to produce limited results as the horse seems to need this minimum to find his place, both mentally and physically, and to move on to more complicated requests.

Connecting the Exercises

Creating a fluid floor plan for your Warm-Up is a great way of keeping the horse's mind in the moment and on the aids. The horse needs to feel unrestricted and unhurried throughout this period, and the most efficient way to do this is to string the five exercises in each Plan together with short interludes of free-walk on a long rein.

\\\ Michael Klimke ///
Michael Klimke

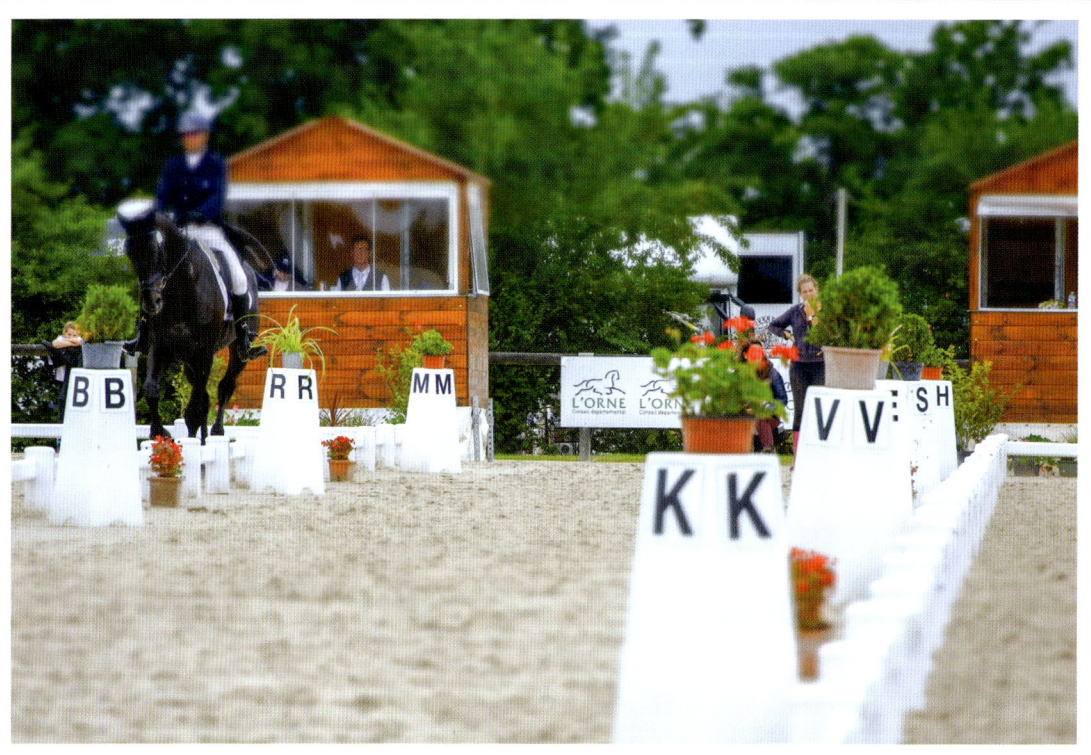

"Most dressage tests are won in the warm-up."

„

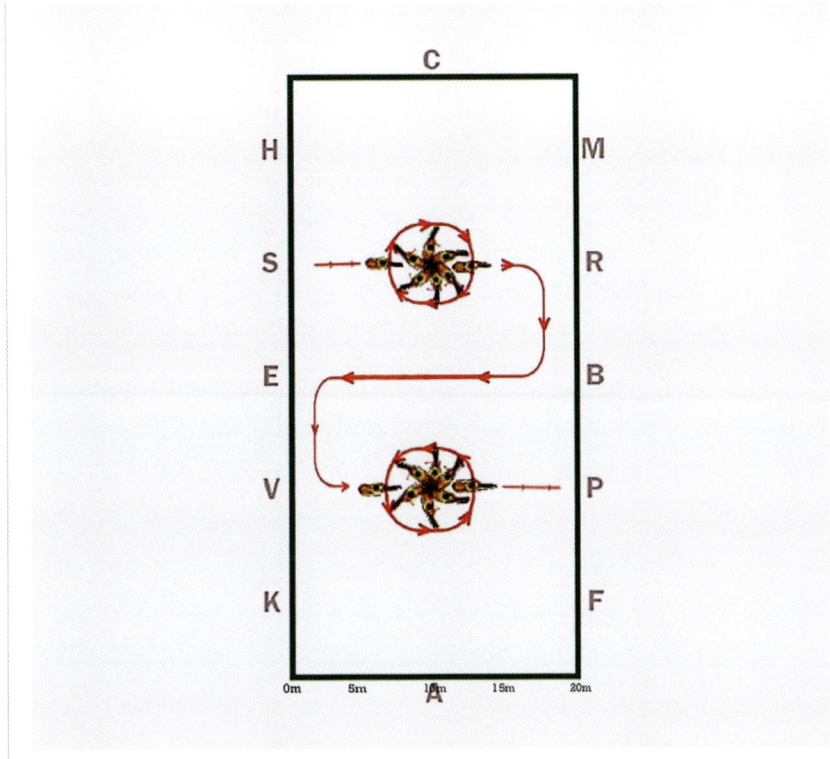

◀ / 5.1 / *Each exercise has a floor plan that shows an ideal way of beginning, performing, and ending the routine.*

After performing an exercise, and hopefully achieving a good response, letting the reins slip into a Long-and-Low or Forward, Down, and Out HNP is both an instant confirmation of achievement for the horse to recognize, and also dissipates any tensions that may have surfaced by releasing his topline completely. After a few free-walk strides and perhaps a change of direction, the rein contact can be re-established and the same exercise can be done in the new direction, or you can move on to one of the other exercises in your Warm-Up Plan.

Variety will keep the horse fresh and positive even if you have to return to the same exercise frequently to solve a problem.

A varied floor plan will keep the horse from getting too focused on the difficult by intermixing it with what he finds easier.

Using Core Warm-Up Exercises for Specific Purposes

Core conditioning with these exercises as a full workout session or to solve a specific issue is an excellent and worthwhile plan as it can help develop a horse without causing stress in between the moments of progress, which can happen all too easily in normal schooling. If it is obvious from the start that going on to more demanding work will only have both horse and rider become even more "blocked," it can be very helpful to spend as much time helping the horse stretch, release, and relax, as he needs. Whole sessions of core conditioning can be very beneficial for a horse like this, and as a result, he can genuinely get past the problem and move on to better things.

Warming Down

Stretching is an excellent way to end a training session, too. As a warm-down, Forward, Down, and Out (The Cat Pose—see p. 186) will not only relax the horse mentally as you offer a long rein, but more importantly, it will fully stretch the back, spine, and core, offering a superb way of "shaking out" any tension before leaving the arena loose, free, and feeling good.

"Everyone has weak spots," says Andrew Peloquin, high-intensity interval training specialist. "Muscles or muscle groups that have trouble keeping up. It's time to turn those weaknesses into strengths."

The Three Exercise Levels: *Release, Coordination,* and *Tone*

For each of the exercises ahead there are three Levels of challenge. Each one will help the horse in a different way. They are *Release, Coordination,* and finally, *Tone the core.*

- **RELEASE LEVEL**—To decompress, stretch, and mobilize the whole body.
- **COORDINATION LEVEL**—To improve posture and balance.
- **TONE LEVEL**—To develop engagement, strength and skill.

1: *Release* Level

Release is the first and most profound Level of the three. It is not first because it is the least, it is first because it is the best. This Level is all about deep stretches, confidence, and freedom.

One of the main objectives of Release Level is to allow a Core Release (see p. 30) to be felt by the horse, not only to free the spine but also to give us the Long-and-Low Outline to work with. All the static (on the spot) and dynamic (free-walk) exercises will align the horse's spine in just the right way for this to happen. With an established Core Release it is possible to then go up to the next Level (Coordination) or use the moment as an opportunity to practice your horse's trickiest exercise from the best starting place of all: softness.

Kyra Kyrklund, Finnish dressage rider and six-time Olympian, says, "I work quite a lot in the walk. What you and your horse can't do

\\\ Dalton Wong ///

Dalton Wong

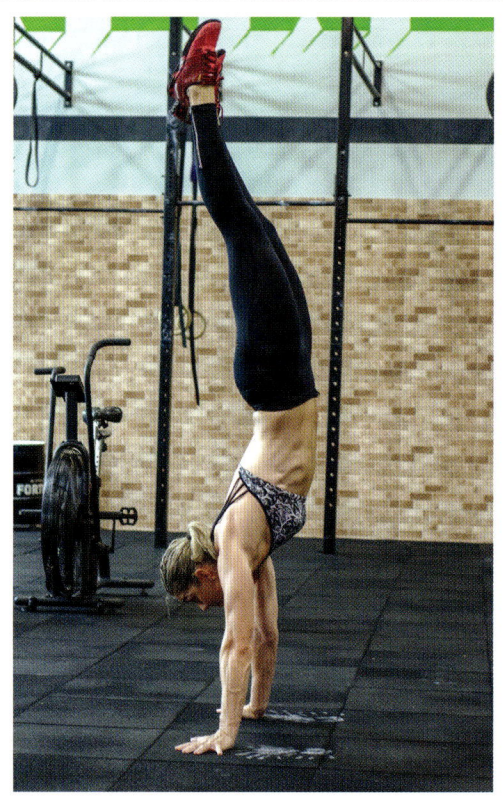

"It is important to work on your weaknesses, not your strengths. Do the stuff you're bad at and the stuff you're already good at can only get better."

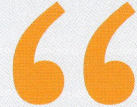

slowly, you can't do at the speed of trot or canter either." All the moving (dynamic) exercises at Release Level are in the free-walk. The free-walk is said to be the "Queen of Gaits"—and she most certainly is. This is the gait from which most of the core can be conditioned. The low intensity, four-time movement naturally gives all the muscles enough stimulation and range of motion to relax, consider things calmly, and then let go and begin to move as nature intended. The walk itself is not the easiest to work with as it can take many forms, which is why it is rewarded so highly in a dressage test (a good walk can win you the class).

There are many advantages to beginning a ride with stretching at the walk. If the horse's core is at all restricted, only the walk gets deep enough to do good without triggering the tension. The higher the impulsion, the more tension will cover the weak areas that we are here to access. The free-walk is therefore a primary conditioning tool. "In the calmness of the walk," taught Nuno Oliveira, "horse and rider can find the time to think and to prepare the quality of the following trot and canter."

The Release Level also gives you valuable, real-time insight into what is strong and weak in your horse on any given day. Some of the exercises will feel easy in both directions, others will be more on one side than the other, and over time, it will be obvious exactly what your horse's best and worst movements are, allowing you to practice the ones needed most.

2: *Coordination* Level

Remember, as Yo-Yo Ma, famed Chinese-American cellist, says, "When a problem is complex, you become tense, but when you break it down

\\\ Dr. Rob Van Wessum ///

Dr. Rob Van Wessum

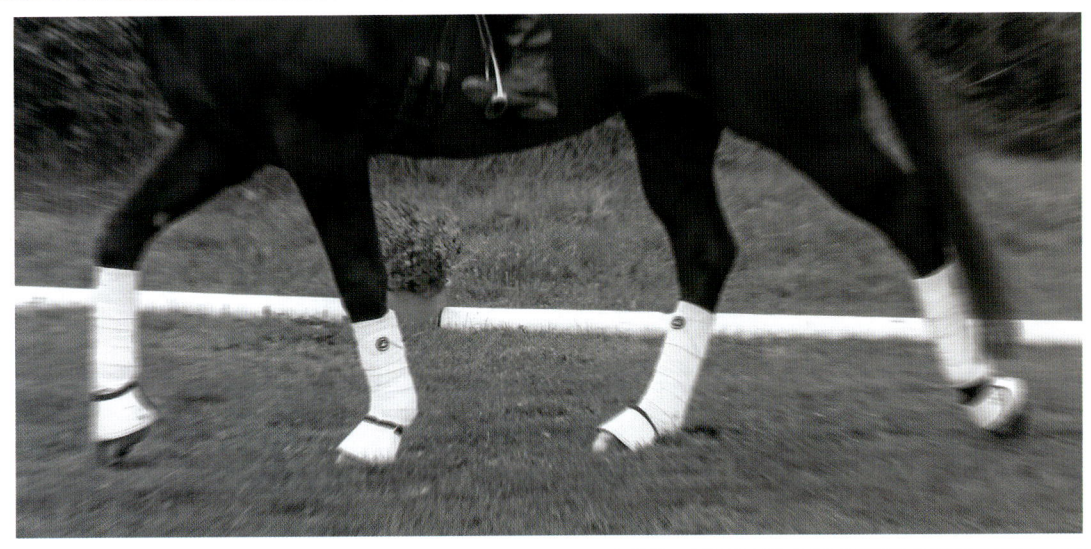

*"The walk has a lot of action;
it really helps develop the horse."*

into basic components, you can approach each element without stress."
Once the horse begins to Release happily and easily during an
exercise, it is time to introduce the next Level, *Coordination*. You will
do the same exercise, yet either with more static steps or in a different
gait. With emphasis upon balance, muscle control, and reflexes, this
Level is designed to develop all-round stability. You will ask the horse
to organize his limbs and string his steps together into the beginning
of a rhythm.

The dynamic Coordination exercises are done in the soft and relaxed
trot d'école—the "schooling trot"—which is as old as the hills for good
reason. The term comes from *Le Cadre Noir,* but it surely goes all the
way back to Greece, as most equestrian wisdom does. This trot is the
supple, chewing-gum gait that can be done all day, and that was its
original purpose.

The *trot d'école* is an extremely useful compromise. As a base for
relaxed core work, we need a naturally balanced, comfortable and
easy gait conducive to low-stress Coordination training, giving the
horse the time he needs to think about his legs: where they are and
what to do with them next.

With any change as fundamental as core training, the horse's body
will go through developments. At this Level, alterations in gait will
be noticed by the rider. Although the gait will alter in a pleasing way
by becoming more comfortable, it often will feel oddly lacking in
power. This is to be expected, as some of the muscles being called into
use are very weak or simply may have never been used. Daily practice
will see fluidity gradually develop as these weak areas strengthen.

3: *Tone* Level

The *Tone* Level is not intended to be the hardest or the fastest. Nothing so crude. It is, though, the most intensive and challenging.

Toning develops ideal posture and great technique from right in the center of the horse's body. Riding the exercises at the Tone Level teaches the horse to be confident and relaxed under light, natural, self-induced impulsion. This can only been done if the horse has developed enough wherewithal from the previous Level (Coordination). As always, if an exercise is ever too tricky, dropping a Level is an easy solution.

In the Tone Level, you will use the *petit galop* for the majority of the dynamic exercises. *Petit galop* is indeed another term from the French School, but alas, *les Français* can't take credit this time, either, because this gait was *the* fundamental training tool of the Roman Cavalry's Hippika Gymnasia School a few thousand years prior. Nevertheless, the gait itself is a super way to develop cantering skills in the most relaxed way possible.

The *petit galop* is just that—a small comfortable canter that is above all easy, unhurried, and relaxing for both horse and rider. Energy levels can vary, yet not at the expense of rhythm, which should be cared for. After achieving results from the previous Level, this gait will allow you to connect the horse's core elements easily while under light impulsion—perfect for toning the body and warming it prior to exertion.

\\\ Bertil Voss ///
Bertil Voss

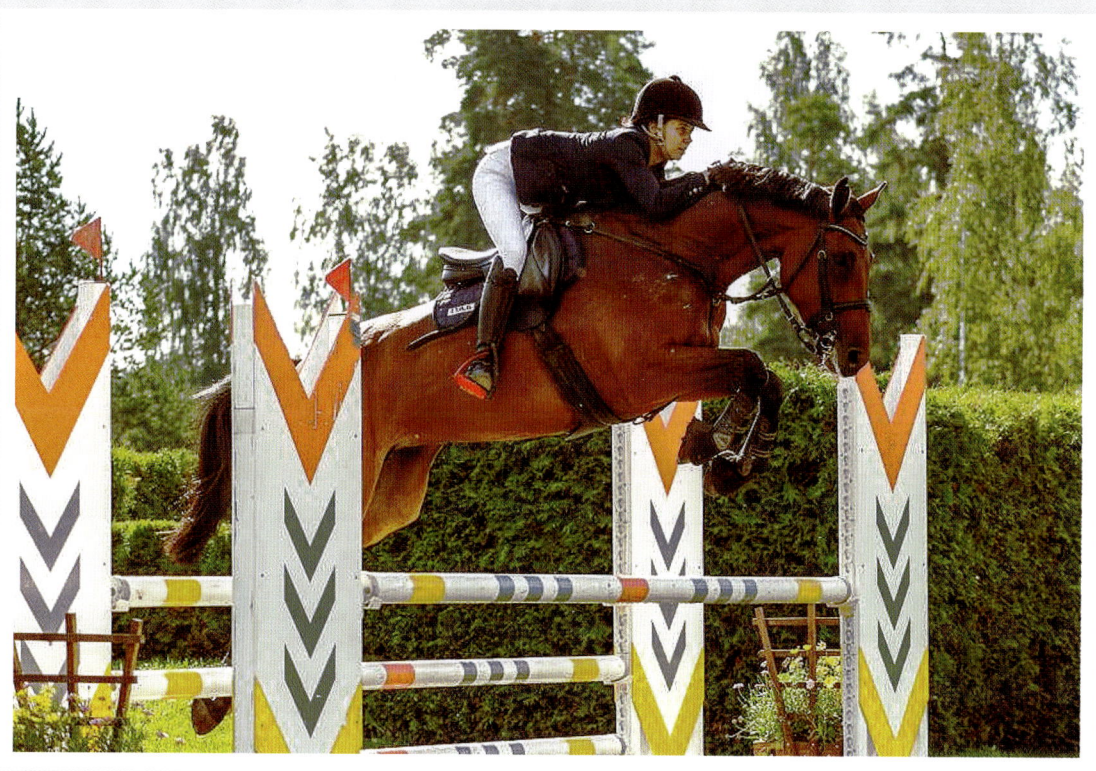

*"You must never rush the horse;
if you do, he will lose
natural balance."*

❞

Throughout, as American dressage Olympian Steffen Peters reminds us: "Keep things simple. You don't want to have to micromanage so many little things."

In all the Levels there is one important rule: Slow is smooth, and smooth is fast!

Head-and-Neck Positions (HNP)

Training a horse to work through the core will develop a very good relationship with your horse's head, neck, and mouth. Different head-and-neck positions (HNP) are crucial for accessing the deeper core structures, as the HNP and the rest of the spine are one wiggly unit. Each HNP has a direct and immediate influence on the rest of the spine.

The core exercises and Levels use HNP as follows:

HNP 1: The Long-and-Low Outline and the Core Release

This is a super HNP for almost all the exercises and a wonderful, loosening posture for everyday work (fig. 5.2).

The Long-and-Low Outline is the simplest and most useful of all the schooling outlines. It is also completely natural. This outline is a direct result of a Core Release (see p. 30) so the horse's mouth, head, and neck are weightless and the back relaxed. One of this HNP's main benefits is that it helps dissolve commonplace tension in the horse's back's main

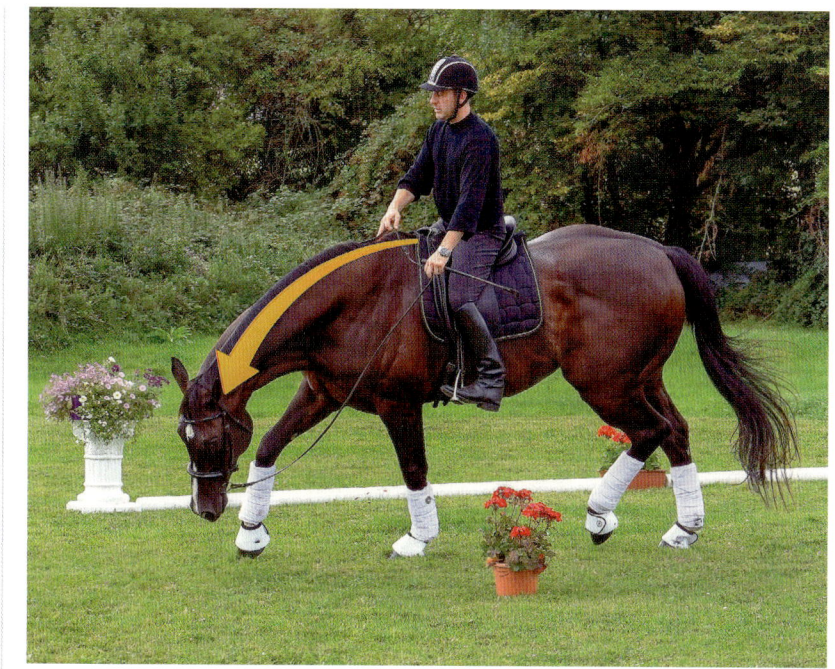

◀ / 5.2 / *Wardance demonstrates the Long-and-Low head-and-neck position (HNP). He is liberated through the back and released through the core.*

muscles, the *longissimus dorsi,* by placing them under gentle traction. Using the horse's on-board biomechanics, this lower frame provides the two Core Powers of Nuchal and Thoracic Lift with the angles they need to round the horse's body completely naturally (fig. 5.3).

In Long-and-Low HNP, the horse's ears should be lower than his withers, and his nose is ideally hanging between chest and knee level. The nose must always be allowed to stretch out as much as it wants, so as long as you are not holding the horse's nose in, you just provide a contact to communicate through. In reality, horses move their heads a lot while finding release or balance, so nose angle should not be obsessed over. Whatever your horse does with his head, it will gradually improve as his core does.

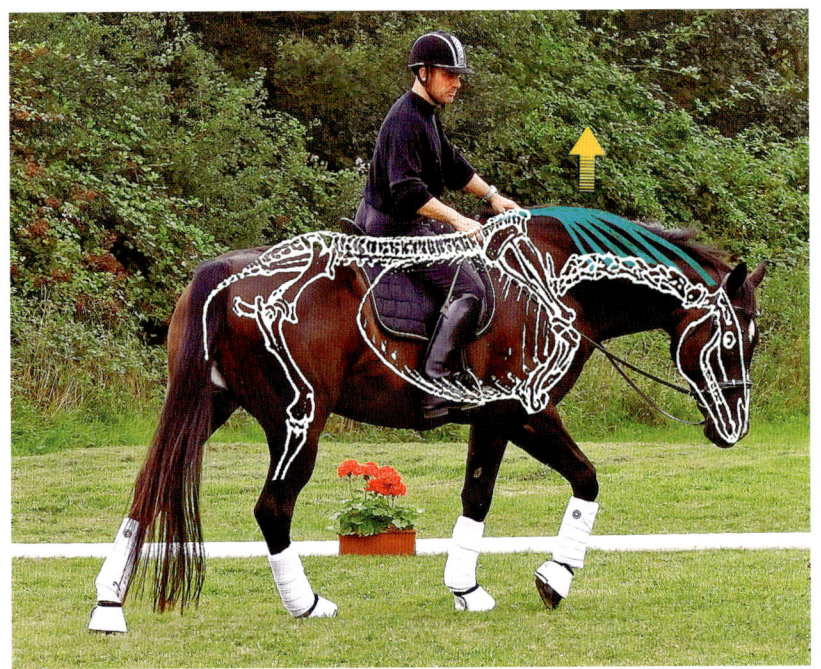

/ 5.3 / *The Nuchal Lift in Long-and-Low HNP. As the horse's head lowers, the Nuchal Lift pulls the spine vertically.* ▶

"Long-and-Low is a test of your training technique," explains British Olympian Carl Hester. "Go into rising (posting) trot and drop the reins. Your horse should stretch down… if he sticks his head up, something needs adjusting in your training."

Long-and-Low requires the horse's back, shoulders, and neck to stretch out, but it does not stretch the whole length of the spine. For that we have the next head-and-neck position.

HNP 2: Forward, Down, and Out (Yoga Cat Pose)

Long-and-Low leads to its big brother: *Forward, Down, and Out* (FDO). This HNP is so important, it has its own exercise (see p. 186)!

Indeed, FDO's party trick is to fully release the horse's spinal column and activate all three Core Powers (see p. 44 for a reminder of these).

By gradually releasing all pressure on the spine, each vertebra has the ideal alignment to begin moving as it was designed through its vertical, lateral, and rotational axes (fig. 5.4). This is a similar effect to that the Yoga Cat Pose has on humans and is a fundamental achievement of muscular release and spinal alignment, and a mainstay of an athlete's warm-up.

FDO performed to the Tone Level is proof of a complete Core Release and a clear test of core condition (fig. 5.5). It is of dramatic benefit to the horse to learn this stretch, yet it is profound; therefore, it will take time to achieve. Many internal mechanisms must self-organize to enable this core-driven posture. A full muscular release cannot be rushed, as

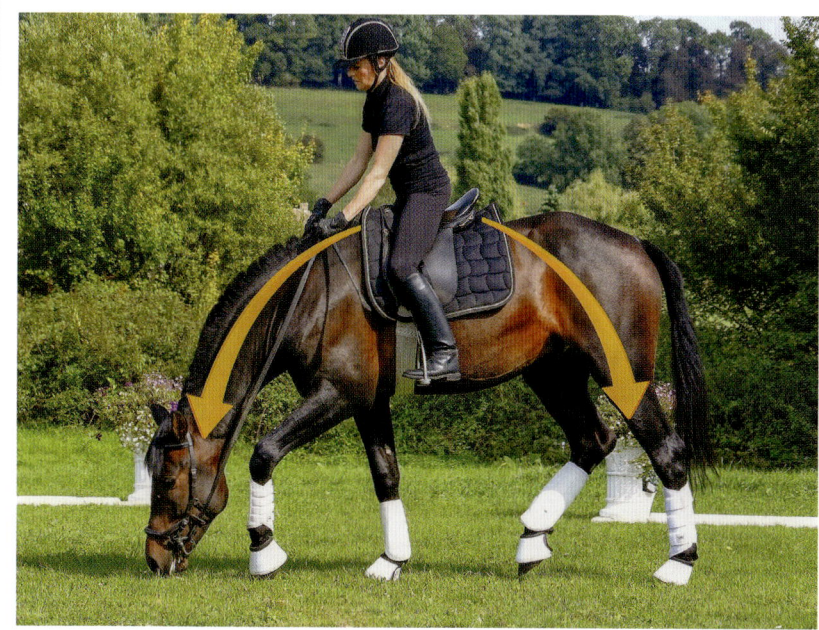

◀ / 5.4 / *The full "grazing" stretch: Bo demonstrates his suppleness in Forward, Down, and Out HNP.*

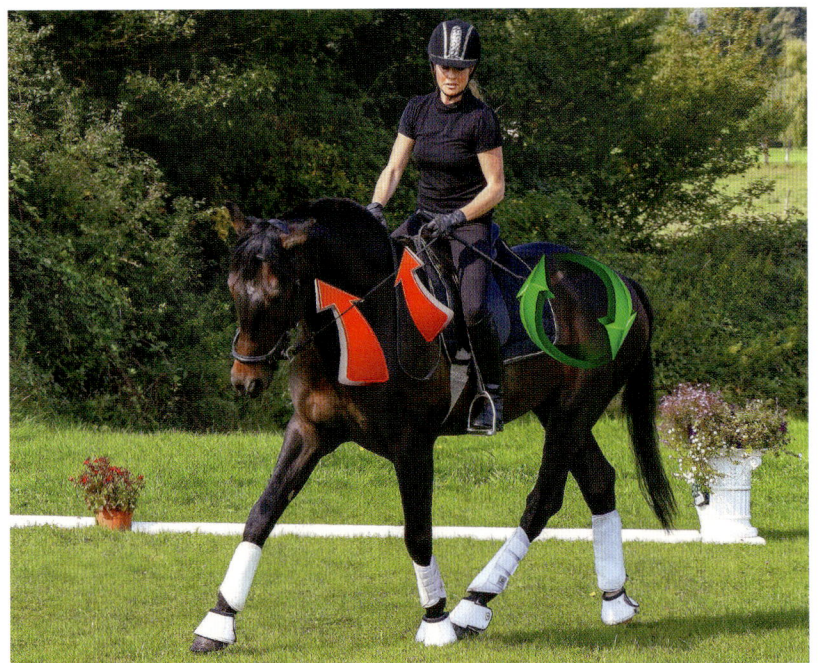

/ 5.5 / *The three Core Powers can develop only when Forward, Down, and Out has released the full length of the spine.* ▶

a horse must trust his body enough to allow the release to happen, and that is quite a brave thing to do for a horse. Our job is to present him with the daily opportunity and encouragement to stretch all the way Forward, Down, and Out—and free himself. Hester says, "When a horse is tired, he'll try to stretch down. Let him do it for a while as it's something you want to encourage. To stretch your horse, lengthen the rein, lower your hand and massage his mouth with the bit by gently squeezing and releasing each rein. Stretch him regularly throughout your training sessions to relax him and reduce the risk of tension."

When your horse is supple enough to perform FDO in walk, trot, and canter, he has achieved full spinal freedom and will be very straight, comfortable, and 100 percent life-affirming to ride.

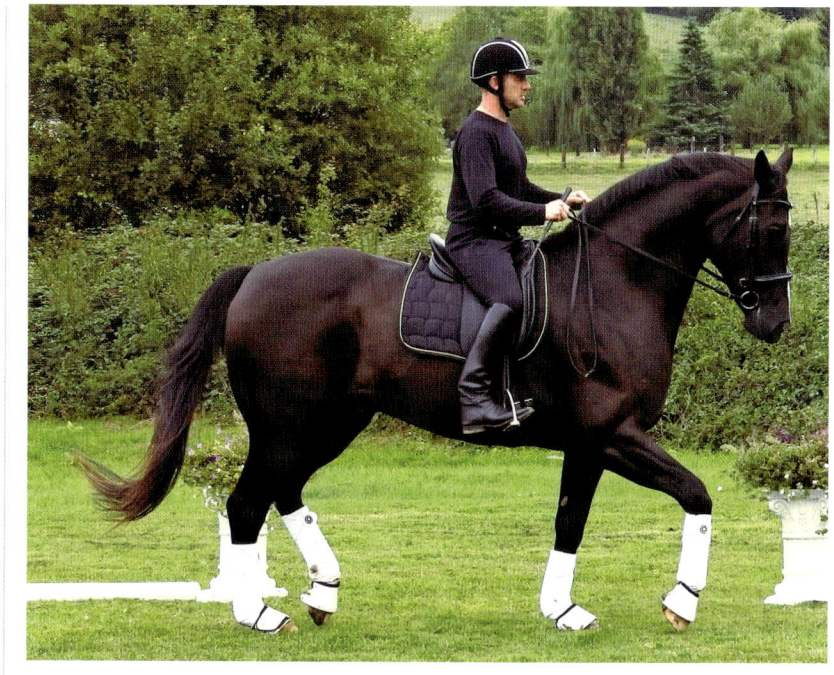

◀ / 5.6 / *The Competition Outline: An alert, supple, and harmonious outline, ideal for all equestrian sport.*

HNP 3: The Competition Outline (Yoga Cow Pose)

When the horse has become stronger and can perform most of the core exercises at Tone Level (see p. 128), you will find that riding in a tension-free Competition Outline, otherwise known as "on the bit," feels natural, uncomplicated, and easy (fig. 5.6). Here is the definition of "on the bit" from the Fédération Equestre Internationale (FEI Rules for Dressage 2018, Article 401):

In all the work, even at the halt, the horse must be "on the bit."
A horse is said to be "on the bit" when the neck is more or less raised
and arched according to the stage of training and the extension
or collection of the pace, accepting the bridle with a light and consistent soft

submissive contact. The head should remain in a steady position, as a rule slightly in front of the vertical, with a supple poll as the highest point of the neck, and no resistance should be offered to the Athlete.

The Competition Outline HNP is in many ways an objective in itself. When the horse's core is sufficiently conditioned it will be possible to spend more and more time in this HNP without tension creeping in, allowing higher and higher levels of performance to be achieved with less and less "effort" from the rider. This is an outline of athleticism, and it will bring success in any discipline.

Yoga-Inspired Warm-Up Aids

The core is an extremely precise and sensitive piece of biomechanics. It also is very adept at defending itself with tension; therefore, if we want to see, feel, and develop core mechanisms, it is important that our aids, ways, and reactions are thoroughly proactive and encouraging.

Seat Aid: Going with the Flow

There is a world of information about sitting in the perfect position on a horse. It is of course a very important component of riding well. For the purposes of the core exercises in this book, your seat has one outstanding role, which is to *go with the horse.* As riders we can all too easily find ourselves in a "blocking" seat, where our weight isn't going forward with the horse's back, but instead, we find ourselves leaning back and down a little, into him. It is easily done, yet nothing will "dip" a horse's back quicker.

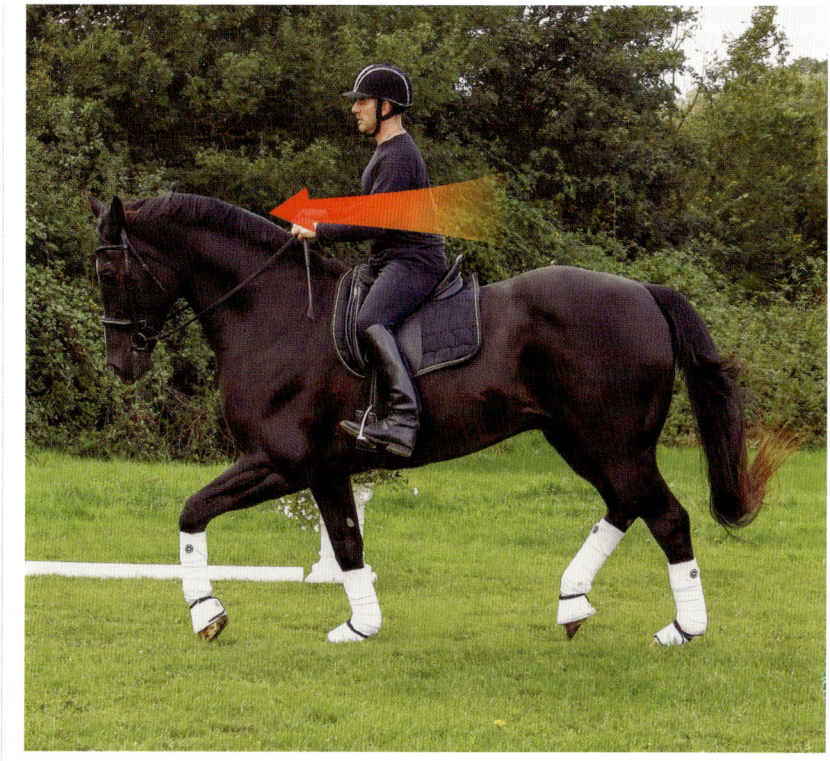

◀ / 5.7 / *The seat going with the flow. The rider's weight should always go with the horse's back, even when slowing down.*

Even from a psychological view, horses seem to cooperate much more when the rider has a ready and ever-so-slightly forward seat, even when slowing down (fig. 5.7). It makes some sense that they will always prefer to feel us following them rather than bracing against their movement, as that seems to be just the sort of contradiction that confuses them.

With the core exercises I'm going to show you, it is helpful to use your seat in a very encouraging way, particularly if you are trying to improve a horse's confidence. Then, when his gaits and paces become more comfortable, sitting in any position is a breeze.

\\\ Isabell Werth ///

Isabell Werth

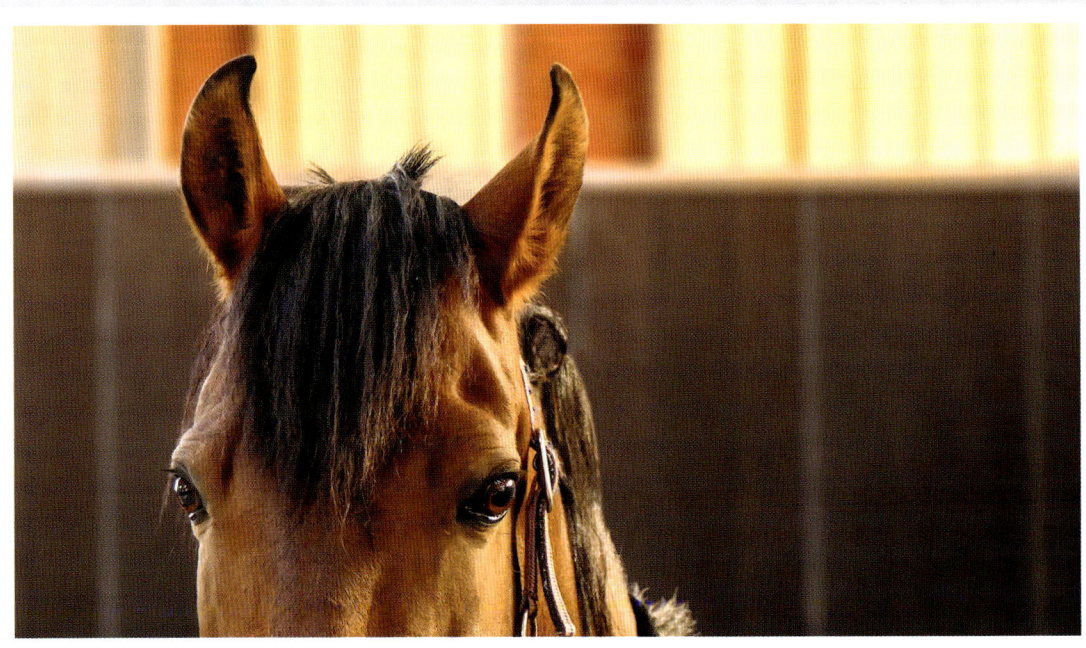

*"Keep him in front of you and flex more.
When you work in flexion he will become
lower behind, up in the neck,
and safe in the contact."*

Rein Aid: The Stretching Flexion

A dressage flexion is commonly considered to be seeing the horse's "inside eye" during a turn, with a uniform bend through poll, neck, and back. This is, of course, correct in a dressage test situation where the training has been theoretically achieved, though to achieve it you have to be clearer and help the horse establish such fine responses and

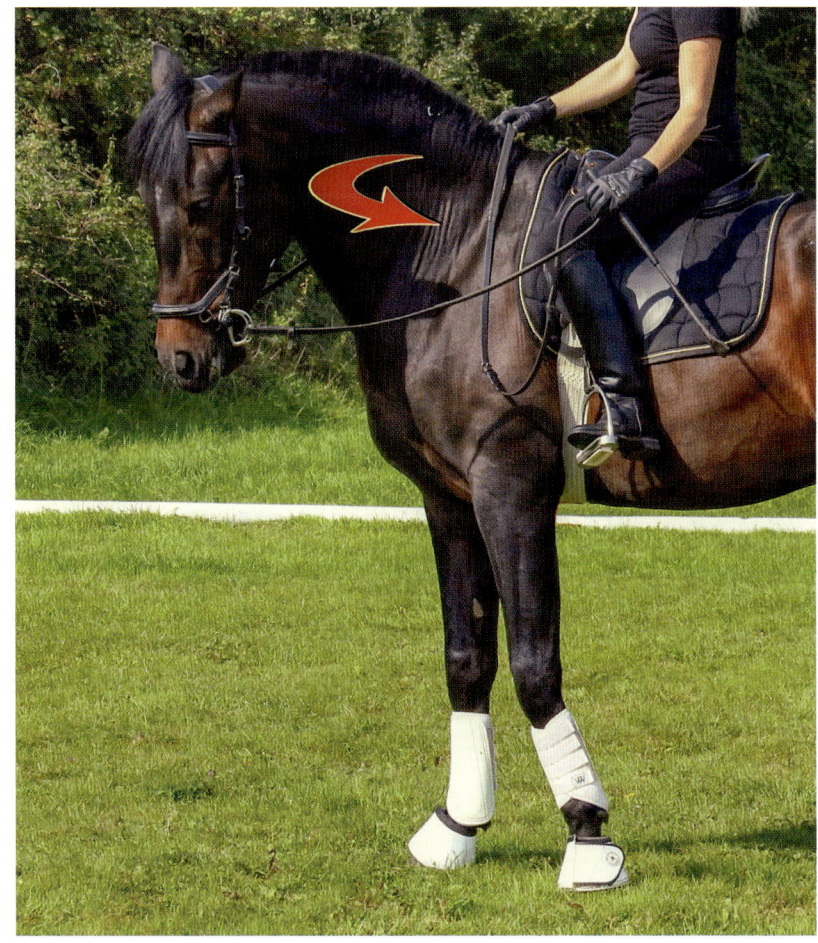

◄ / 5.8 / *The Stretching Flexion: During low-impact exercises, this rein aid creates the ideal amount of flexion needed to help align the horse's spine.*

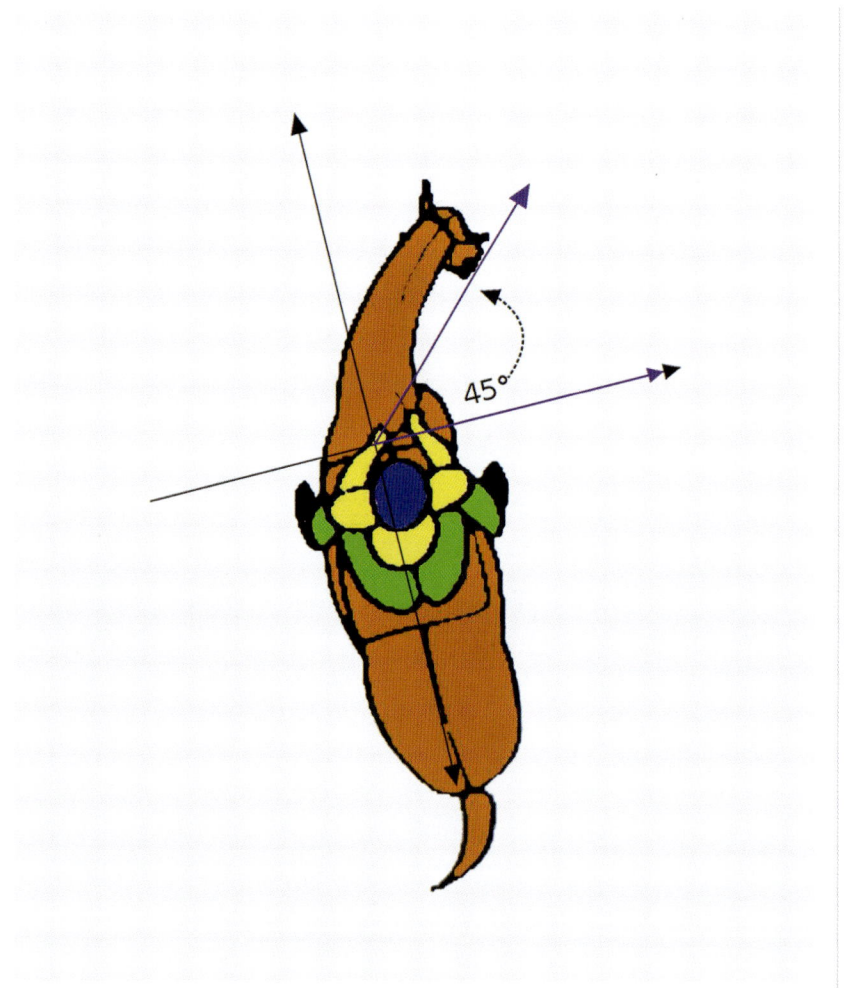

/ 5.9 / *The angle required to release the core and allow the horse to stretch into a soft, Long-and-Low HNP is approximately 45 degrees.* ▶

results. In this sense, training dressage movements to improve dressage is a little like learning to skydive after leaving the plane.

Your job with this aid is to simply hold the inside rein contact still, keeping the neck at 45–50 degrees during the movements that require it—the rest is done by Mother Nature (figs. 5.8 & 5.9).

When alignment happens and the core releases, the horse will round to the inside rein automatically, dropping your inside contact. It is as simple and wonderful as that.

Rein Aid: Hold, Not Pull

Four-time Olympian Steffen Peters reminds us, "When we touch a horse on the inside rein, he should bend to the inside. The horse must answer to this."

When you create the Stretching Flexion, the way in which you *hold* the rein is important if you are to help release the horse. When your horse shows he would like to round himself, it is very important that he is encouraged by immediately rewarding with a forward hand, allowing the horse to stretch into his newfound roundness as much as he wants to (fig. 5.10).

While creating the inside flexion you should:

/1/ Use a "rubbery" inside rein contact.
/2/ Shorten the rein to the right length and *hold* the Stretching Flexion at 45 degrees—don't take or give (for now).
/3/ Wait for the horse to react to the leg part of the aid (whatever that exercise requires), then—when he rounds just a little and begins to release his core—you can reward him by giving him the inside rein.

When the horse's core is strong enough he will be able to become round from your leg aid only, leaving you nothing to do with the inside rein in corners—as it should be.

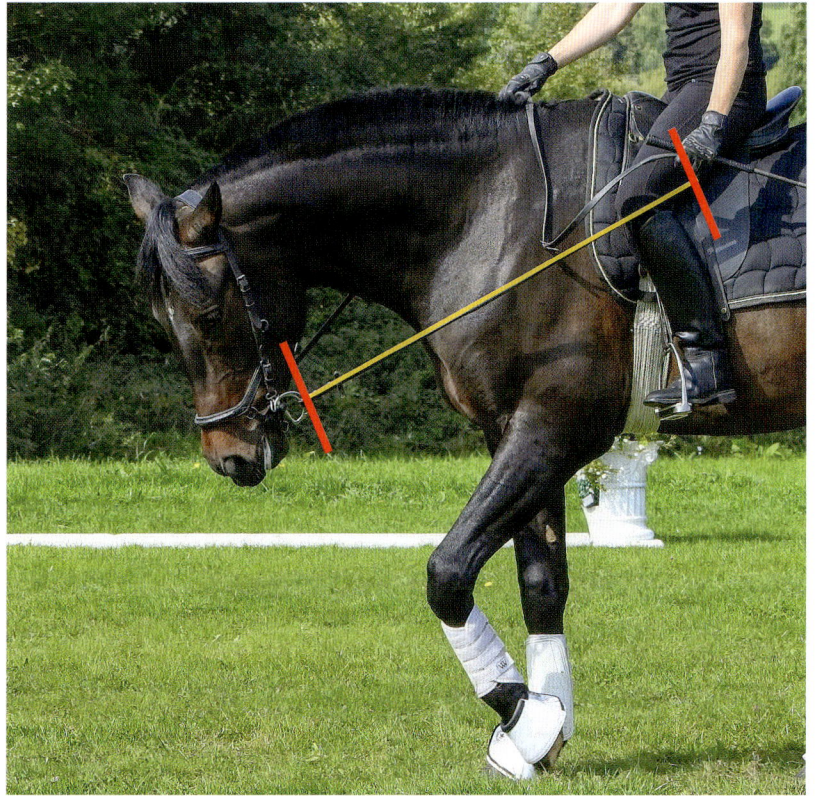

/ 5.10 / Holding the rein is different than pulling. The horse must not feel trapped, so you must never pull. Hold and give are the only rein aids that will help a horse align and release. ▶

Rein Aid: "Framing" the Outside of the Horse

In your Warm-Up Plan, it helps to keep things simple. For example, if your horse is not responding to your inside leg, there is little point giving any outside aids as there is nothing on the outside to "catch"—nothing to *Frame*—and we risk overloading the horse with aids that he can't process.

When the horse does become more supple and can move sideways easily, away from your light inside leg aid, you need to Frame the

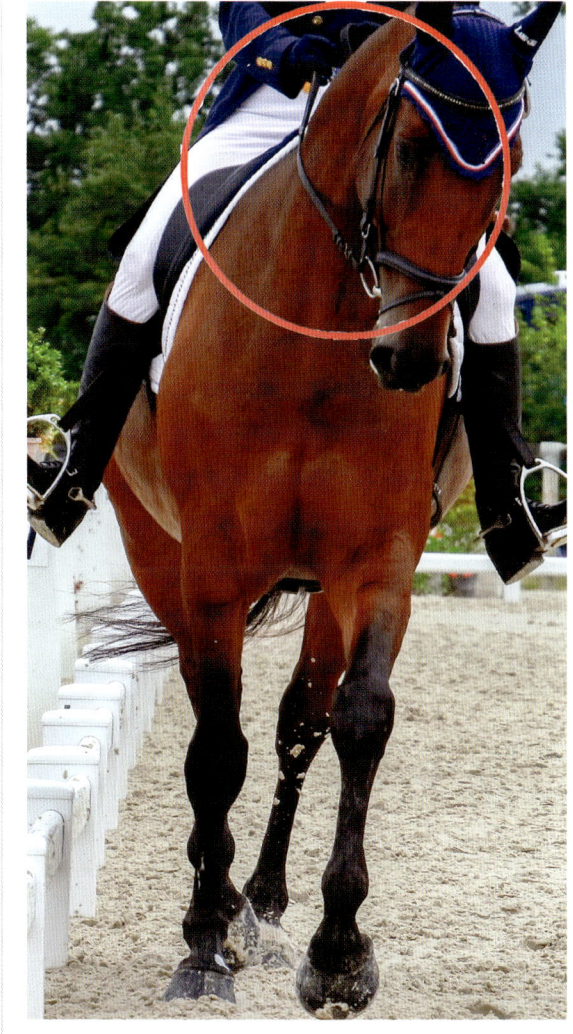

◀ / 5.11 / *Framing the horse with the outside rein: When the horse has a strong core, we can channel the outside of his body and do not need the inside rein.*

lateral movement somehow or the horse will yield to the leg and you will go sideways when you ask for bend.

Framing the outside of the horse with your outside rein is the solution. If you provide a good, firm outside rein contact, it allows you to channel and Frame the shoulder, sending the balance forward and preventing it from sliding sideways (fig. 5.11). The Perfect Pirouette (Yoga Thread the Needle—see p. 250) is the very exercise to practice this important understanding between horse and rider.

Framing will eventually bring superb steering to your steed.

Mind Aid: Variety—Keep Him in the Zone

Here it helps for us to consider the words of Paulo Coelho de Souza, the Brazilian novelist: "When you are enthusiastic about what you do, you feel this positive energy. It's very simple."

The whip and spur aids create *reactions,* but we don't want reactions, we want *understandings.* There is no understanding in a reaction; it simply delivers discomfort that the horse moves away from. From an educational point of view alone, this method is a poor teacher because the victim becomes desensitized to its significance. This is why tools like the whip and spur become "necessary" equipment. When the horse moves away from the spur, he is not more likely to listen to the leg next time than the last. Only showing him, then encouraging and rewarding his attempts, will do that.

By using a little "herbie psychology" you can motivate the horse proactively to try things, keeping your friend relaxed and receptive in the Alert Learning Zone (see p. 76).

One of our best tools in training may be repetition, but it can very easily be taken too far. The endless circles with countless non-respondent aids are all too familiar and would turn anyone into a sleepwalker. No, it is our job to keep our horses entertained, alert, and learning how to *do* things, rather than how to avoid them. As Mary Poppins famously said, "In every job that must be done, find the fun and the job's a game!"

Mind Aid: The Tidbit Reward

If you want your horse to learn quickly, you must appeal to his mind in its special "herbie" terms. There is one power in the universe that has a special psychological hold over our horses: their favorite snacks (fig. 5.12).

Whether an actual carrot, a mint, or yesterday's ciabatta, the road to the horse's heart and mind has many flavors and this can be a critical

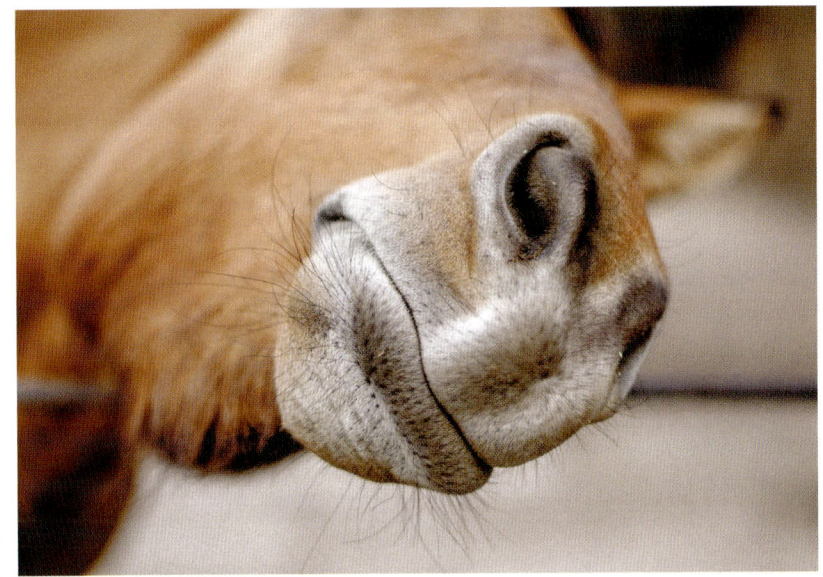

◀ / 5.12 / There is power in a tidbit! The instantaneous gift of a favorite snack tells the horse he did well in a way that can't be matched with a pat.

educational tool when used wisely. Immediately administering a treat when he *just* did something really well translates in his mind as a positive, friendly, and above all, *memorable* act worthy of repetition. Voila, suddenly you have a very attentive dance partner! This is, of course, completely natural. Horses exist in real-time and do not really associate a pat with the half-pass they did 30 seconds ago. Timing is everything in "Herbie World."

Training with treats has a wonderful side effect: As the horse is deciding to perform for a tidbit, the progress that you make in a training or warm-up session becomes, in his eyes, his idea. It is a win-win.

There must be a word of warning though: For your equine friend, this concept can become an obsession, and you risk being seen as nothing more than a walking Pez dispenser. So please, use this Mind Aid wisely, or you may awaken a hungry, slathering monster.

Mind Aid: The Tapping Stick

There are subtler ways to get the horse on team and in the game. Horses don't need a penalty; they need an explanation. We must remember that they haven't seen the latest Ingrid Klimke video and don't have a clue what we want or expect, so we need a *kind* way of inducing a horse to move, and that is simple: become a fly (fig. 5.13).

The horse's skin is so sensitive that you never need anything that causes pain. He can feel a fly landing on his haunches and knows to within half a millimeter where it is to swish away, so it is not as

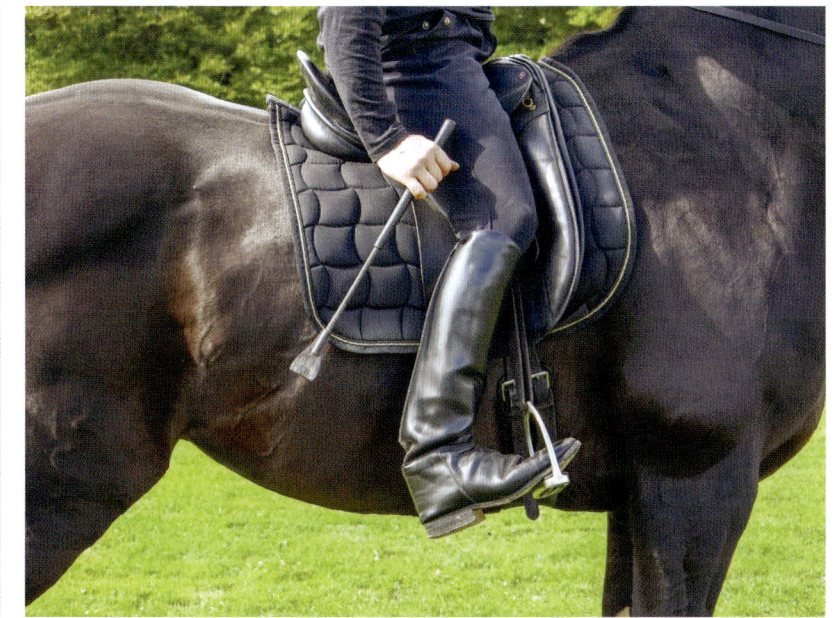

◄ / 5.13 / The Tapping Stick: No pain—you only want to give the horse a repeating signal. Reward and its timing are excellent positive reinforcements, yet motivating a horse to try something new often involves a different approach.

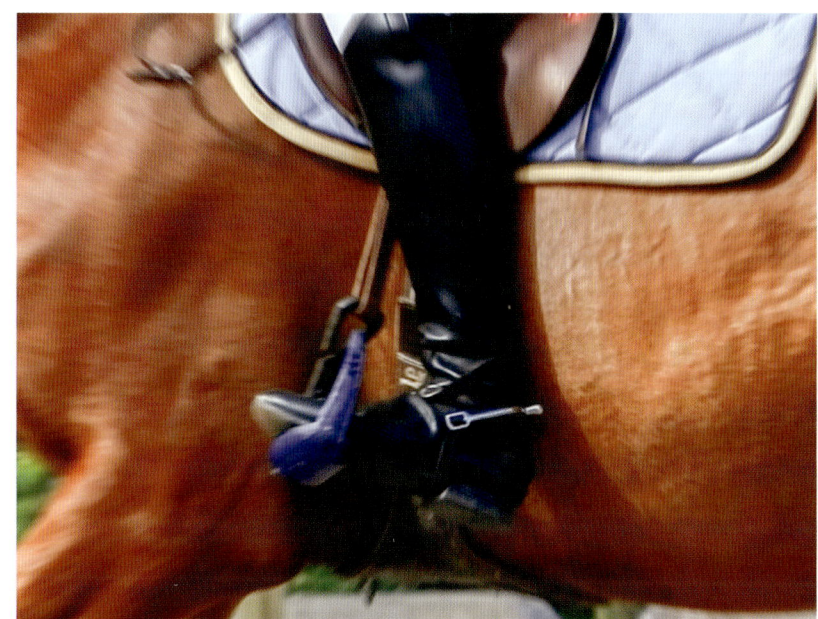

◄ / 5.14 / The spur is an inefficient and uncomfortable aid that causes apprehension and does not promote understanding or goodwill.

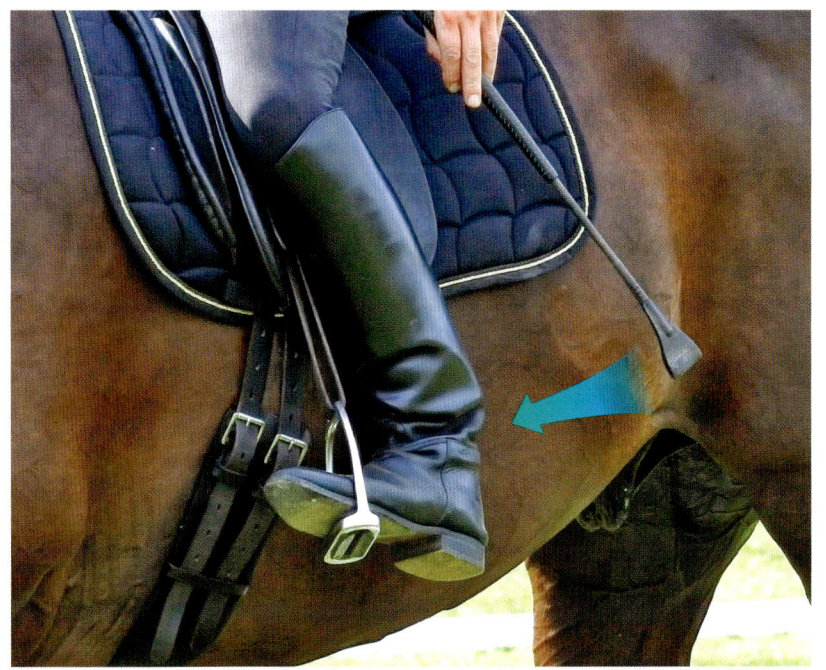

/ 5.15 / *The Tapping Aid: No negativity, just a signal that repeats until the horse moves away from it, just like it was a fly.* ▶

if he can't feel your leg, let alone the spur (fig. 5.14). He certainly does feel it, but he is simply not sure what it *means*.

A much more intelligent solution is to use a bat or crop (the kind used for jumping that has no sting in its tail). With this you can repeatedly tap the horse in the same rhythm as your leg aid (fig. 5.15). At some point the horse does as he would do with anything "annoying" and moves away from it, at which point both aids stop and you can give a reward. This is a very efficient way for the horse to learn without resentment or pain, and it works very well indeed.

This is the basis behind Exercise 5: The Driving Seat (see p. 211) and is an excellent way to reduce the need for that military hardware

■■ Core Conditioning for Horses

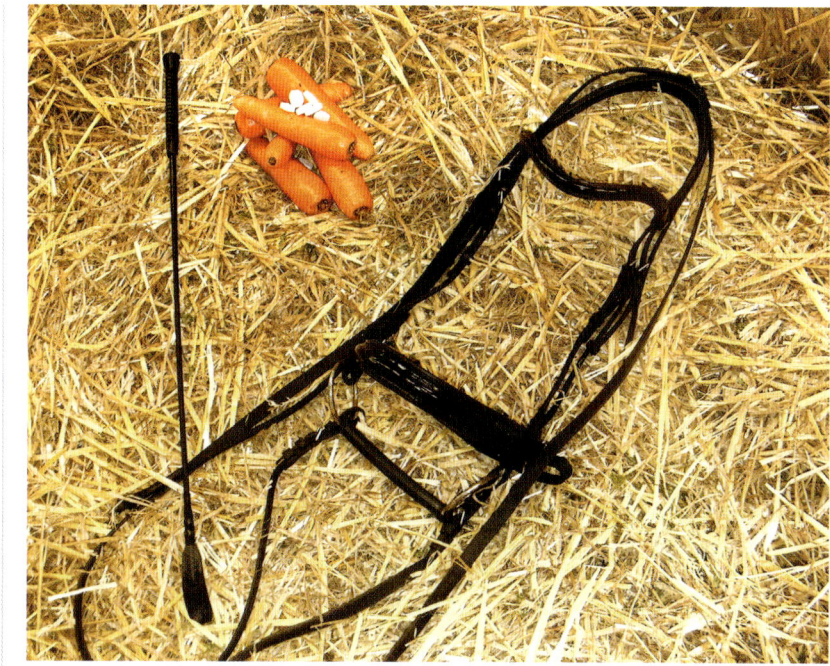

◄ / 5.16 / *The only artificial aids you need: A mild bit, a short stick, and the horse's favorite snack.*

we talked about early in the book. This is simpler, kinder, faster, and makes our horses happier for all the right reasons.

Tapping the stick can also be used to teach a horse to keep going on his own. If there is a tendency to drop out of pace when the rider stops using her legs, instead of using the legs to keep him going, try tapping until the horse restores the original gait. It works every time. ■

\\\ Dan Millman ///

Dan Millman

"The secret of change is to focus all
of your energy not on fighting the old,
but building the new."

6

10 Core Exercises for the Horse

Getting Started

So, now you have a Warm-Up Plan and Core Score, and we've discussed how to ride "yoga-style." Now let's look at the 10 Core Exercises for the Horse. In the pages ahead, you'll find both the core exercises along with their human yoga equivalents so that I may illustrate the effects accurately and you may see the inspiration behind my prescribed movements for the horse.

Let's revisit the four Core Warm-Up Plans and their primary effects, as well as the exercises in each:

CONNECTION: mobility, cooperation, communication, and education.

- **Core Release Volte** (Yoga Half-Moon Pose), p. 156
- **Turn on the Forehand** (Yoga Half Split Pose), p. 169
- **Forward and Back** (Yoga Balancing Table to Tiptoe Chair Pose), p. 198
- **The Rounding Rein-Back** (Yoga Garland Pose), p. 223
- **The Perfect Pirouette** (Yoga Thread the Needle Pose), p. 250

FLEXIBILITY: suppleness, straightness, range of motion, and better HNP.

- **Core Release Volte** (Yoga Half-Moon Pose), p. 156
- **Turn on the Forehand** (Yoga Half Split Pose), p. 169
- **Forward, Down, and Out** (Yoga Cat Pose), p. 186
- **Limbering Leg Yield** (Yoga Revolved Triangle Pose), p. 238
- **La Giravolta Longe** (Yoga Revolved Half-Moon Pose), p. 274

WELLNESS: maintenance, good health, support, and calming.

- **Core Release Volte** (Yoga Half-Moon Pose), p. 156
- **Forward, Down, and Out** (Yoga Cat Pose), p. 186
- **The Rounding Rein-Back** (Yoga Garland Pose), p. 223
- **Limbering Leg Yield** (Yoga Revolved Triangle Pose), p. 238
- **La Giravolta Longe** (Yoga Revolved Half-Moon Pose), p. 274

AGILITY: Sport mode!

- **Turn on the Forehand** (Yoga Half Split Pose), p. 169
- **Forward and Back** (Yoga Balancing Table to Tiptoe Chair Pose), p. 198
- **The Driving Seat** (Yoga Chair Pose), p. 211
- **The Rounding Rein-Back** (Yoga Garland Pose), p. 223
- **Forward, Down, and Out to Competition Outline**
  (Yoga Cat to Cow Pose), p. 264

Results You Can See

To help demonstrate how the core exercises based on yoga principles should be performed, I'd like to introduce two lovely equines found wandering around my farm. Meet Wardance and Bo (figs. 6.1 & 6.2).

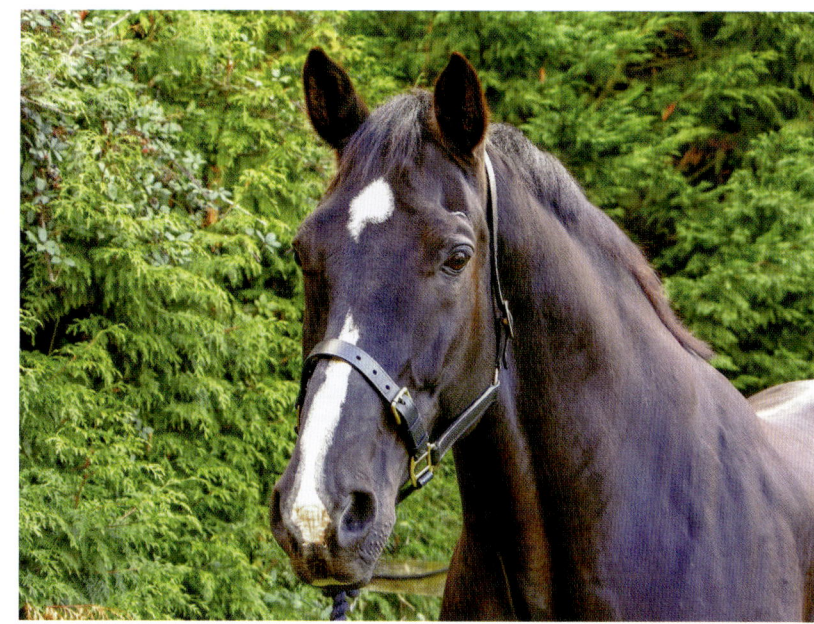

◂ / 6.1 / *Wardance, a German Hanoverian.*

/ **6.2** / *Bo, a Spanish Pura Raza Espagola (PRE).* ▶

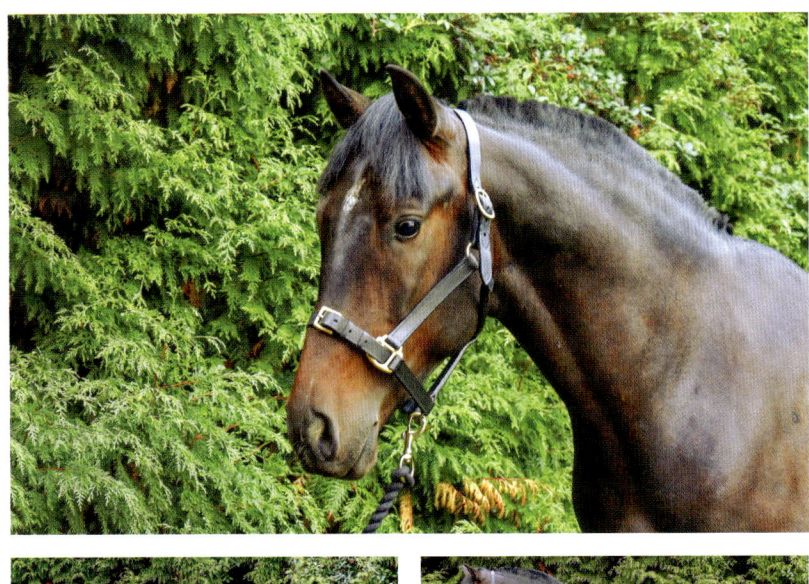

/ **6.3** / *Wardance (left) is 17 hands tall and built for power, but lacks agility.* ▶

/ **6.4** / *Bo (right) is 16.1 hands and born to dance but easily becomes tense.* ▶

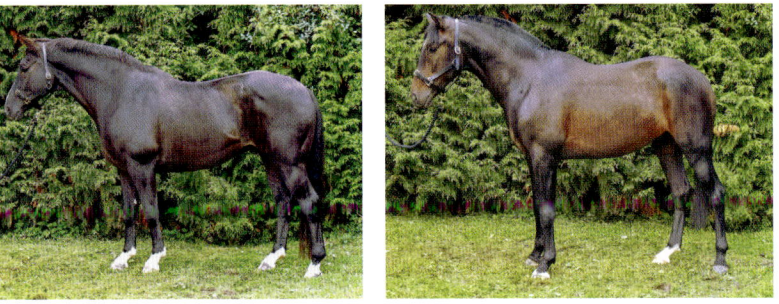

Wardance is 12 years old and a fully formed 17-hand Hanoverian gelding. He has been doing the yoga-inspired warm-up exercises for two years (fig. 6.3). He has done very little for a horse of his age and has an irrational fear of chickens. Working with him is pure entertainment, as he is like an inquisitive puppy.

Bo is a 16.1-hand, just-turned-five-year-old Yeguada Andalusian dancing machine (fig. 6.4). He is a goofy kid with a heart of gold who likes naps and Flamenco. He came to me unbacked and unfettered, and after some core work from the ground, he began a starter program using the Wellness Plan exercises after backing and has now been under saddle for one year.

WARDANCE SUMMARY:

- **Riding Style:** Powerful and a big mover, typical of the breed.
- **Core Score:** 1 (at time of writing).
- **Strengths:** Good walk and canter.
- **Weaknesses:** Can tend to hollow and become unbalanced in a strong trot or canter.
- **Objective:** Strengthen the core further to Core Score 0 using the Agility Plan.

BO SUMMARY:

- **Riding Style:** "Olé!"
- **Core Score:** 2
- **Strengths:** Young and open, has an unrestricted back, and is 100 percent enthusiastic.
- **Weakness:** When tense, he can get hollow with choppy gaits, typical of the breed.
- **Objective:** Core strengthening to develop roundness and agility to Core Score 1, using the Wellness Plan as his daily Warm-Up.

Ready? *Andiamo!* ◾

/ 6.5 / *The Core Release Volte is an exercise so simple and helpful, the horse wants to do it. The volte aligns the spine to release the core and stretch the back in two directions simultaneously.* ▶

Exercise 1

⸎ / The Half-Moon Pose
⸎ / The Core Release Volte

This is the simplest, gentlest, and most useful back stretch of all (fig. 6.5). This exercise is both easy to do and master, and it almost immediately gives the core its freedom.

The Yoga *Half-Moon Pose* is a completely natural and very kind exercise that gently stretches the back and sides of the human body. The horsey equivalent is the *Core Release Volte,* which gives the horse the same benefit as the human version, and shows the horse how easy it is for him to release and bend through the body a little more each day. All horses and ponies can master this exercise, no matter what their age, education, or history.

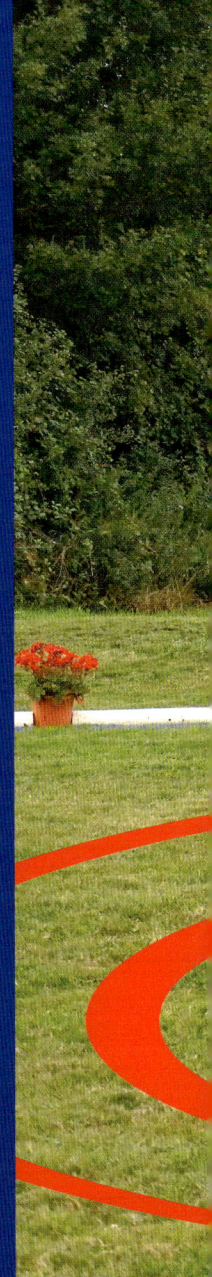

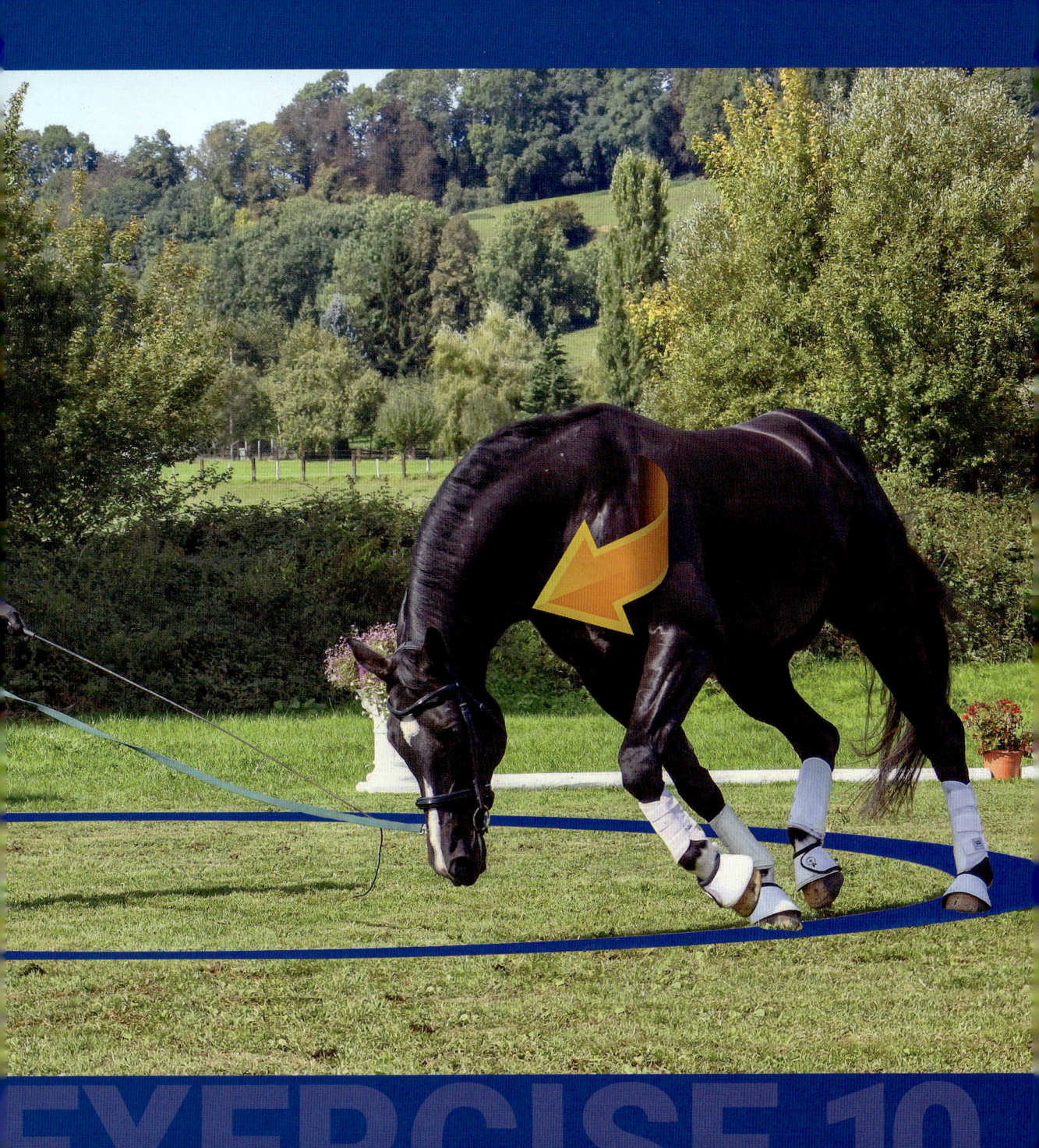

EXERCISE 10

🧘 / The Revolved Half-Moon Pose

The *Revolved Half-Moon Pose* challenges your balance and mental focus. As the weight distribution requires good spinal flexibility, this exercise can be gradually mastered to strengthen the whole body (fig. 6.77).

This pose helps a human:

• Tone the whole body.
• Stretch limbs and back.
• Improve coordination and balance.

"The Revolved Half-Moon Pose stretches the sides of the body, hamstrings, calves, groin, and spine," explains Australian yoga instructor Jacqueline Buchanan. "On a deeper level, it reduces anxiety, stress, and sluggishness, thanks to how it elevates your heart above your head."

/ **6.77** / *The Revolved Half-Moon Pose is a challenging pose of fine balance, coordination, and relaxation through your back.* ▶

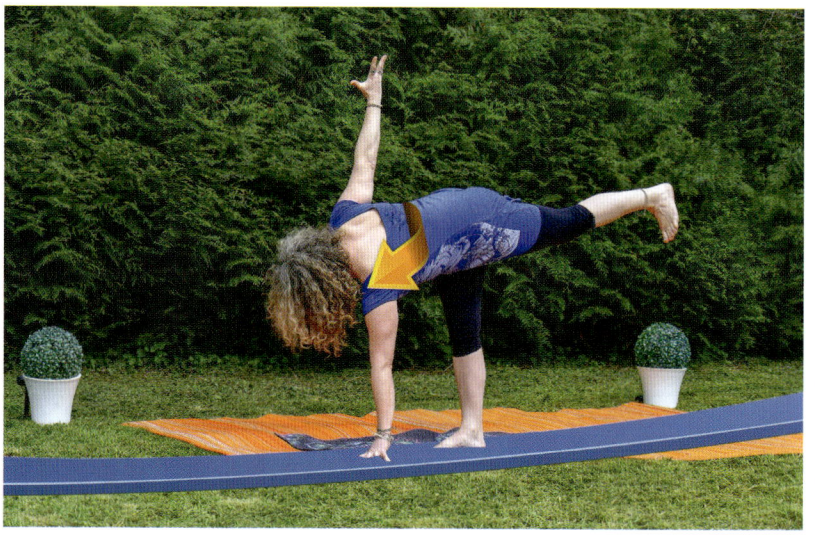

/ La Giravolta Longe

La Giravolta is a very old exercise from Classical European equitation that we don't see anymore, which is a shame because it's terrific. This unmounted exercise gives the horse a chance to practice with different solutions to his physical challenges, yet without a human wobbling about on top. One thing at a time.

La Giravolta Longe is really just shoulder-in on a longe circle. This simple exercise has incredible benefits to a horse. It precisely aligns the spine, releases the core, and allows the horse to stretch, first into Long-and-Low, then gradually Forward, Down, and Out (which the horse will look for all on his own). This critical angle of spinal alignment can reset the horse's deepest geometry, however horrible, and turn training around gently, simply, and permanently.

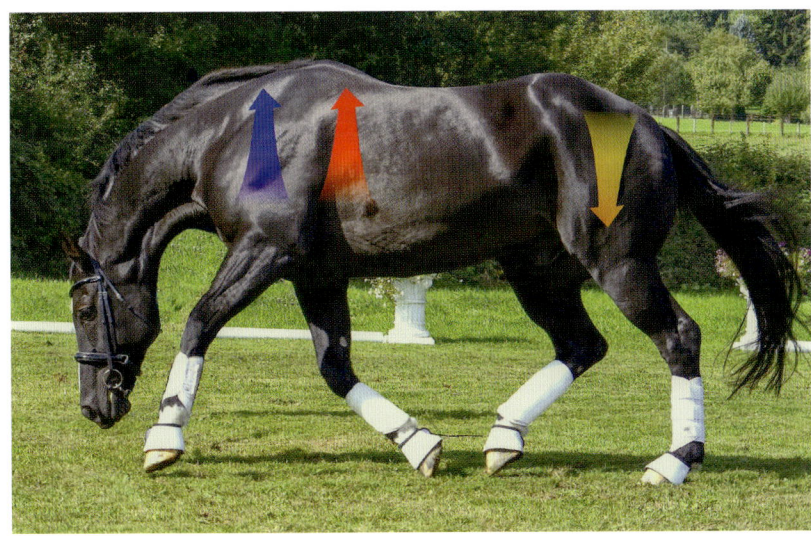

◄ / 6.78 / *Wardance in La Giravolta: The exercise's angles create perfect spinal alignment; then the horse can learn to use his Core Powers to perfect his own posture before you complicate matters by climbing on board.*

This exercise helps the horse to:

- Learn to bend well and not fall in/out.
- Coordinate upper body to the limbs.
- Manage the center of gravity better.
- Find more relaxed and smoother paces.

The Classical Schools of Equitation understood the alignment properties of shoulder-in, and in particular, how effective shoulder-in on a circle can be to help a stiff horse to soften. "The shoulder-in *(l'Epaule en Dedans),*" wrote its inventor French dressage master François Robichon de La Guérinière, "has so many benefits that I regard it as the alpha and omega of all exercises for the horse,

/ 6.79 / *La Giravolta keeps it simple. With a slow and relaxed gait, the Giravolta's use of the volte is kind, relaxing, and deeply liberating for the horse.* ▶

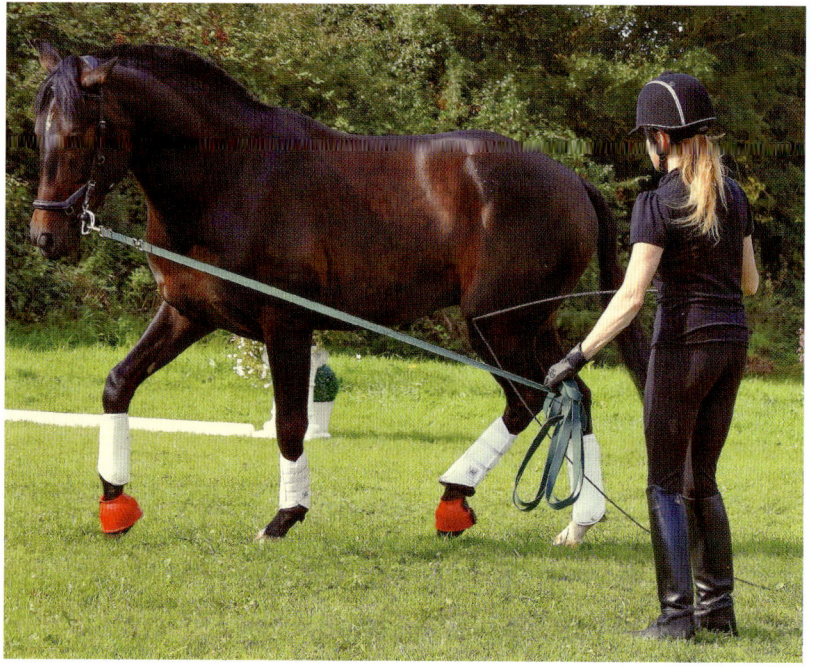

which are intended to develop complete suppleness and perfect agility in all its parts. This is so true that a horse trained according to this principle and spoiled afterward either in the school or by some ignorant person can be restored to full agility if a horseman puts him back into this exercise for few days."

La Giravolta's alignment puts the horse's outside foreleg in the track of the inside hind leg, on a slow and relaxed 6-meter (20-foot) volte (fig. 6.79). The Stretching Flexion (see p. 139) on this volte is the recipe for this elusive sweet spot.

This exercise helps solve these issues under saddle:

- Rough gaits.
- Crookedness.
- High head.
- Unpredictable movement or temperament.
- Blocked mouth.
- Blocked back.

By removing your weight from the equation and doing this on the longe, the horse can learn for himself how best to bend, stretch, and coordinate through this exercise's levels. At the achievement of Tone Level, the horse should be supple, straight, and very easy to ride (fig. 6.80).

What It Does Inside the Horse's Body

- Aligns the spine and limbs at the optimal curvature.
- Releases the core.

- Releases tension in the *longissimus* muscle.
- Fully activates the three Core Powers of Nuchal Lift, Thoracic Lift, and Pelvic Tilt.
- Rounds the horse's back from the core's deepest points.

Core Score, Level, and Head-and-Neck Position

If your horse has a Core Score of:

- **0–1**, do this exercise at the **TONE LEVEL.**
- **2–3**, do this exercise at the **COORDINATION LEVEL.**
- **4–5**, do this exercise at the **RELEASE LEVEL.**

/ 6.80 / *Retraining posture: By isolating the horse's precise spinal alignment, La Giravolta allows the rest of the body to fall into a relaxed and comfortable frame.* ▶

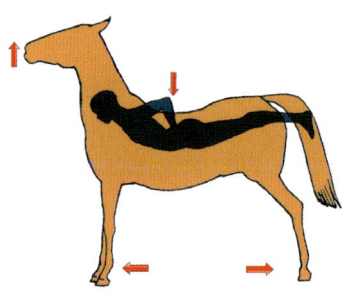

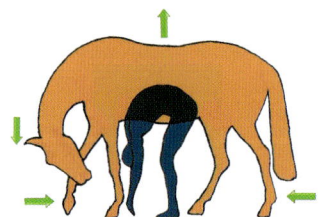

The most important premise of this exercise is to help the horse self-align. Only then can he relax his defensive or tense musculature and round into the stride. As the improvement in posture is naturally found through alignment, there is no need for straps, elastics, or any kind of restrictive equipment.

- **RELEASE LEVEL** (Free-Walk in Long-and-Low HNP): In the free-walk we are simply aiming for a smooth Core Release from the Stretching Flexion (see p. 139). As soon as the horse finds stability in Long-and-Low, he is ready to go into the *trot d'école*. If your horse has a known back issue, this is the Level that will slowly alleviate the discomfort of tension and put his movement on a better road.

- **COORDINATION LEVEL** (*Trot d'École* in Long-and-Low to Forward, Down, and Out): Create a low-intensity, two-time *trot d'école* while maintaining shoulder-in on the longe volte. As with Release Level, at Core Release and Long-and-Low HNP, allow the horse to find his way into the Forward, Down, and Out position. When the horse is consistently in Forward, Down, and Out at this Level, gradually introduce the Tone Level.

- **TONE LEVEL** (*Petit Galop* in Long-and-Low to Forward, Down, and Out HNPs): The art form in this exercise is the *petit galop*. At this point of the horse's core training, he will have excellent balance and suppleness. The *petit galop* will tone, hone, and tighten the core like no other exercise. All three Core Powers can be activated from the La Giravolta's Tone Level in Forward, Down, and Out. You will not believe what your horse can eventually do by mastering La Giravolta Longe.

How to Do It

OVERVIEW: La Giravolta Longe is very, very simple to do. Just longe your horse, stand still, and spin on the spot while the horse makes a nice circle around you. What is crucial for a good Giravolta is that the horse must choose his own speed. You must not rush or drive; the exercise requires a slow, balanced gait that is directed, flexed, and bent by the human, yet maintained and balanced by the horse (fig. 6.81). You need only a bridle, longe line, longe whip, and leg protection. No flash, side-reins, elastics, or any other restraint. You are going *au naturel.*

- **STEP /1/** Begin longeing in walk on an 8–10-meter (25–30-foot) circle until the horse is settled, then pick up a light trot for a few circles until a rhythm is established. Then gradually shorten the longe line to bring the horse onto a 6-meter volte. This puts 3 meters (10 feet) between you and the horse—the

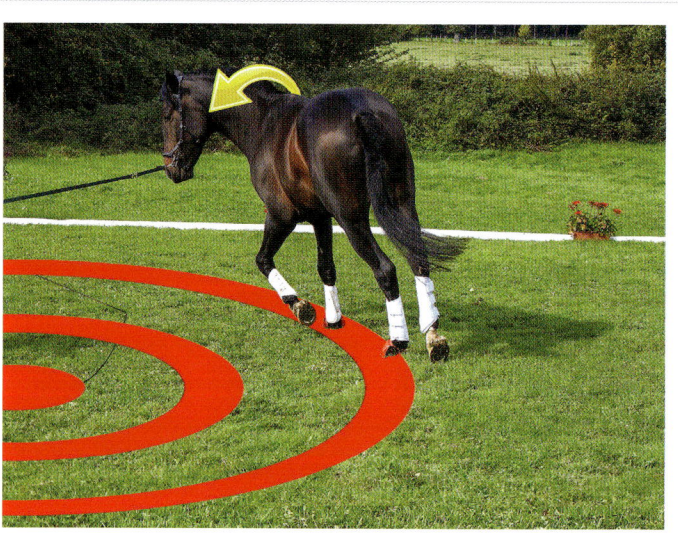

/ 6.81 / Bringing the HNP to the inside, we place the horse's body into alignment, releasing the core and naturally dropping the outline into Long-and-Low or Forward, Down, and Out. ▶

perfect distance to hold the whip so it points at his side, roughly where your leg would be when riding. This will help him understand the intention of your leg aid when mounted, and promote bend through his back. Maintain the same whip distance for the whole circle (fig. 6.82). It is best to hold the whip's tail with the handle, as you don't want to use the "whipping" part at all. It is an unnecessary threat, as well as a distraction.

- **STEP /2/** The angle you set is critical. With the longe whip held pointing at the horse's shoulder to prevent the shoulder from falling toward you, bring his head slightly farther in to make a Stretching Flexion (fig. 6.83).
- **STEP /3/** Hold this body angle until the horse's core releases and he lowers his head and begins to look for a soft, Forward, Down, and Out HNP. When established, the entire exercise can be performed in Forward, Down, and Out, giving unparalleled spinal flexibility and all the benefits that this brings to the ride.

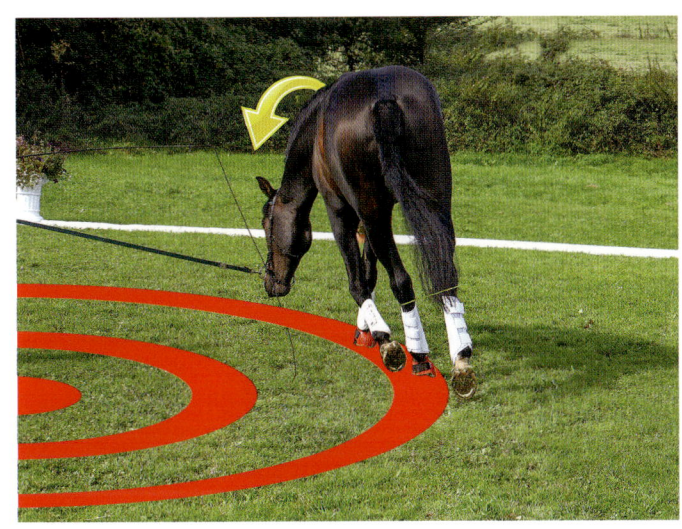

◀ / 6.82 / *Standing still in the center, use the whip to ask for more forward activity and for the horse to keep his shoulder to the outside of his neck flexion.*

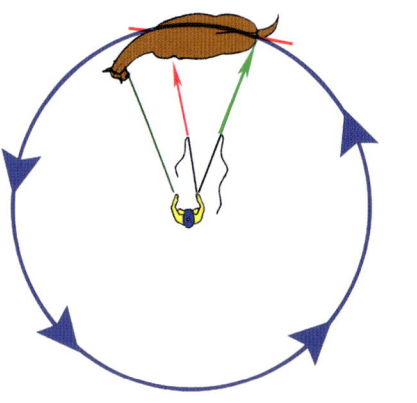

/ 6.83 / *Standing still in the center, use the whip to ask for more forward activity and for the horse to keep his shoulder to the outside of his neck flexion.* ▶

The goal of La Giravolta is for the horse to discover how to relax and learn how to balance himself really, really well, using his core.

Common Problems and Solutions

- ***No Core Release.*** The volte may be too big. When the circle is too large, the shoulder-in angle can't be maintained, therefore the horse's spine will not align and the core cannot release. It will be necessary to make a guiding contact on the fleshy shoulder with the end of the longe whip to explain that—because you need the inside Stretching Flexion to help him—the horse must keep his body out on the volte.
- ***Dropping out of the gait. Lazy chap!*** You choose the gait and he has to keep it—that is a rule. If the horse drops the gait, consider whether he is ready for it at all, and if so, do the minimum amount of gesturing with the longe whip to induce an upward gear change to restore the original gait. There is never any need to whip the horse; touching with the whip to guide is all you should do and all you need.

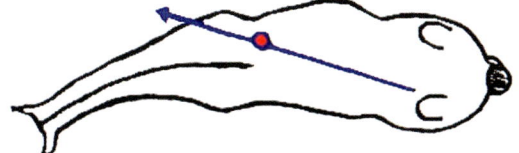

◄ / 6.84 / During La Giravolta, your aim is to gently help the horse align his inside hind on the same line as his outside fore, creating ideal shoulder-in alignment.

- ***The horse makes an egg-shaped circle.*** They always try this! Be firm and make the whip point at the inside shoulder all the time. When the horse comes into contact with it by falling in, he teaches himself not to fall across the circle. This is an incredibly valuable lesson.

Core Score Zero Goal

A Core Score 0 horse performing La Giravolta Longe is like watching a ballet. The horse is completely light to the hand and perfectly balanced in any gear. This is a beautiful thing to accomplish with a horse and an excellent way to begin a sensitive and cooperative riding session.

Viva La Giravolta! ∎

END OF EXERCISE 10
The Revolved Half-Moon Pose / La Giravolta Longe

\\\ Xenophon ///
Xenophon

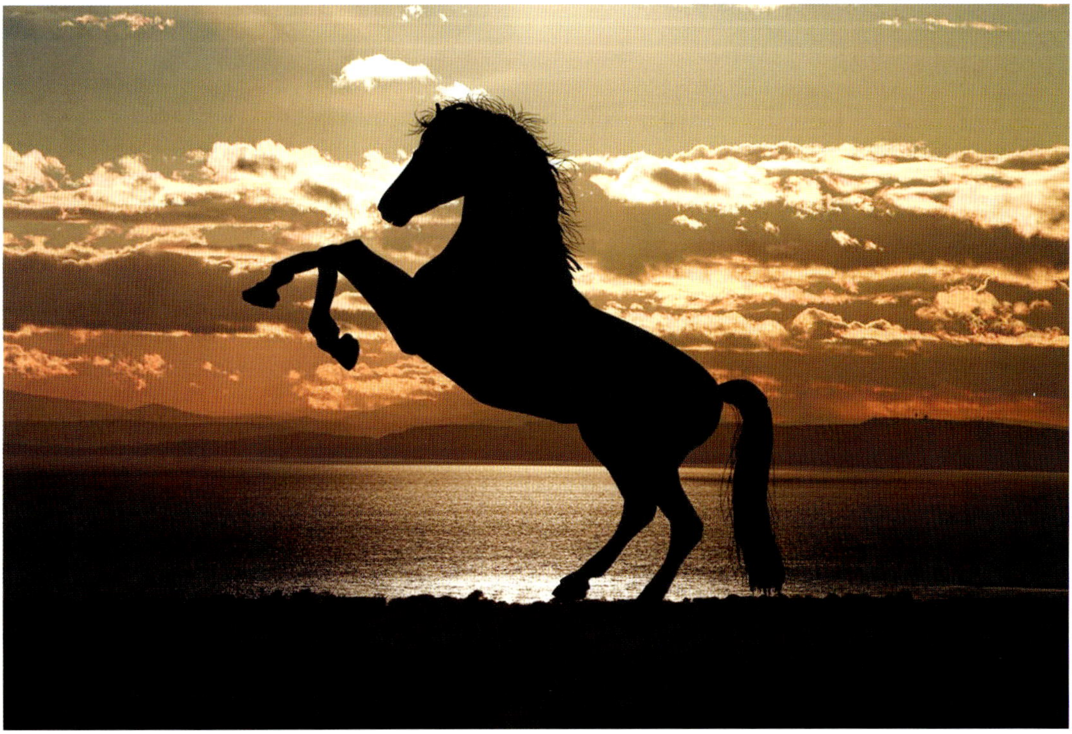

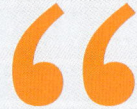

"Ride the horse in such a way
that it will be pleased with itself and want
to create a proud and delightful appearance."

7

Happy Bendy Horsey!

A well ridden, daily yoga-inspired warm-up will serve your horse in three ways:

- Bring his core into good condition.
- Strengthen his posture so it is unaffected by a rider.
- Make him feel alert, entertained, and understood before work begins.

In many ways, these aspects are the most important considerations for any riding horse, as his well-being depends upon a balance between them. Whatever you plan to do in your training session, it stands the best chance of success if you can encourage all three ways to become day-to-day habits.

Practice Makes Perfect

Wherever your starting point, core conditioning will improve any horse and rider's partnership if practiced daily.

Teaching your horse to perform these core conditioning exercises will take time, and they may feel quite sticky to begin with. Very few horses will find these exercises easy in the beginning, and it is to be expected—this is why they are going to be good to incorporate. Just as when any of us are learning a new skill, thoughtful repetition will bring improvements quickly. Of course, it depends upon the horse's very unique physical condition and consequent Core Score (see p. 82), yet with all horses, the body will need to acclimate to a new posture, even when it is more efficient.

If in any doubt about how a horse may react, it is best to bring in an experienced horse person to give additional advice specific to the individual horse. Always consider safety first. With some Core Score 4–5 horses, it is best to seek professional consultation before deciding upon an exercise program of any kind. There may well be chronic pain in the back that should be identified and treated before any physical activity is asked.

Wherever the starting point, when the horse begins to move better in your Warm-Up Plan, it is a message to you that he feels more confident not only in himself, but in you, too. The 20-minute Core Conditioning Warm-Up will unlock your horse's abilities to carry you and at the same time bring you closer together as a team. As his job gets easier, so will yours, making more magical moments

\\\ George W. Loomis ///
George W. Loomis

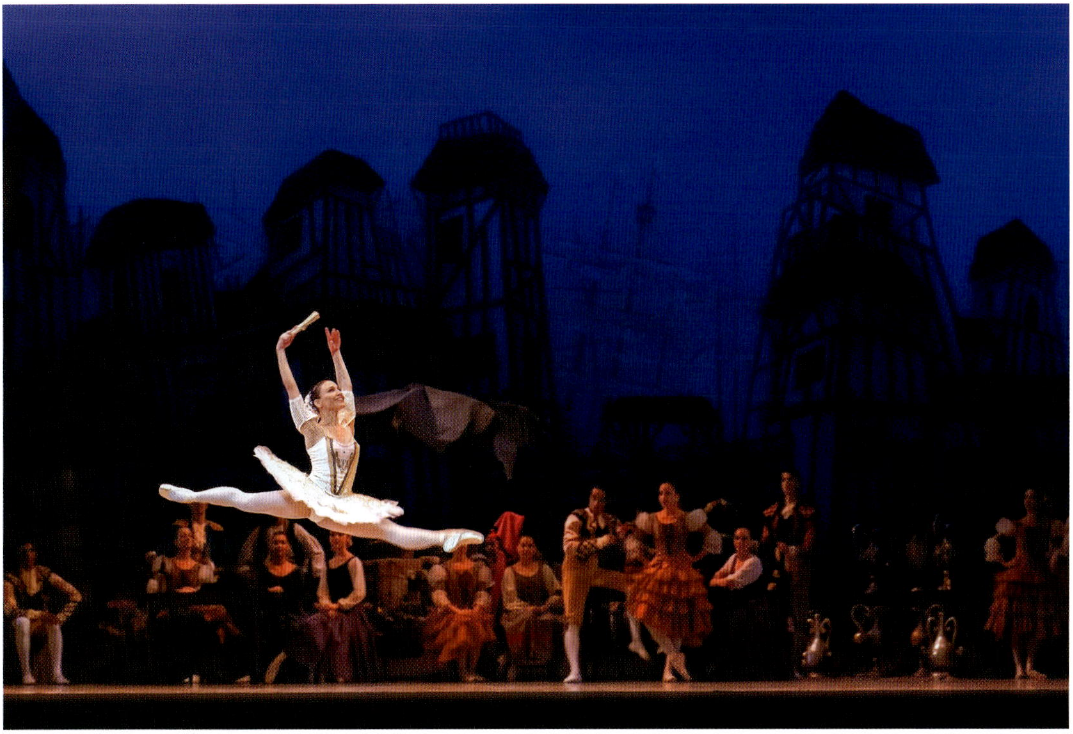

"Don't practice until you get it right, practice until you can't get it wrong."

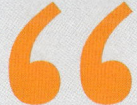

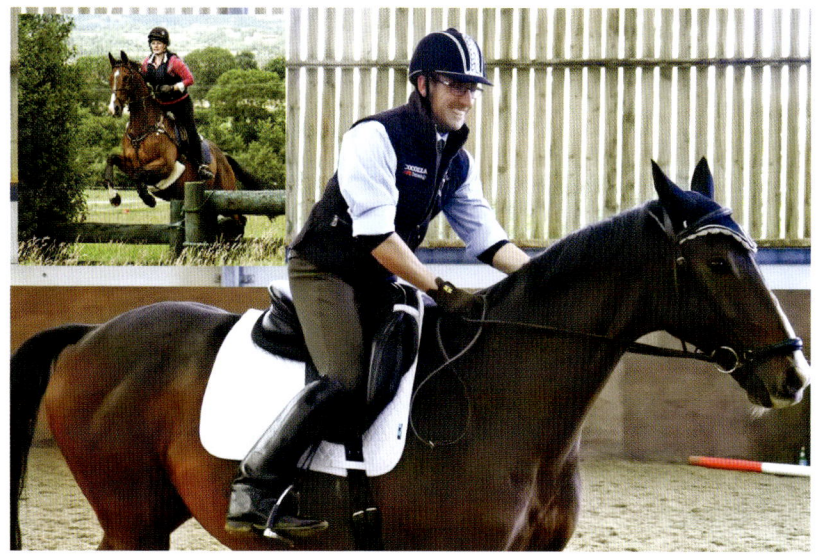

The author with Dana's Ollie, a Core Story kissing spine sufferer (see p. 174), now fully recovered and having a pain-free and fun life (inset). ▶

where everything falls into place and you can really connect. This is where the adventure really begins. What is more, as your partner he will feel understood, respected, and free, which are, of course, the most important things of all.

May your horse be with you. ■

acknowledgments

/ thank you to: /

- Bertil Voss BHSI
- Four Dimensional Digital Imaging (4DDI) Equine
- Dr. Hilary Clayton, FRCVS
- Sarah Le Jeune, DVM
- Gerd Heuschmann, DVM
- Doychin Lyudov, DVM
- Ivana Ruddock-Lange at Whole Horse Dissection
- Jayne Grimshaw
- Rosario D'Onofrio
- Philippa Dimmock
- Emilia Frisk
- Nigel and Maggie McNeil-Smith
- Dawn and John Wagstaff
- Carolyn Elizabeth Darley Miller
- Randi Thompson

- The Melkkilä Stable
- Janna Maari
- Alison Robertson
- Aleksi Kallioniemi
- Tiia Tuulivaara and Kanada
- Debbie Isaacson and Chaussette
- Dana Marie Ewans and Oliver
- Dr. Jean-Marie Denoix
- Michael Dam, DVM
- Dr. Jean-Pierre Pailloux
- Fabrice Rue
- Eric Cleary
- Xavier Ribard
- Remy Bourdais
- Guerric and Aline Paris
- François Rohmer

- Carl Sanderson
- Marc and Huw Lee
- Giovanni Battista Tomassini
- John Gibbon
- Rolland Dowson
- Robert Van Wessum, DVM
- Grace Fairburn
- Conte Gian Carlo Cocozza
- Contessa Stella Cocozza
- Visconte James Cocozza
- Sarah Watson-Wright
- Naomi Wright
- Molly Sivewright, FBHS
- Heather Moffat
- Sally Swift
- Jeremy Houghton-Brown
- Gloria Leverett

acknowledgments

/ thank you to: /

- *François Baucher*
- *Kelly Gledhill*
- *Lorraine Lockert*
- *Jochen Schleese*
- *Frank Stübben*
- *Bill Steinkraus*
- *Randy Frantz, DVM*
- *François Robichon de la Guérinière*
- *Franke Sloothaak*
- *Alois Podhajsky*
- *Gustav Steinbrecht*
- *Pippa Francis*
- *Dr. Richard Coomer, BCVSP*
- *Klaus Balkenhol*
- *La Fédération Française d'Équitation*
- *La Commission Européenne*
- *La Fédération Équestre Internationale*
- *Deutsche Reiterliche Vereinigung*
- *The United States Dressage Federation*
- *The American Morgan Horse Association*
- *The British Horse Society*
- *The American Trakhener Association*
- *CIRALE Deauville*
- *Xenophon*
- *Le Cadre Noir*
- *British Dressage*
- *Horsetalk.co.uk*
- *The Chronicle of the Horse*
- *Eurosport*
- *Dressage Today*

This book was made possible only with the patience and expertise of *Rebecca Didier*, *Martha Cook*, and *Caroline Robbins*, and all the team at Trafalgar Square Books. Thank you so much.

I would like to give a very special mention to the following individuals—they have made the impossible possible and helped no end.

Thank you:
Terri and *Iris Walker*, *Helen Newitt*, *David Lewin*, *Paul Barber*, *Tony* and *Mary Humphreys*, *Marina Kallioniemi* and *Pena*, *Dr. Nathalie Parsy*, *Veronica* and *Jenny Lee*.

index

/ page numbers in *italics* indicate illustrations /

A

Abdominal muscles. *See* Core muscles
Agility Warm-Up Plan, 109–10, 153
Aids. *See also* Leg aids
 artificial, 144, *147–48*, 217–19, *220*, 282–83
 mind aids, 144–49
 rein aids, 139–144
 release of, *147*, 148
 from seat, 136–37
 yoga-inspired, 136
"Alert" mental state, 76, 78
Ali, Muhammad, 18
Anticipation, negative, 32
Apt, Marla, 225
Art, *10*, 80
Ashe, Arthur, 116
"Asleep" mental state, 76, 78
Athleticism, 10–12, *13*, 28–30, 81, 89
Attention, of horse, 76

B

Back, of horse. *See also* Core muscles
 anatomy, 29–30, *40*, 42, *42*, *56–58*, 57, 61–62
 evolutionary context, 9–12
 flexibility of, 30–32, *31*
 head position and, 27
 pain in, 111, 288
 rider's effects on, 10–19
 rounding of, 49–50
 weakness of, 14–15
Backing process, *14*
Backing up, 225–27, 237
Balance
 development of, 162, 172, 190, 195, 203, 231, 242, 268, 284
 of lift and thrust, *38*
 nuchal ligament in, 49, *192*
 rear end in, 42–43, *43*
Balancing Table Pose, 200–201, *200*
Bend, *31*, *86*, 93
Biomechanics and Physical Training of the Horse (Denoix), 190
Blocking, 136–37
Bo, *153–54*, 154–55
Body language, 20–21, 24
Body sections, 39–43, *39*
Bracing, with seat, 136–37
Breeds, training approaches and, 24–25
Buchanan, Jacqueline, 276

C

Canter, 128
Carrying role, of core, 37
Cat Pose, 133, 186–89, *188*, 266, *267*
Cat to Cow Pose, 265–66, *267*
Cavalry horses, 26
Cervical spine, 40, *40*
Chair Pose, 212–13, *212*
Choudhury, Bikram, 102
Churchill, Winston, 23
Classical School, of training, 25–26, *25–26*
Coelho de Souza, Paulo, 144
Communication, by horses, 20–21
Competition Outline
 overview, 135–36, *135*, 241
 exercises using, 268–273, *268*
Conditioning, 3, 30, 117, 125, 288
Confusion, effects of, 35
Connection Warm-up Plan, 107–8, 152
Contact, 90, *91–92*, 131, 140–41, 191–92
Cooperation, horse's instinct for, 32
Coordination, *75*, 89, *257*, *262*
Coordination Level, for exercises, 123, 125–27
Core conditioning
 benefits of, 117
 challenge levels, 123–130
 as full training session, 122
 Head-and-Neck Positions in, 130–36
 practice of, 288
 in Warm-Up, 70, *70*
Core muscles. *See also* Back, of horse
 back and, 19
 development of, 25, 30
 function of, 1, 37–43, *39*, 173, *173*
 pathologies in, 58–60
 release of, 30–32
 in resistance, 54–56
Core Powers
 overview, 44–45, *44*
 blocking of, 58
 Nuchal Lift, 48–50
 Pelvic Tilt, 50–54
 Thoracic Lift, 45–48
Core Release, 123, 130–32
Core Release Volte exercise
 overview, 159–164, *159–160*
 execution of, 154–167, *156*, *164–65*
 in Forward, Down, and Out exercise, 195
 yoga pose inspiration, 158–59, *158*
Core Score assessment
 overview, 82
 chart for, 96–99
 examples of, 110

non-ridden indicators for, 100–106
ridden indicators for, 83–95
Core Story case histories
Dana and Ollie, 174, 176, 178, 180
Debbie and Chaussette, 228, 230, 232
Doychin Lyudov, 204
Marina Kallioniemi, 256, 258
Core Warm-Up plans, 107–10
Covey, Stephen R., 59
Cow Pose, 266, *267*
Crandell, Jason, 248
Crookedness, 86, *87–88*, 88, 90

■■ D
Da Vinci, Leonardo, 8, 9
Dana and Ollie case history, 174, 176, 178, 180
Dancer's warm-up, 68–69, *69*
Dashama, 71
De La Guérinière, François Robichon, 24–25, 278–79
Debbie and Chaussette case history, 228, 230, 232
Decarpentry, Albert, 225
Denoix, Jean-Marie, 190
"Difficult" horses, 32–35
Dressage, 120, 125, 135–36, 175, 177, 245
Driving Seat exercise
overview, *210*, 211, 213–17
execution of, 217–220, *218–220*
yoga pose inspiration, 212–13
Dujardin, Charlotte, 219, 221
Dynamic exercises, 72

■■ E
Eastern traditions, of physical development, 30
Emotional stability, 78
Evolutionary history, of horse, 10–13, *13*
Exercise
dynamic, 72
low-impact, 30

■■ F
Fairburn, Grace, 58
Fédération Equestre Internationale, 135–36
Feel, in riding, 22
Figure eight, in Core Release Volte, 160
Fish, Hazel, 68
Flexibility Warm-Up Plan, 108, 152
Flexion, 93, 139–141, *139–140*
Floor plans, defined, 119, 121, *121*
Fly, tapping stick aid as, 146

Focus, 76
Forehand. *See also* "Sitting" posture
function of, *39–40*, 40–41
weight distribution onto, 31, 48, *51*, 52
Forelegs, weight-bearing on, *259*
Forward, Down, and Out exercise
overview, 186, *187*, 189–194
execution of, 189–194, *189–191*, *194*
yoga pose inspiration, 188–89, *188*
Forward, Down, and Out HNP
discussed, 132–34, *133*, 160
as release, 121
in warm-down, 122
Forward, Down, and Out to Competition Outline exercise
overview, *264–65*, 265, 268–270, *268*, *272*
execution of, 270–73, *271–72*
yoga pose inspiration, 266, *267*
Forward and Back exercise
overview, *198–99*, 199, 202–7, *203*
execution of, *202*, *206–7*, 207–9
yoga pose inspiration, 200–202, *200–201*
"Framing" of horse, 142–44, *143*, 181. *See also* Head-and-Neck Positions
Freedom of movement, 9
Free-walk, 119, 121, 125
Front end. *See* Forehand

■■ G
Gaits, regularity of, 89, 177
Garland Pose, 223–25, *224*
Gaulthier, Veronique, 201
Gillespie, Barry H., 64
"Going with" the horse, 136–37, *137*
"Grazing" stretch, *133*
Gribbons, Anne, 226
Guérinière, François Robichon de La, 24–25, 278–79
Gymnasium of the Horse, The (Steinbrecht), 53

■■ H
Half-Moon Pose, 156, 158–59, *158*
Half-Split Pose, 169–171, *170*
Haunches, turn on, 254. *See also* Hindquarters
Head-and-Neck Positions (HNPs)
overview, 130–36
back position and, 27
as Core Condition indicator, 83, 90–91, *91–92*, 96–99
restrictive equipment and, 26–28, *27–28*

Herriot, James, 33
Hess, Christopher, 195, 197
Hester, Carl, 70, 132, 134, 207–8
Hindquarters
engagement of, *53*, 171–72, *171*, 175, *175*
function of, *39*, 42–43, 185
handling of, 104–6, *105*
HNPs. *See* Head-and-Neck Positions
Hollowing, of back, 57–58, *58*, 61
Holmer, Matilda, 61–62
"Hoof Lift," 104–6, *105*
Hope, Rosie, 196

■■ I
Iliopsoas muscles, *173*
Impulsion, 125, 128, 185
Inflammation, 62
Injuries, prevention of, 68–69
Inside aids. *See* Outside/inside aids

■■ J
Jumping, improving, 205

■■ K
Kallioniemi, Marina, 256
Kissing spines
case histories, 178, 180, 204, 256
described, 61, *61–62*
Kleven, Helle Katrine, 19, 49
Klimke, Michael, 120
Kyrklund, Kyra, 123, 125

■■ L
La Giravolta Longe exercise
overview, *274*, *275*, 277–281, *277–78*, *280*
execution of, 282–85, *282–85*
yoga pose inspiration, 276, *276*
Lateral aids, 214
Lateral movements, 242–47, 255
Le Jeune, Sarah, 56
Lead changes, 163–64
Leaning, *89*
Learning Zone, 76, 78–80
Leg aids
in Driving Seat exercise, 213–14
outside/inside, 139–144, 263
Legs, of horse
protection of, 185
weight-bearing strain on, 58, *259*
Leg-yield, 241, 245
Lengthening, of stride, *202*, 205, *206*, 209

Lifting role
  of core, 37, *38*
  of shoulder, 47
Limbering Leg-Yield exercise
  overview, 238, *239*, 241–45, *241–42*, *244*
  execution of, 245–49, *246–47*
  yoga pose inspiration, 240–41, *240*
Litwicki, Becky, 253
Long-and-Low Outline HNP
  benefits of, 121
  in Core Release, 30, 130–32, *131*, 160, *160*
  flexion in, 140, *140*
Longe, exercises on, 274–285
Longissimus dorsi muscles, 56–57, *57*, 61–62, 131
Loomis, George W., 289
Lumbar spine, *52*, 242
Lyudov, Doychin, 204

■ ■ M
Ma, Yo-Yo, 125, 127
Mehdi, Shirin, *189*
Mental state, 76–79
Middle back, *39*, 42, *42*
Military School, of training, 25–27, *25*, *27*, 62–63
Millman, Dan, 150
Mind aids, 144–49
Mindset, of horse, 83, 93–95, *94*, 214
Mood, 100–101, *100–101*
Morris, George, 80
Mouth, of horse, 83, 90–91, *91–92*, 96–99
Movement
  communication role, 21, 24
  freedom of, 9
Multifidus muscles, 58, *173*
Muscle development/distribution, 103–4, *103–4*

■ ■ N
Nature, 11
Neck. *See also* Head-and-Neck Positions
  anatomy, 40, *40*
  as Core Condition indicator, 83, 90–91, *91–92*, 96–99
  "Nervous" mental state, 76, 78
Nguyen, Jaclyn, 241
Nose position, in Long-and-Low Outline, 131
Nuchal Lift
  discussed, 48–50
  in exercises, 161, *161*, 191, *192*

and Head-and-Neck Positions, 131, *132*
Nuchal ligament, 49, *49*, 50

■ ■ O
Ogle, Marguerite, 266
Older horses, 113
Oliveira, Nuno, 27, 29–30, 125
"On the bit," 135–36, *135*
Outside/inside aids, 139–144, 181, 253–55, 260–63

■ ■ P
Pace, maintaining, 149, 284
Pain
  in core muscles, 54, 56–60
  effects of, 32, 95
  in horse's back, 111, 288
  training to avoid, 66
Peloquin, Andrew, 122
Pelvic Tilt
  discussed, 43, 50–54, *51–53*
  in exercises, *171*, 229, 242
Pelvis, rotation of, 42, *52*, 185
Pena case history, 204
Perfect Pirouette exercise
  overview, 250, *251*, 253–260, *253–54*, *257*
  execution of, *259–262*
  yoga pose inspiration, 252–53, *252*
Pessoa, Fernando, 45
Peters, Steffen, 141
Petit galop, 128
Phelps, Laura, 159
Physical Therapy for Horses (Kleven), 19, 49
Pilates, Joseph, 102
Podhajsky, Alois, 34, 104, 185, 237
Politz, Gerhard, 255
Posture
  in Core Score, 82
  development of, 102, 227, *227*, 229, 274–285
  equipment for positioning of, 26–28, *27–28*
  horse's mindset and, 214, *215*, *277*
  in motion, 1
  as non-ridden core indicator, 102–4, *103–4*
  rider's effects on, 14–15, *15–16*
Practice, importance of, 288–290
  Preparation, importance of, 68. *See also* Warm-Up
Preventative work, 63, 111, 113

■ ■ R
Range of motion, *74*, 268
Ray, Amit, 73
Reactive horses, 78, 144
Rear end. *See* Hindquarters
Regularity, of gaits, 89
Rein aids
  framing with, 142–44, *143*
  holding, vs. pulling, 141, *142*
  in stretching flexion, 139–141, *139–140*
Rein-back, 225–27, 237
Relaxation, benefits of, 76
Release
  of aids, *147*, 148
  through core, 31, 50, 121, 133–34, 140–41
Release Level, for exercise, 123–25
Repetition
  benefits of, 72, 144, 146, 231, 288
  pitfalls of, 144–45
Resistance, 32–35
Restrictive equipment, 26–28, 62–63
Revolved Half-Moon Pose, 274, 276, *276*
Revolved Triangle Pose, 238, 240–41, *240*
Rewards
  release of aids as, 148
  stretching exercises as, 192–93
  treats as, 145–46, *147*
Rib cage, 40, *40*, 42, 46, 173
Ridden mindset, 83, 93–99, *94*, 214
Rideability, 82, 83, *84–85*, 85, 96–99
Ridge Morris, Megan, 78
Riding and riders
  biomechanical effects of, 14–19
  feel in, 22, 24
Rolling, 106, *106*
Rounding Rein-Back exercise
  overview, *222*, 223, 225–231, *225*, *227*, *229*
  execution of, 231–37, *233–35*
  yoga pose inspiration, 224–25, *224*

■ ■ S
Saddle contact area, 42, *42*, 50, 60
Safety considerations, 288
Savoie, Jane, 164
Schils, Sheila, 241–42
Schwartz, Jerry, 191–92
Seat aids, 136–37, *137*, 213
Self-carriage, 26
Serratus ventralis, 47, *47*
Shankar, Ravi, 212–13
Shortening, of stride, *202*, 205, 209

Shoulder-in, 277–283
Shoulders
- anatomy, 47, *47*
- control of, 255, *260*
- flexibility of, 45–46, *46*
- function of, *41*
- in Limbering Leg-Yield exercise, 242
- overdevelopment of, 104

Silent language, of horses, 20
Simek, Barbora, 202
"Sitting" posture
- benefits of, 50, *51*, 85–86
- in exercises, 203, *203*, 225, *225*

Soundness, 83, 89, 96–99
Spine. *See also* Back, of horse
- anatomy, 29–30, *39–40*
- flexibility of, *16*, 17, *31*

Spinous processes, 60–61
Spondylosis, 61, *61–62*
Spurs, 144, *147*, 148
Stability, development of, 127
Stadler, Peter, *29*
Stance, of horse, 10
State of mind, 76–79
Static stretches, 72
Steering, 40, *41*
Steinbrecht, Gustav, 53
"Stepping Under," 179, *179*
Stiffness, in core muscles, 54. *See also* Tension
Stoicism, 58
Straightness, 86, *87*, 88
Stretching. *See also* Warm-Up
- benefits of, 122, 191–92, 195, 197
- Long-and-Low Outline in, 130–32
- in motion, 190
- in Release Level, 123

Stretching Flexion
- described, 139–141, *139–140*
- in exercises, 160, 182, *182*, 279, 281

Stride
- Lengthening/shortening of, *202*, 205, *206*, 209

"sitting" into, *51*
Submission, 27
Suppleness
- as Core Condition indicator, 83, 85–88, *86–88*, 96–99
- importance of, 58

"Survival" mental state, 76, 78
Suspension, 40, *41*

T

Tapping Stick aid, 146–49, *147–48*, 217–19, *220*
Teamwork, horse's instinct for, 32
Tension
- avoiding triggers of, 30, 74, 125
- in back muscles, 57–58, *58*, 130–31
- effects of, 32
- release of, 134

Thoracic Lift, 45–48, 131, 191
Thoracic sling, 40, *40*, 45–46, *45–48*, 229, 259
Thoracic spine, *189*, 242
Thread the Needle Pose, 250, 252–53, *252*
Thrust, 37, 42–43, *43*, 51
Thrusting role, of exterior muscles, *38*
Tidbit rewards, as aid, 145–46
Tiptoe Chair Pose, 201–2, *201*
Toning Level, for exercises, 123, 128, 133
Topline, 104, 193
Training
- goal of, 19
- inspired by human fitness techniques, 65
- physical effects of, 14–15, *15–16*
- psychological considerations, 15
- schools of, 24–27, 62–63

Transitions, 217
Traurig, Christine, 76
Treats, 145–46
Trot, 127, 132
Trot d'école, 127
Truex, Van Day, 11
Turn on the Forehand exercise
- overview, *168*, 169, 171–181, *171*, *175*, *179*
- execution of, *181–84*, 182–85
- yoga pose inspiration, 170–71, *170*

U

Ueshiba, Morihei, 67
Understanding, vs. reaction, 144
United States Dressage Federation (USDF), 175, 177, 245
Unmounted exercises, 111, 274–285
Unridden core indicators, 101–6
Uphill stride/positioning, 53, *53*. *See also* "Sitting" posture

V

Van Wessum, Rob, 126
Variety, 121–22, 144–45
Voss, Bertil, 77, 129, 216

W

Walk, benefits of, 125
Wardance, 154, *154*, 155
Warming Down, 122
Warm-Up
- aids in, 136–149
- benefits of, 68–70, 287
- connection of exercises in, 119, 121, *121*
- core conditioning and, 70
- exercise plans for, 107–10, 152–53
- as feedback period, 119
- leg-yield in, 245

Way of going, assessment of, 81–99
Wellness Warm-Up Plan, 109, 111, 152
Werth, Isabell, 138
Westlake, Susan, 50
Whip aids, 144, 146–49, *147–48*, 282–83
Willingness, *94*. *See also* Ridden mindset
Wong, Dalton, 124

X

Xenophon, 286

Y

Yoda, 55
Yoga, 3, 72–79, *78–79*, 112
Young horses, 111, 113

Z

Zakharova, Svetlana, *69*